Advances in General and Cellular Pharmacology

VOLUME 1

A Continuation Order Plan is available for this series. A continuation order will bring delivery of each new volume immediately upon publication. Volumes are billed only upon actual shipment. For further information please contact the publisher.

Advances in General and Cellular Pharmacology

VOLUME 1

Edited by

Toshio Narahashi
Duke University Medical Center

and

C. Paul Bianchi
University of Pennsylvania School of Medicine

PLENUM PRESS · NEW YORK AND LONDON

Library of Congress Cataloging in Publication Data

Main entry under title:

Advances in general and cellular pharmacology.

Includes bibliographies and index.
1. Pharmacology. 2. Cells, Effect of drugs on. I. Narahashi, Toshio. II.
Bianchi, Carmine Paul, 1927-   [DNLM: 1. Pharmacology–Periodicals. 2.
Cells–Drug effects–Periodicals. W1 AD612]
RM300.A38 1975   615'.1   75-38640
ISBN-13: 978-1-4615-8200-7   e-ISBN-13: 978-1-4615-8198-7
DOI: 10.1007/978-1-4615-8198-7

©1976 Plenum Press, New York
Softcover reprint of the hardcover 1st edition 1976
A Division of Plenum Publishing Corporation
227 West 17th Street, New York, N.Y. 10011

United Kingdom edition published by Plenum Press, London
A Division of Plenum Publishing Company, Ltd.
Davis House (4th Floor), 8 Scrubs Lane, Harlesden, London, NW10 6SE, England

Contributors

J. Thomas Bigger, Jr.
Departments of Medicine and Pharmacology
College of Physicians and Surgeons
Columbia University
New York, N.Y. 10032

Seymour Ehrenpreis
New York State Research Institute for Neurochemistry and Drug Addiction
Ward's Island
New York, N.Y. 10035

Syogoro Nishi
Department of Physiology
Kurume University School of Medicine
Kurume, 830, Japan

Achilles J. Pappano
Department of Pharmacology
University of Connecticut Health Center
Farmington, Connecticut 06032

Douglas R. Waud
Department of Pharmacology
University of Massachusetts Medical Center
Worcester, Massachusetts 01605

Francis M. Weld
Department of Medicine
College of Physicians and Surgeons
Columbia University
New York, N.Y. 10032

Preface

Knowledge of the mechanism of action of drugs at cellular, subcellular, or molecular levels is of vital importance not only in giving the basis of interpretation of the systemic action of drugs but also in improving existing drugs; in designing new forms of drugs; and in giving the basis of therapeutic applications. Classical pharmacology, concerning the action of drugs at integrated levels, does not necessarily give sufficient information as to the mechanism of action of drugs. A variety of sophisticated concepts utilizing the methods of physics, chemistry, biophysics, biochemistry, and physiology must be synthesized to understand the mechanism of action. Only since the last decade, however, have these techniques been fully applied to pharmacological investigations. It is of utmost importance to realize that a new dimension of pharmacological research has indeed emerged as a result of such a multidisciplinary approach; this approach is encompassed in general and cellular pharmacology.

Such recent studies of drug actions have led to a number of important findings. Certain chemicals and drugs were found to possess highly specific actions on cellular functions, so that they are widely being used as powerful tools for the study of a variety of physiological and pharmacological problems. Our knowledge of the cellular mechanisms of drug action has provided the basis for interpreting the systemic effects of the drugs and insight into the molecular mechanism involved.

For example, the puffer fish poison tetrodotoxin was shown to cause a highly specific inhibition of the sodium conductance increase in nerve membranes, thereby blocking impulse conduction. This stimulated research along this line and led to important contributions as to the mechanism of action of some other neuroactive toxins or agents such as batrachotoxin and local anesthetics. Applications of intracellular microelectrode techniques to cardiac pharmacology have unveiled a variety of important features concerning the mode of action of antiarrhythmic and other cardiac drugs. Recent developments and applications of biochemical and physiological techniques have made it possible to clarify the nature of cholinergic and adrenergic receptors in the postsynaptic membranes, a contribution with an immense pharmacological impact and importance.

General and cellular pharmacology is a multidisciplinary field requiring integration of many fields of knowledge at a high level to achieve an appropriate understanding of drug action. It has developed rather recently and will continue to be a fertile field where a number of challenging accomplishments are expected to be made in the coming years. General and cellular pharmacology represents a modern-day approach to the mechanism of cellular drug action and provides a virgin field for many stimulating achievements in the future.

This new series of books, *Advances in General and Cellular Pharmacology*, is intended to provide a forum for this field. Each expert is to contribute an in-depth review on his own field from his own point of view. Therefore, one should not expect comprehensive review articles from this series of books, but to find newer approaches and techniques with solid theoretical and experimental bases.

Toshio Narahashi
C. Paul Bianchi

Contents

3 **Pharmacology of Heart Cells During Ontogenesis** 83
ACHILLES J. PAPPANO

4 **Analysis of Dose–Response Relationships** 145
DOUGLAS R. WAUD

1

Cardiac Cellular Pharmacology: Automaticity in Cardiac Muscle— Its Alteration by Physical and Chemical Influences

FRANCIS M. WELD AND
J. THOMAS BIGGER, JR.

I. AUTOMATICITY IN HEART MUSCLE

The heart rhythmically and spontaneously activates itself many times in a minute. The process responsible for this behavior has been termed the "normal automatic mechanism" and is a property of only a few cell types in the heart. Cells in the sinoatrial node, atrioventricular rings, and ventricular specialized conducting tissues possess the capacity for automaticity of this type whereas ordinary atrial and ventricular muscle cells do not. This mechanism not only is the basis for normal cardiac rhythmicity but also can generate arrhythmias in the heart. Although the normal automatic mechanism is complex and probably varies somewhat in different types of

FRANCIS M. WELD · Department of Medicine, and J. THOMAS BIGGER, JR. · Departments of Medicine and Pharmacology, College of Physicians and Surgeons, Columbia University, New York, New York. Supported in part by National Institutes of Health Grants HL-12738, HL-70204, HL-50269, and HL-05864.

1

automatic cells and in different species, much is now known about the cell membrane behavior which underlies automaticity and about alterations in this behavior caused by a variety of physical and chemical influences. In this chapter, it is our intention to discuss the factors which generate and modify the automaticity brought about in heart muscle by spontaneous diastolic depolarization.

Early observations on the excitatory process in frog and tortoise heart were reviewed and extended by Burdon-Sanderson and Page (1880). Using external electrodes in a capillary electrometer system, they confirmed the inseparability of ventricular contraction and electrical activity and noted that cardiac rate was dependent upon temperature. With the first photographs of cardiac electrical activity (Burdon-Sanderson and Page, 1884), spontaneous atrial depolarization was delineated, as were induced atrial and ventricular depolarization, atrioventricular conduction delay, and intraventricular conduction delay.

Meek and Eyster (1914), without the benefit of intracellular microelectrodes, described the general behavior of the different cardiac pacemaker tissues in a way which has scarcely been improved upon to the present time. They delineated the progressively slower inherent firing rates possessed by the specialized cardiac pacemaker tissues "from above downward." This hierarchy of automaticity progressing from sinoatrial node to ventricular tissues results in control of cardiac rhythm by the "highest" center (i.e., the sinoatrial node) unless its inherent rate is depressed by influences such as the vagus nerve. Their concept of the hierarchy of pacemakers is still valuable in the analysis of pacemaker activity today.

Prior to microelectrode studies, arguments arose as to the nature of spontaneous rhythmicity—some authors favoring slow depolarization in pacemakers (Arvanitaki, 1938; Rijlant, 1936), others, oscillatory behavior (Bozler, 1943). The introduction of glass capillary microelectrodes allowed measurement of transmembrane voltage in single muscle cells (Ling and Gerard, 1949). The first demonstration of the time–voltage course of a cardiac pacemaker cell was by Draper and Weidmann (1951) in Purkinje fibers from sheep and dogs and by Trautwein and Zink (1952) in cells of the frog sinus venosus. These studies showed that automatic cells undergo spontaneous membrane depolarization during phase 4. In true pacemaker cells this process brings transmembrane voltage to the critical firing threshold to initiate a regenerative action potential. In potential pacemaker cells, such as those in the peripheral Purkinje system, spontaneous diastolic (phase 4) depolarization may or may not reach the critical firing threshold under normal circumstances. In still other cardiac cell types, such as working atrial and ventricular muscle, no spontaneous membrane depolarization occurs following repolarization of the action potential, since these cells totally lack the membrane conductance properties capable of generating normal automatic behavior.

In the classical electrophysiological sense, automaticity resulting from spontaneous phase 4 depolarization depends on the four variables illustrated by the diagrams in Figure 1, where the transmembrane voltage–time course of a single cardiac Purkinje cell is shown. In each panel of Figure 1, a normal spontaneous action potential is shown as a solid line; the effects of modifying one of the four classical electrophysiological determinants of automaticity is shown in dashed lines. Figure 1A shows that a more rapid rate of phase 4 depolarization results in a more rapid attainment of the critical firing threshold ($V_{threshold}$) and thus a more rapid rate of spontaneous discharge. Slowing phase 4 depolarization has the opposite effect. Figure 1B shows that if the transmembrane voltage change during phase 4 depolarization is small, transmembrane voltage can fail to reach the threshold voltage, and thus abolish automaticity. Figure 1C reveals that a change to a more positive threshold voltage will result in a slowing of firing rate, while the converse is true for a shift to a more negative threshold voltage. Figure 1D reflects the different intervals between successive action potentials resulting from changes in maximum diastolic voltage: increases in maximum diastolic voltage slow the spontaneous firing rate; decreases in maximum diastolic voltage enhance spontaneous firing. Although these classical features of automaticity are conceptually simple, they are themselves determined by complex interactions between both passive and active membrane behavior.

Hoffman and Cranefield (1960) outlined the possible ionic causes for spontaneous phase 4 depolarization: (1) The resting membrane could show a gradual loss of potassium conductance. This would cause transmembrane voltage to move in a positive direction, toward zero, since the potassium equilibrium potential (see equation 7) is about -100 mV for usual intra- and extracellular potassium concentrations (140 mEq/liter and 3.5 mEq/liter, respectively). (2) A gradual increase in membrane conductance to sodium ions during diastole could equally well explain the spontaneous phase 4 depolarization, since the sodium equilibrium potential is about $+30$ mV (inside of the cell positive). (3) A decrease of electrogenic sodium pumping in the course of diastole would also result in spontaneous phase 4 depolarization, owing to a time dependent decrease in outward (repolarizing) current. (4) Finally, there might be other membrane ionic conductance changes (e.g., calcium) responsible for spontaneous phase 4 depolarization. There is now reasonable evidence that all four of these proposed mechanisms play a role in spontaneous phase 4 depolarization in one or more cardiac cell types. We will attempt to show in subsequent sections that the individual mechanisms contribute variably to pacemaker currents in different cell types, and—perhaps equally important—in the same cell type under different circumstances.

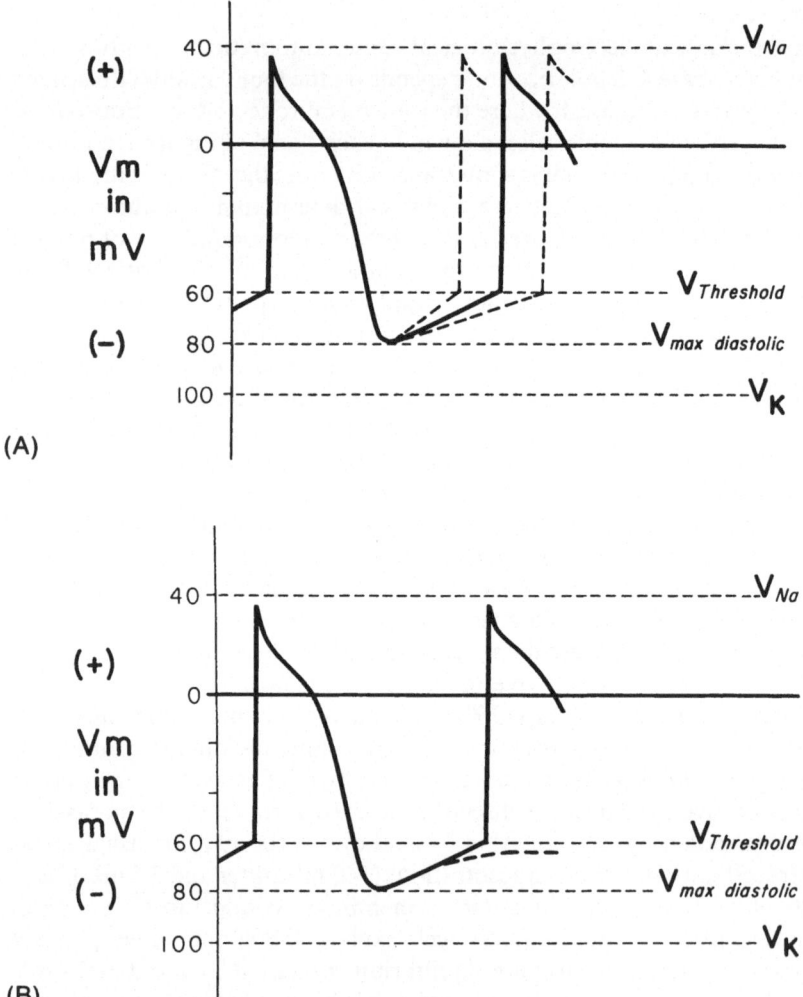

Figure 1. Electrophysiological determinants of automaticity. The solid lines of each panel represent the action potentials of an automatic fiber. The dashed lines represent changes caused by alterations in the following determinants of automaticity. A: Rate of phase 4 depolarization. B: Magnitude of phase 4 depolarization. C: Threshold voltage (critical firing threshold). D: Maximum diastolic voltage. Symbols: V_m = transmembrane voltage; V_{Na} = sodium equilibrium potential; V_K = potassium equilibrium potential; $V_{threshold}$ = threshold voltage; $V_{max\ diastolic}$ = maximum diastolic voltage; absicissa is time (uncalibrated).

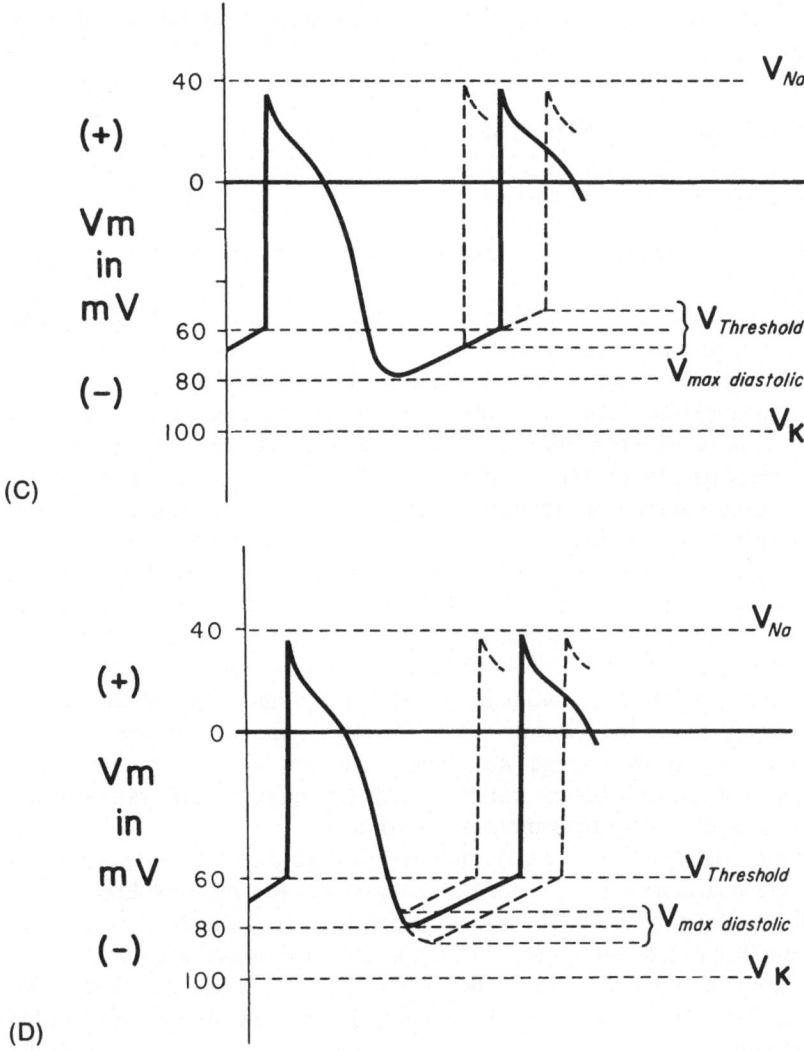

(C)

(D)

II. CHARACTERISTICS OF THE "RESTING" MEMBRANE IN CARDIAC CELLS

To understand the genesis of phase 4 depolarization and its expression in the whole heart, it is valuable to understand cardiac cable properties and transmembrane ionic gradients and conductances. The purpose of this section is to review some of the aspects of these topics which are germane to cardiac automaticity.

A. Membrane Cable Properties

1. Membrane Equivalent Circuit

The cable properties of cardiac cells have been recently reviewed (Freygang and Trautwein, 1970), and the resultant implications concerning cardiac cellular electrical behavior outlined (Bigger and Weld, 1976). Cardiac cable properties have been studied in Purkinje fibers, ventricular muscular trabeculae, and in sinus node (Weidmann, 1952, 1970; Bonke, 1973a). The resting Purkinje fiber membrane has electrical characteristics of conductance (reciprocal of resistance) and capacitance which determine the membrane's voltage response to current (charged ion flow). Although it is an oversimplification, the membrane model in Figure 2 illustrates most passive and active electrophysiological characteristics of the membrane. R_1 and R_2 represent the membrane's electrical resistance to ionic current flow owing to the physicochemical structure of the membrane and internal structure of the fiber bundles. For a cardiac cell membrane resting at a voltage substantially negative to the critical firing threshold, R_1 and R_2 may be considered constant for very small (e.g., 1 mV) displacements of transmembrane voltage away from the resting value. However, membrane resistance is determined largely by voltage- and time-dependent ionic conductances, so that R_1 and R_2 cannot be accurately regarded as having static values under conditions of changing transmembrane voltage.

From a morphologic standpoint, R_1 probably resides in the surface membrane across which ionic transfer from perfusing solutions directly into the cell interior can occur. R_2 represents, at least in part, the resistance of the intercellular clefts which separate apposing cardiac cell membranes and lead to the exterior of the multicellular fiber bundles (Falk and Fatt, 1964; Fozzard, 1966; Freygang and Trautwein, 1970). The extensively folded sarcolemmal membrane of individual Purkinje cells and fiber bundles (Mobley and Page, 1972) is probably responsible for the larger capacitance of Purkinje strands per cross-sectional area compared to other cardiac tissue types. C_1 is the capacitance of the sarcolemmal membrane containing R_1, probably located at the outer margins of fiber bundles. C_2 probably represents the capacitance of the more deeply located cell membranes and the membranes lining the deep intercellular clefts.

Capacitance is an inherent property of the surface and cleft membranes, reflecting the ability of the membrane to store electrical charge when subjected to voltage differences across its inner and outer margins. Capacitance

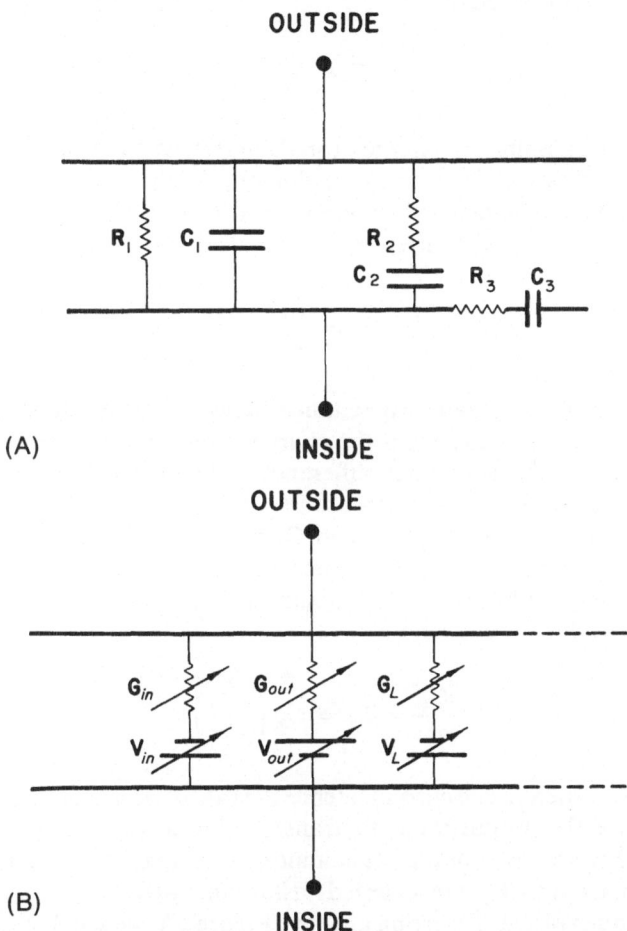

Figure 2. Electrical equivalent circuit for Purkinje cell membrane. A: R_1 and C_1 represent that portion of resistance and capacitance oriented in parallel. C_2 is that portion of membrane capacitance linked in series to a portion of membrane resistance, R_2. R_3 and C_3 are longitudinal (myoplasm, disk) resistance and capacitance. B: Active electrical equivalent for ionic conductances (reciprocal of resistance) and electrical driving forces. All the elements of this diagram are represented by R_1 in (A). G_{in} and V_{in} are the ionic conductances and driving forces for ions with a positive equilibrium potential. G_{out} and V_{out} are the ionic conductances and driving forces for ions with a negative equilibrium potential. G_L and V_L are the conductances and driving forces for unidentified background currents. Arrows indicate that values are not fixed, but vary according to time and voltage dependence of the conductances and determination of driving forces by the difference between equilibrium potentials and transmembrane voltage. The polarity of background current is shown as inward owing to predominantly negative transmembrane voltage.

is mathematically defined as

$$C = \frac{Q}{V} \tag{1a}$$

where Q is the amount of charge stored, and V is the voltage difference across the membrane. When a voltage difference exists across a cardiac cell membrane, the capacitance of the membrane will thus store electrical charge, and equation (1a) can be written more specifically as

$$C_m = \frac{Q_m}{V_m} \tag{1b}$$

where C_m is total membrane capacitance between intracellular and extra-cellular spaces (C_1 and C_2), Q_m is the charge stored in this capacitance, and V_m is the transmembrane voltage difference. When capacitance is large per unit area of membrane, a transmembrane voltage change caused by applied current flow will be slow, since C_1 and C_2 must be fully charged before the membrane's maximum voltage difference can be attained. The rate of trans-membrane voltage change can be obtained by mathematically differentiating equation (1b), which then yields

$$\frac{dQ_m}{dt} = I_m = C_m \left(\frac{dV_m}{dt} \right) \tag{2}$$

where I_m is transmembrane current. Hence the rate of transmembrane voltage change is directly proportional to transmembrane current and inversely proportional to the membrane capacitance. Note that equation (2) is valid only if both C_1 and C_2 are charged instantaneously during a change in transmembrane voltage. Referring again to Figure 2A, we see that the voltage across C_1 will always equal the transmembrane voltage regardless of the magnitude of dV_m/dt. However, the rate of charging of C_2 is limited by R_2, the portion of membrane resistance (R_m) between intracellular and extra-cellular spaces ($R_m = R_1 + R_2$). For slow transmembrane voltage changes, the voltage across both C_1 and C_2 equals V_m at any instant. For fast voltage changes, only the voltage across C_1 is instantaneously equal to V_m, with subsequent time course of charging of C_2 depending on the current crossing R_2.

It is important to show that the rate of transmembrane voltage change during phase 4 depolarization is slow enough to permit essentially instan-taneous charging of both C_1 and C_2 to a value equal to V_m, and thus show that equation (2) is valid for spontaneously depolarizing cells. Since voltage drops across elements of a parallel electrical circuit are equal, the identical transmembrane voltage will appear across R_1, across C_1, and across R_2C_2 of Figure 2A. The rate of charging of C_2 is limited by the series-linked resistance, R_2. What we wish to prove is that the limitation in rate of charging of C_2 is insignificant during the slow voltage changes of phase 4 depolarization so that we can consider C_2 always charged to V_m. During a linear depolarization of the cell membrane from -90 mV to -70 mV in 1 sec, the magnitude of the current flowing through the membrane ionic conductances to charge a C_m of 10 μF/cm^2 is calculated from equation (2) as only 2 $\times$ 10^{-7} A/cm^2. Let us assume the worst, i.e., that all current must flow through R_2 before charging either portion, C_1 or C_2, of total membrane capacitance. If this magnitude of current does not produce a significant voltage drop across R_2, then we can be confident that a measured transmembrane voltage difference appears across C_2 as well as C_1, and that equation (2) is valid. Using the experimentally determined value for R_2 of 300 Ω-cm^2 (Fozzard, 1966), the voltage drop across R_2 caused by a current of 2 $\times$ 10^{-7} A/cm^2 is calculated from Ohm's law as 0.06 mV. Thus, we can safely assume that the series-linked resistance, R_2, is not a significant impediment to charging of C_2 at the slow rates of transmembrane voltage change encountered during action potential phase 4 depolarization.

Equation (2) pertains to a cell or a cellular syncytium where all areas of membrane are undergoing the same conductance changes. In reality, however, groups of pacemaker cells may be contiguous with others with lesser pacemaker properties, and in such situations spatial voltage gradients clearly exist. In such cells or fibers, the voltage at one point in the cell membrane is influenced by passive (electrotonic) spread from neighboring areas of cell membrane which are at different transmembrane voltages. Two values of the cell membrane, its space constant and its time constant, determine the magnitude and spatial distribution of a "local" voltage displacement arising from local current flow.

2. Space Constant (λ)

This is the distance from a point source of voltage displacement (or current polarization) at which intervening membrane resistance ($R_1 + R_2$ of Figure 2A) and core resistance (R_3) are equal. Cable theory predicts that the original polarization, ΔV_0, will fall according to

$$\Delta V = \Delta V_0 e^{-x/\lambda} \tag{3}$$

where ΔV is the measured voltage displacement, x is the distance from the source of voltage displacement at which the measurement is made, and e is the base of natural logarithms. The space constant of cardiac Purkinje fibers is about 2 mm (Weidmann, 1952; Fozzard, 1966). This relatively large value indicates that the intercellular connections (intercalated disks) must have a very small resistance to current flow. The space constant of dog, sheep, and calf ventricular muscle is about 1.0 mm (Kamiyama and Matsuda, 1966; Weidmann, 1970) and that of atrial muscle is about the same (Bonke, 1973a). The space constant in the sinoatrial node is small, about 0.5 mm, which may reflect both the extremely small size of individual cells and also their arrangement in small clusters within a single basement membrane, embedded in a thick collagen stroma. In such a cluster, there are no typical intercalated disks. However, intercellular contacts within and between clusters do exist (Kawamura, 1961; Torii, 1962), and they allow current spread over a considerable distance despite the complex geometrical arrangement of the fibers.

3. Time Constant (τ)

The time constant of a resistive–capacitive circuit is equal to the time taken to reach 0.63 of a voltage change caused by onset of a constant polarizing current in the circuit. In a cardiac cell we could estimate the time constant of the membrane if we could observe the voltage–time course of transmembrane voltage *at* the site of application of a current pulse. Cable theory provides that

$$\Delta V = \Delta V_0 e^{-t/\tau_m} \tag{4}$$

where t is the time after onset of current flow, and

$$\tau_m = R_m C_m \tag{5}$$

where R_m and C_m are membrane resistance and capacitance, respectively. It is not usually possible to measure the membrane voltage deflection at precisely the point of current application, so other methods have been used to calculate the membrane time constant: Hodgkin and Rushton (1946) and Weidmann (1952) utilized the time course of voltage response to an intracellular rectangular current pulse at various distances from the site of current application; alternatively, τ_m can be calculated from the slope of the line relating half-rise time of the electrotonic potential to distance from site of current application. [The slope of this line is approximately $2\lambda/\tau_m$ (Hodgkin and Rushton, 1946; Bonke, 1973a)]. The dc time constant measured by these methods is about 20 msec for sheep Purkinje fibers (Weidmann, 1952), 4 msec for sheep or calf ventricular muscle (Weidmann, 1970), and 3 msec for rabbit crista terminalis or atrial trabeculae (Bonke, 1973a). The larger time constant for Purkinje fibers results from a greater cross-sectional membrane capacitance, which in turn is probably a result of the extensive infolding of the Purkinje cell membrane (Mobley and Page, 1972), rather than a higher capacitance for a given area of unfolded surface membrane.

Both space constant and time constant are important determinants of automaticity. The larger the space constant, the greater the area of distribution of a local voltage disturbance. Since the area of involved membrane is crucial in determining whether or not a local response will become regenerative (Fozzard and Schoenberg, 1972), space constant becomes a major determinant of excitability. Similarly, a shorter time constant means that a local current disturbance requires less time to cause a given voltage displacement.

4. Membrane Geometry

The geometry of fiber connections is important for the initiation of excitation in a pacemaker focus and for the successful propagation of the resultant action potential. Geometrical considerations become particularly influential in diseased hearts, or under adverse environmental conditions, when an automatic focus may be surrounded by partially depolarized fibers with reduced excitability.

There are several geometrical determinants of automaticity. First, the length of a cell or bundle of cells with active pacemaker properties must be sufficient to overcome the "neutralizing" effect of local circuit currents from adjacent nonpacemaker membrane. For point-polarized Purkinje fibers, this liminal length is approximately $0.1-0.2 \times \lambda$, or about 0.3 mm (Fozzard and Schoenberg, 1972). Second, the number of side-to-side connections and branching within a pacemaking syncytium or fiber bundle will tend to suppress pacemaker activity confined to a very small area (e.g., just greater than the liminal length) by virtue of the increased availability of local stored capacitative charge to antagonize a transmembrane voltage change. Third, once a propagating response has been generated from a pacemaker cell or group of cells, the geometry of the local tissue is an important determinant of successful propagation.

When the cardiac impulse conducts in a fiber whose diameter is decreasing as a function of distance (e.g., the peripheral Purkinje fiber), it becomes more susceptible to block. As fiber diameter decreases, its core resistance, r_i (the resistance of a unit length of fiber core in Ω/cm), rises as the inverse square of the radius. In this circumstance, r_m (the resistance of a unit length of membrane in Ω-cm), increases as the reciprocal of fiber radius. Therefore, the space constant ($\lambda = \sqrt{r_m/r_i}$) will decrease as the fiber radius decreases, favoring decreased conduction velocity. However, as the radius decreases, c_m (the membrane capacitance per unit fiber length in $\mu F/cm$) also decreases, which means that local circuit current has less capacitance to fill as the membrane depolarizes. Interactions between active and passive determinants of conduction also occur. For example, just as predicted by the model in Figure 2A, the Purkinje membrane capacitance is frequency dependent: Carmeliet and Willems (1971) have shown that the membrane capacitance encountered by a normal action potential propagating in a bovine Purkinje fiber is about one fourth that encountered by a slowly propagating action potential in Sr-Tyrode solution. Since so many variables interact with conduction, it is often difficult to predict the precise effect of a given geometry on propagation of the cardiac action potential. One site where cable-like strands show pronounced tapering is in the distal Purkinje fibers. It is interesting that when unidirectional conduction block occurs at this site, the impulse usually blocks in the orthograde direction, i.e., when conduction is proceeding into smaller and smaller fibers. Unfortunately, the Purkinje fibers also anastomose with the ventricular muscle syncytium near this site so that the precise mechanism of block in the distal Purkinje fibers remains uncertain.

B. The Basis of Resting Transmembrane Voltage

1. Neutral Ionic Pumping

All cardiac cells are dependent upon oxidative metabolism to establish and maintain their transmembrane ionic gradients. Since the cell membrane is permeable to sodium and potassium, the ATPase-dependent membrane cation pump must continuously extrude sodium from the cell interior in exchange for potassium in order to avoid an increase in intracellular sodium or a decrease in intracellular potassium concentration. This cation pump can be inhibited by metabolic poisons such as ouabain, 2,4-dinitrophenol or sodium cyanide, and it appears to be highly selective since it cannot extrude lithium from the cell interior (Trautwein and Schmidt, 1960; Vassalle, 1970).

2. Equilibrium Potential

The tendency of an ion to diffuse from a higher to a lower concentration establishes an electrical force exactly equal and opposite to the chemical (diffusion) force. This electrical force, called the equilibrium potential, is given by the Nernst equation for each ionic species (e.g., potassium) as

$$V_K = -\frac{RT}{F} \ln \frac{[K]_{in}}{[K]_{out}} \tag{7}$$

where V_K is the potassium equilibrium potential, R is the universal gas constant, T is absolute temperature, F is Faraday's constant, $\ln'$ is the natural logarithmic function, and $[K]_{in}$ and $[K]_{out}$ are the ion's concentration (more properly, specific activity) at the inner and outer membrane surfaces. The intracellular potassium concentration (about 140 mEq/liter) is much higher than extracellular potassium concentration (about 4 mEq/liter), resulting in a potassium equilibrium potential of about -100 mV (inside negative). Sodium is distributed across the membrane with an opposing, and less steep, concentration gradient. The resultant equilibrium potential for sodium ions is about $+40$ mV (inside positive). It is important to realize that this electromotive force for an ionic species would exist even if the membrane were impermeant to that ion. If a cell is incapable of maintaining its transmembrane ionic gradients, the ionic equilibrium potentials will shift toward zero.

3. Ionic Electrical Driving Force

The electrical driving force on an ion equals the difference between the equilibrium potential and the transmembrane voltage—for potassium ions, $V_m - V_K$. If a membrane separates different concentrations of a single ionic species to which it is selectively permeable, then the transmembrane voltage is exactly equal to that ion's equilibrium potential, at which the chemical (diffusion) and electrical forces on the ion are equal and opposite. When transmembrane voltage is different from the ionic equilibrium potential, a net transmembrane flow of that ion occurs since chemical (diffusion) and electrical forces on the ion are no longer balanced.

4. Membrane Ionic Conductances

The conductance (reciprocal of resistance) of a membrane for an ionic species is an expression of the electrical "ease" with which the ion can cross the membrane in response to an electrical driving force. Ionic conductance and electrical driving force define transmembrane ionic current (e.g., for potassium and sodium) through Ohm's law:

$$I_K = g_K(V_m - V_K) \tag{8a}$$

$$I_{Na} = g_{Na}(V_m - V_{Na}) \tag{8b}$$

The relationships of equations (8a) and (8b) have been exploited by the use of voltage clamp circuits (Figure 3) in order to evaluate time and voltage dependence of ionic conductances: Experimental conditions are chosen to maximize and/or minimize the transmembrane conductance of the ionic species

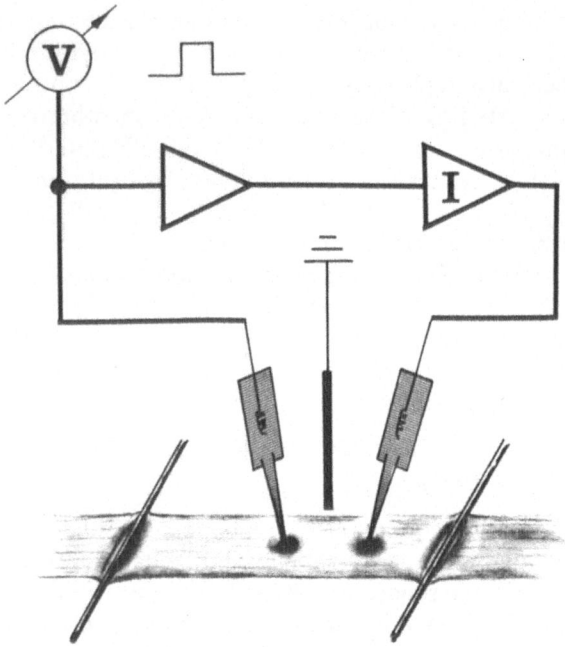

Figure 3. Diagrammatic representation of voltage-clamp circuit. A Purkinje fiber segment is electrically isolated by two crush injuries. Intracellular microelectrodes are separated by a grounded shield. Variable voltage source, V, represents the command voltage which determines holding and test clamp voltages. The voltage signals from command and from left-hand microelectrode are summed (dot) and amplified (empty amplifier symbol); the resultant signal causes current output from the power amplifier, I, to bring the transmembrane voltage to a value such that the voltage measured at the summing point remains constant.

to be studied; transmembrane voltage (V_m) can be clamped to any value and current is measured as a function of time. The ionic species carrying the current can be inferred by the clamp voltage at which the current under investigation reverses polarity; reversal should occur at the ion's equilibrium potential (Hodgkin and Huxley, 1952d). Changes in ionic composition of the perfusion fluid and specific ion blockers are also very useful experimental tools.

For the resting membrane net transmembrane current is zero by definition; the most important ionic conductances are those of sodium and potassium; thus,

$$I_{m\,\text{resting}} = I_K + I_{Na} + \cdots = 0 \tag{9}$$

At rest, g_K is much larger than g_{Na} ($g_K/g_{Na} \approx 20$). We can relate membrane conductances and ionic electrical driving forces to R_1 in Figure 2A, as shown in Figure 2B. For simplicity, all ions having a negative equilibrium potential are lumped into a single outward ionic conductance, G_{out}, and electrical driving force, V_{out} ($V_{out} = V_m - V_{equilibrium}$). The same convention is used for inward currents and background currents. Background current is a term for the current residual once the time-dependent currents are accounted for. Hodgkin and Huxley (1952d) used the term "leak current" for this component of membrane current.

5. Resting Transmembrane Voltage

As noted above, resting membrane potassium conductance is much greater than resting membrane sodium conductance. In order that net resting transmembrane current is zero [equation (9)] the electrical driving force on sodium ions must be larger than that on potassium, as predicted by equations (8a) and (8b). This condition is met by, and is the reason for, a resting transmembrane voltage much closer to the potassium than to the sodium equilibrium potential.

Inspection of equations (8a) and (8b) reveals that resting transmembrane voltage will not change, if the ratio of g_K to g_{Na} does not change, as long as transmembrane ionic concentration gradients (and, therefore, the ionic equilibrium potentials) do not change. This concept is illustrated by the hypothetical fibers of Figures 4A and 4B; both are resting spontaneously at the same transmembrane voltage, where, by definition, net transmembrane ionic current is zero. In fiber A, however, both inward and outward ionic conductances are greater than in fiber B, and greater metabolic activity must be expended in maintaining ionic concentration gradients. It is actually conceivable that a marginally oxygenated or substrate-limited cell could profit from a decrease in membrane conductance since it would be able to maintain its ionic gradients at a lower metabolic cost.

The fibers depicted in Figures 4C and 4D simply demonstrate the transmembrane voltage changes which are induced by decreases in net outward and inward currents, respectively. Both fibers begin with resting transmembrane currents and voltages as in Figure 4A. In Figure 4C inward ionic current flow is decreased, and this results in a shift of transmembrane voltage in the negative direction, indicated by the arrow. Consequently, the magnitudes of the opposing currents will once again approach each other [equation (8)], and become exactly equal when the transmembrane voltage reaches a new, steady state at a more negative level [equation (9)]. The same series of events is shown for a decrease in outward ionic conductance in Figure 4D.

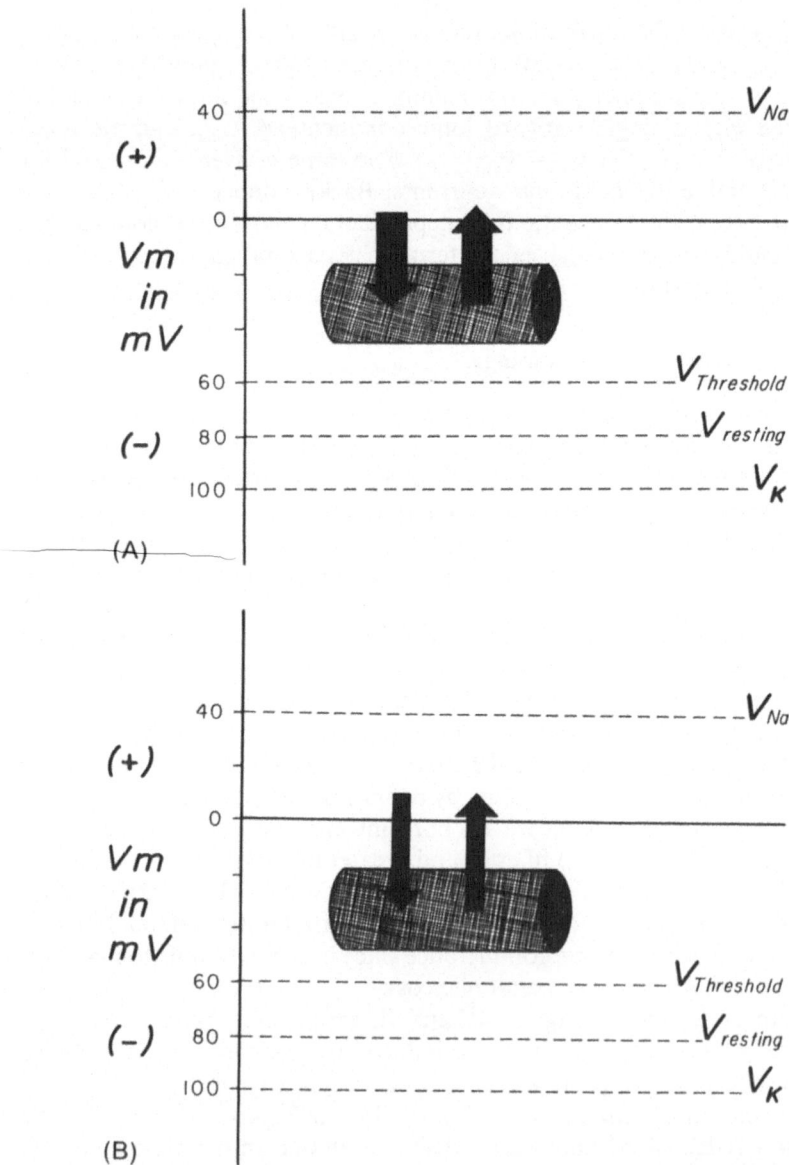

Figure 4. Determination of resting transmembrane voltage by diastolic ionic currents. Magnitude of currents is diagrammatically represented by width of arrows crossing membrane of schematic fiber. A and B: Resting transmembrane voltage is identical in each case despite larger currents in panel A, because resting transmembrane voltage is determined by net transmembrane current, which is zero in both cases. C: When inward ionic current is reduced, a corresponding net

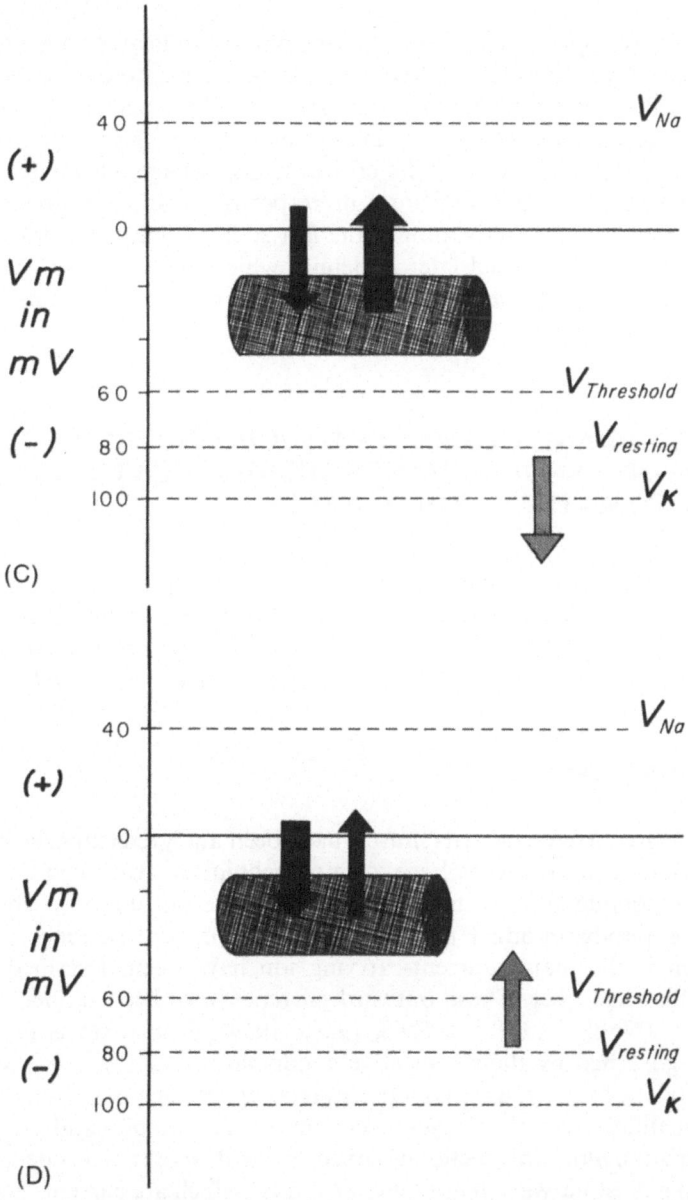

outward current ensues, which in turn will cause the resting transmembrane voltage to move in a negative direction, toward, but never beyond, V_K. Conversely, when outward current is reduced, a net inward current ensues and the resting transmembrane voltage shifts in a positive direction, toward V_K. As the membrane slowly depolarizes the threshold voltage will usually shift in the positive direction as well (see text). Symbols as in Figure 1.

One can easily appreciate that the transmembrane voltage change in Figure 4C is potentially antiautomatic, because it carries the membrane further away from the critical firing threshold for fast inward sodium current. Conversely, the situation in Figure 4D promotes automatic firing, since depolarization brings the membrane closer to its critical firing voltage. However, the increased excitability resulting from a more positive resting transmembrane voltage is limited by inactivation in the fast sodium channel at these more positive voltages (discussed later in detail), which in turn moves threshold voltage in a positive direction and decreases maximal inward sodium current on activation.

III. MEMBRANE CURRENTS WHICH UNDERLIE SPONTANEOUS PHASE 4 DEPOLARIZATION IN AUTOMATIC CARDIAC CELLS

In this section we will discuss the ionic conductances which contribute to spontaneous depolarization in diastole. Net transmembrane current in diastole is the algebraic sum of outward, inward, and background currents [see Figure 2B; equations (8) and (9)]; each of these will be considered.

A. Outward Currents

Outward currents in heart muscle have been analyzed extensively using both current clamp and voltage clamp techniques. Although only one potassium conductance seems to be present in the membrane of the squid giant axon (Hodgkin and Huxley, 1952d), four outward currents in which potassium is the major current-carrying ion have been described in the cardiac Purkinje fiber. These outward currents have been termed i_{K_1}, i_{K_2}, i_{x_1}, and i_{x_2} (Noble and Tsien, 1968, 1969a, 1969b; Hauswirth $et\ al.$, 1972); they are governed by their respective conductances, g_{K_1}, g_{K_2}, g_{x_1}, and g_{x_2}. The behavior of these four conductances is complex, each possessing its own special qualities, such as voltage-dependent gating variables and/or rectifier characteristics. Since this section is concerned with spontaneous depolarization during diastole, we will not review i_{x_1} or i_{x_2}, which are currents activated in the plateau voltage range.

1. Instantaneous Voltage-Dependent Potassium Current (i_{K_1})

Early experiments using intracellular current pulses in cardiac fibers revealed time-dependent and time-independent components of potassium conductance (Hutter and Noble, 1960; Hall *et al.*, 1963; Carmeliet, 1961). The time-independent potassium conductance has been termed g_{K_1}. The current governed by this conductance, i_{K_1}, has been termed a background current because of its time independence. It is of great interest that g_{K_1} is strikingly nonlinear; it rectifies very strongly in an inward direction (Hall *et al.*, 1963; Deck and Trautwein, 1964; McAllister and Noble, 1966; Noble and Tsien, 1968) during membrane depolarization, resulting in less potassium current than expected if g_{K_1} rectification is essentially that of the linear current–voltage relationship of the 'leak' current in squid giant axon (Hodgkin and Huxley, 1952*d*). The mechanism of inward-going rectification in heart muscle is uncertain but results in conductance with time and voltage dependence strikingly different from classical Hodgkin–Huxley theory. The rectifier mechanism of g_{K_1} results in a large g_{K_1} when outward currents are applied, but a small g_{K_1} when inward currents are applied to the resting Purkinje fiber membrane (Noble and Tsien, 1968). Haas and Kern (1966) gathered direct evidence that i_{K_1} is carried by potassium ions in Purkinje fibers by measuring radioactive potassium flux in sodium-free solutions as a function of clamp voltage; the current–voltage relationship constructed by this method agreed with previous electrical methods (Hall *et al.*, 1963; McAllister and Noble, 1966; Arnsdorf and Bigger, 1972). Although this important potassium current is considered to be instantaneously voltage dependent, we must realize that a rapid time-dependent process cannot be excluded (since it is impossible to measure time dependence of cardiac membrane currents with time constants as short as about 10 msec). Quantitatively, i_{K_1} is the largest outward ionic conductance of the cardiac cell membrane in the voltage range of phase 4 depolarization.

Using values of transmembrane current and voltage after relatively long voltage clamp steps, such as those in Figures 5 and 6, we have plotted the "steady-state" current–voltage relationship for a shortened Purkinje fiber in Figure 7. For V_m between -90 and -60 mV, the steady-state current–voltage relationship is composed primarily of i_{K_1} and background inward currents. Since i_{K_1} makes a large contribution, V_m rests at -80 mV (near the reversal potential of i_{K_1}, about -100 mV). The term i_{K_1} figures prominently in the expression of automatic behavior, since an increase in i_{K_1}, an outward current, will cause the fiber to hyperpolarize. Conversely, a decrease in i_{K_1} will move resting transmembrane voltage to more positive values, closer to the critical firing threshold for fast inward sodium current. This shift, as discussed previously, favors the development of automaticity, since less depolarizing current is needed to elicit a regenerative response (Figures 1 and 4).

The decrease in slope conductance of i_{K_1} as the membrane is depolarized (inward-going rectification) is manifest in the steady-state current–voltage relationship of Figure 7; as the membrane is clamped to voltages more and

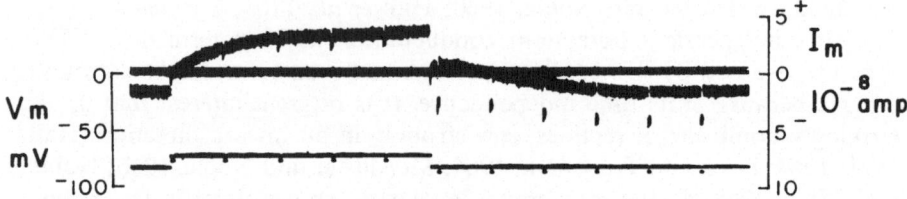

Figure 5. Activation and deactivation of pacemaker current (i_{K_2}). Purkinje fiber segment (2 mm) voltage clamped from -83 mV to -75 mV for 10 sec and back to -83 mV. Time base represents zero reference for both current and voltage; time tics at 100 msec and 1 sec. Transmembrane voltage (V_m) is bottom trace, with corresponding transmembrane current (I_m) recorded at top. On depolarization to -75 mV, outward current slowly increases as i_{K_2} activates. On repolarization to -83 mV, there is a gradual "tail" of current owing to deactivation of i_{K_2}. Four mV hyperpolarizing voltage-clamp steps of 50 msec duration are superimposed on the holding and test clamps at 2-sec intervals. Note the current response to these small hyperpolarizing steps at -75 mV compared to the much larger currents necessary to hold the same step at -83 mV (so-called inward rectification at the more positive voltage). During the return voltage clamp to -83 mV the small hyperpolarizing voltage clamp steps show a progressively smaller current response, indicating that membrane conductance is decreasing during the observed gradual current change. Thus, the gradual current change following the clamp back to -83 mV represents a diminution of an outward current rather than an increasing inward current.

more positive to resting V_m, the slope conductance decreases and then actually becomes negative (Deck and Trautwein, 1964; Noble and Tsien, 1968). Alterations in the rectifier function for i_{K_1} could have an important effect on excitability. For example, a decrease in the intensity of inward-going rectification in Figure 7 would result in a smaller dip toward negative current in the neighborhood of the critical firing threshold. Thus, more inward

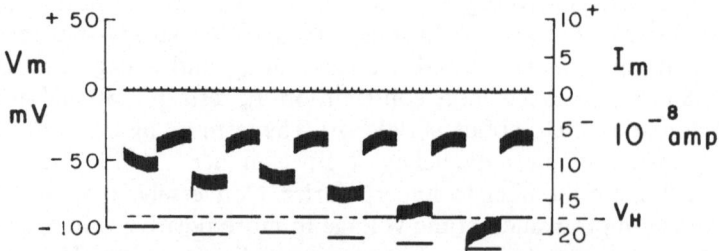

Figure 6. Reversal potential for the pacemaker current (i_{K_2}). Same convention as in Figure 5, but a different Purkinje fiber and time tics at 1 sec. Dotted line drawn through holding clamp (V_H) near -85 mV. The responses to a series of clamps negative from V_H are shown. Note that the direction of the slow current change during the negative clamps reverses at voltages slightly negative to -100 mV, close to the calculated potassium equilibrium potential for the external potassium concentration of 4 mEq/liter. See text.

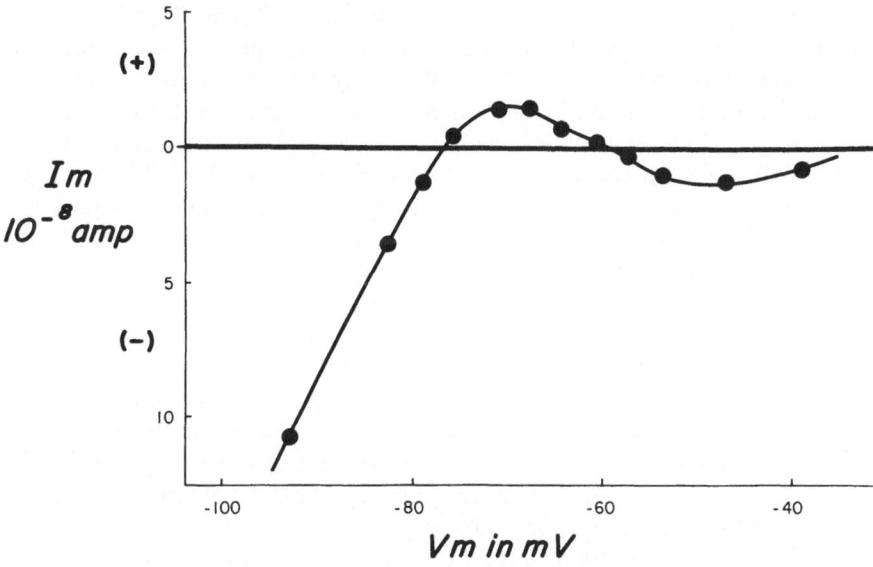

Figure 7. "Steady-state" current–voltage relationship in a sheep Purkinje fiber, where transmembrane current is measured after long (10 sec) test voltage clamps. Note the marked decrease in membrane slope conductance at transmembrane voltages positive to –80 mV, with negative slope conductances for about 20 mV positive to –70 mV (so-called inward rectification). See text.

(depolarizing) current would be required to bring the membrane to the threshold voltage. This would cause slowing or cessation of spontaneous automaticity.

2. Potassium Pacemaker Current (i_{K_2})

Weidmann (1951) measured membrane slope conductance changes during spontaneous phase 4 depolarization in Purkinje fibers by injecting square pulses of current into a fiber and measuring the resultant transmembrane voltage deflections. He found that the induced voltage displacements were larger as phase 4 depolarization progressed and concluded that membrane conductance decreased during spontaneous depolarization. Similar changes in slope conductance were later found in sinoatrial node cells during phase 4 depolarization (Dudel and Trautwein, 1958). These changes suggest that the pacemaker potential in these two cell types is the result of a decrease in an outward current during diastole. The two major ionic species with a transmembrane distribution which could produce an outward current are potassium and chloride. Subsequent studies have indicated that chloride ion distributes passively across the membrane and contributes little to membrane conductance in the voltage range of pacemaker depolarization (Carmeliet, 1961; Dudel et al., 1967c). The suggestion that a time-dependent decrease in potassium conductance is the major mechanism for pacemaker depolarization in Purkinje fibers evolved from several laboratories, but proof awaited studies with the voltage clamp, where V_m could be held constant. Deck and Trautwein (1964), using a voltage clamp technique adapted to cardiac cells (Deck et al., 1964), found that membrane repolarization was followed by a time-dependent decay of outward current which reversed its polarity as the membrane voltage was clamped negative to about -100 mV. Vassalle (1966) demonstrated the applicability of this current change to actual phase 4 depolarization by voltage clamping a Purkinje fiber to its maximum diastolic potential at the moment phase 3 repolarization was complete. He, too, noted a fall in outward membrane current which reversed polarity near the calculated potassium equilibrium potential. The major characteristics of this Purkinje fiber pacemaker current are illustrated in Figures 5 and 6. Figure 5 shows a 2-mm Purkinje fiber segment clamped from a test voltage of -75 mV to a holding voltage of -83 mV; a time-dependent change in transmembrane current results. By periodically superimposing 4-mV, 50-msec hyperpolarizing voltage clamps during the test and holding voltage clamps, it is shown that membrane conductance falls during the observed current change at -83 mV, thereby identifying this current change as a decreasing net outward current rather than an increasing net inward current. The records in Figure 6 are from a different Purkinje fiber segment subjected to test clamp voltages negative to a holding voltage of -85 mV. The slow current change is fully deactivated at -100 mV, since test clamps more negative than -100 mV do not produce any increase in the slow current following return to the holding clamp. Equally important is the observation that the slow current change reverses sign at a test clamp slightly negative to -100 mV. The reversal potential for the ion responsible for the current change is therefore very close to the calculated potassium equilibrium potential, indicating that the ionic species carrying the current is, in all likelihood, potassium. Experiments by others have previously shown that this reversal voltage follows the predicted equilibrium potential for potassium as external potassium concentration is varied (Noble and Tsien, 1968; Peper and Trautwein, 1969). Thus we can be reasonably confident that the time-dependent current change responsible for spontaneous phase 4 depolarization in cardiac Purkinje fibers is caused by the time-dependent decay of a potassium current, called i_{K_2} by Noble and Tsien (1968). Time-dependent decay of an outward potassium current has also been incriminated in frog sinoatrial node automaticity, but the reported voltage clamp records are not shown (Lenfant et al., 1972).

A full understanding of the potassium current, i_{K_2}, is crucial to the comprehension of spontaneous phase 4 depolarization. To measure i_{K_2}, an arbitrary holding voltage is chosen, usually within the activation voltage range for this current. Our holding voltage of -85 mV in Figure 6 is within the activation range of i_{K_2}, since clamp steps returning to this holding level from more negative levels do result in slow activation of outward current. (Current increases in an outward, or positive, direction during the holding clamp.) Test voltage clamp steps negative to -100 mV fail to increase the magnitude of outward current change on return to -85 mV. The i_{K_2} curve is defined by the amount of current change on return to a constant holding voltage from many different test voltages. By exploring test voltages throughout the activation range of i_{K_2} (-90 to -50 mV), instead of only the range negative to -100 mV as in Figure 6, we can derive the full S-shaped i_{K_2} current–voltage relationship seen in Figure 8. Unlike the construction of the steady-state current–voltage relationship in Figure 7, the points which make up this i_{K_2} current–voltage relationship represent current change and are absolute values of current; there is no zero reference for current.

It is important to recall that i_{K_2} represents an outward current which decreases following action potential repolarization. Notice also that the time

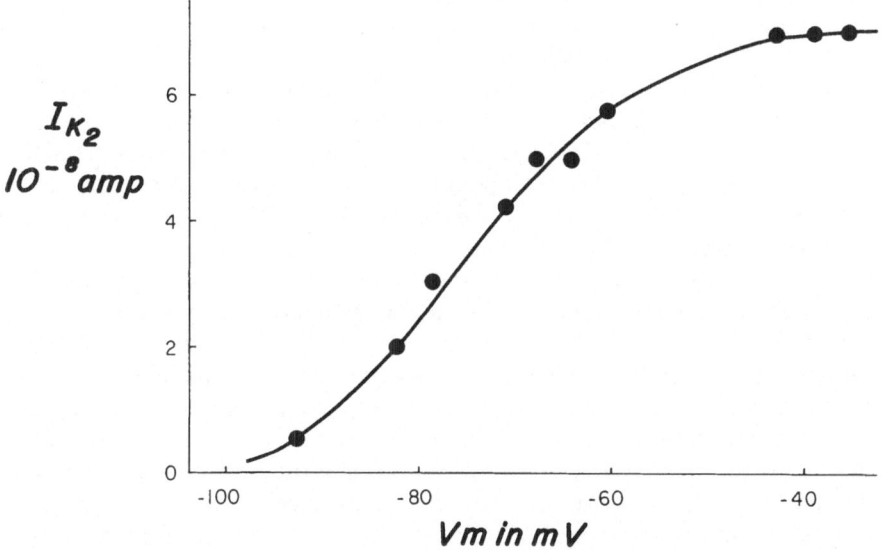

Figure 8. Potassium pacemaker current–voltage relationship. Holding voltage for this fiber was -85 mV. i_{K_2} is measured as the amount of current change which occurs with time following return to the holding voltage from various test voltage clamps. Note that i_{K_2} is negligible below -90 mV and is fully activated at about -50 mV.

course of change of i_{K_2} (in Figures 5 and 6) is much slower (seconds) at −83 mV than the phase 3 repolarization of an action potential (tens of milliseconds). This means that repolarization of an action potential proceeds to completion before an appreciable amount of i_{K_2} deactivates and that the subsequent slow deactivation of i_{K_2} can produce pacemaker depolarization.

To assess the interaction of i_{K_2} and the steady-state current–voltage relationship, we aligned the voltage axes and added the observed amount of deactivated i_{K_2} at each transmembrane voltage to the steady-state current–voltage curve in Figure 9. In the steady state, at a transmembrane voltage of −90 mV, all of i_{K_2} is essentially deactivated, so that i_{K_2} makes no significant contribution to the steady-state current–voltage curve. Conversely, in the steady state at −50 mV, i_{K_2} is fully activated, so that at this voltage the full amplitude of the i_{K_2} curve is contributing to the steady-state current–voltage relationship. The dashed curve in Figure 9 represents the current–voltage relationship during action potential repolarization, which is rapid enough so that i_{K_2} remains essentially fully activated, yet slow enough so that all other transmembrane currents (e.g., i_{K_1} and i_{x_1}) practically reach their steady-state values. The separation between this calculated curve and the steady-state current–voltage curve at −90 mV is 8×10^{-8} A, a value nearly equal to the full amplitude of the i_{K_2} current. (The dashed curve is essentially equal to the steady-state curve plus full activation of i_{K_2}.) The dashed curve crosses the zero current axis at the maximum diastolic voltage.

Using the steady-state current-voltage relationships (solid line) and the steady state plus i_{K_2} (dashed line) in Figure 9, we can demonstrate the properties of these curves which will determine phase 4 depolarization. First, it is clear that deactivation of a larger i_{K_2} will cause a larger phase 4 depolarization. Second, the membrane slope conductance ($\Delta I/\Delta V$) of the steady-state curve between the maximum diastolic and resting voltages will determine how much voltage change will occur with any given deactivation. Figure 10 shows the importance of slope conductance in determining the magnitude of phase 4 depolarization: panel A shows a diagrammatic steady-state current–voltage relationship with a higher slope conductance than the current–voltage relationship of panel B, and consequently the same amount of i_{K_2} deactivation causes less spontaneous phase 4 depolarization in panel A than in panel B. Third, the position of the zero-current intercept of the steady-state curve relative to the critical firing threshold is a major factor determining whether or not spontaneous automaticity is produced. Figure 11 shows the steady-state current–voltage relationships for two hypothetical fibers; if repolarization carries the membrane of fiber A to a maximum diastolic voltage negative to threshold, the subsequent deactivation of i_{K_2} will by definition cause the membrane to reach threshold voltage, whereas fiber B will not be automatic, regardless of the magnitude of i_{K_2}, because its steady-state curve crosses the current axis negative to the threshold voltage. Fourth, the

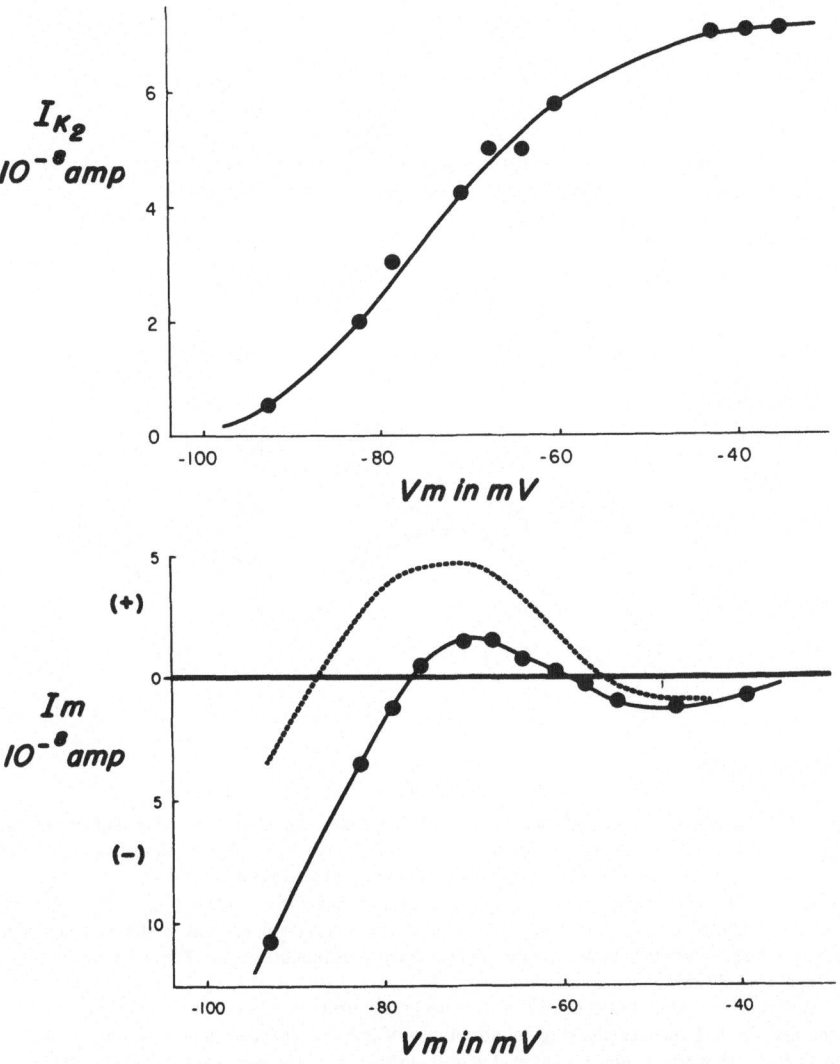

Figure 9. Contribution of i_{K_2} to the steady-state current–voltage relationship. The upper curve is i_{K_2} vs. V_m; the lower solid curve is the steady-state current–voltage relationship. Both curves from same fiber. Note alignment of the voltage axes, but different Purkinje current scales. The dotted curve represents the change in the steady-state curve which would occur if i_{K_2} were fully activated at all voltages. All transmembrane currents except i_{K_2} rapidly approach their steady-state values during action potential repolarization, but i_{K_2} remains nearly fully activated (i.e., changes much more slowly than the rate of repolarization). Therefore, the dotted curve is a fair representation of the membrane current–voltage relationship during spontaneous action potential repolarization in the voltage range near V_H (but it does not reflect changes in driving force for potassium or in i_{K_2} rectification at V_m different from V_H).

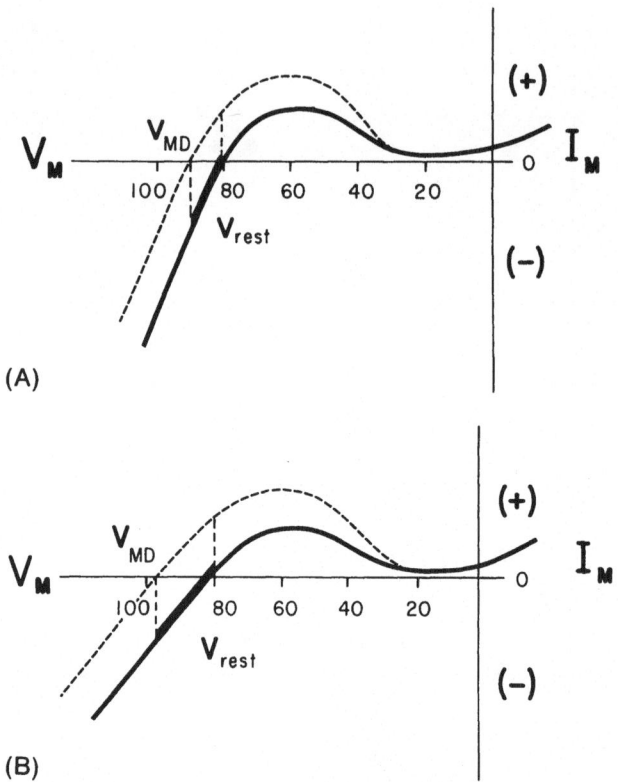

Figure 10. The effect of membrane slope conductance on the magnitude of phase 4 depolarization. In both panels, the solid curves indicate the steady-state current–voltage relationship and the dashed curves the current–voltage relationship during phase 3 repolarization.

A: Resting voltage of -80 mV and a maximum diastolic voltage (V_{MD}) of -90 mV. After action potential repolarization is complete, the pacemaker current (difference between solid and dashed curves) will deactivate, and produce spontaneous phase 4 depolarization from -90 mV to -80 mV.

B: Another fiber in which resting voltage and magnitude of pacemaker current are identical to the fiber in A. However, the slope conductance of the steady-state current–voltage relationship in B is less, and so the maximum diastolic voltage is more negative (close to -100 mV). Also, the same amount of pacemaker current deactivation causes a greater magnitude of spontaneous phase 4 depolarization.

position of the i_{K_2} current–voltage relationship on the voltage axis can shift to either a more positive or a more negative voltage.

In Figure 9, most of the i_{K_2} curve is positive to the resting transmembrane voltage; thus, a shift of this i_{K_2} curve to a more positive value on its voltage axis will result in a relatively small increase in the magnitude of diastolic

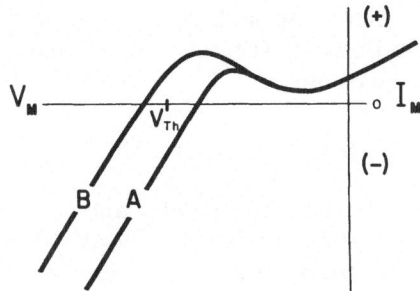

Figure 11. Steady-state current–voltage relationships and automaticity. Two hypothetical fibers, A and B, have steady-state curves which cross the current axis on either side of the threshold voltage, V_{Th}, which is the same for both fibers. The two outward currents i_{x_1} and i_{K_2} carry the membrane to a voltage negative to the threshold value during action potential repolarization. Fiber A will be automatic because as i_{K_2} deactivates, V_{Th} will be attained. The current voltage curve of fiber B will not permit automaticity since the intersection of the steady-state curve is at a transmembrane voltage negative to threshold, V_{Th}.

depolarization. If, however, the initial curve lay at a more negative position on the voltage axis, then a shift of the i_{K_2} curve in the depolarizing direction on the voltage axis would cause a large increase in the magnitude of diastolic depolarization. Conversely, if the entire i_{K_2} curve is initially placed at voltages positive to the resting transmembrane voltage, then a shift to a still more positive voltage range will not increase phase 4 depolarization any further.

The behavior of i_{K_2} has been successfully reconstructed using a single gating variable of the Hodgkin–Huxley type and a rectifier function (Noble and Tsien, 1968; Hauswirth *et al.*, 1972). The i_{K_2} can be separated from both the instantaneous membrane potassium conductance (i_{K_1}) and the conductance which is primarily responsible for action potential repolarization (i_{x_1}) (Hauswirth *et al.*, 1972). The mathematical description of i_{K_2} is given as

$$i_{K_2} = g_{K_2}(V_m - V_K) \qquad (10)$$

where g_{K_2} is the conductance of this slow potassium membrane channel. The conductance is governed by the gating variable of the channel, s, which can vary from 0 to 1 so that

$$g_{K_2} = s(\bar{g}_{K_2}) \qquad (11)$$

where $\bar{g}_{K_2}$ is the maximum obtainable pacemaker potassium conductance, and s follows classical (Hodgkin and Huxley, 1952*d*) first-order kinetics

$$\frac{ds}{dt} = \alpha_s(1 - s) - \beta_s(s) \qquad (12)$$

where α_s and β_s are activating and deactivating voltage-dependent rate constants, respectively. Equation (12) can be integrated to give s as a function of time (s_t) during a step clamp

$$s_t = s_\infty - (s_\infty - s_0)e^{-k_s t} \tag{13}$$

where s_∞ is the steady-state final value of s, and s_0 is the value of s at the instant prior to the voltage clamp step. For steady-state voltage conditions, $ds/dt = 0$ in equation (12) and the value of s_∞ is given by

$$s_\infty = \frac{\alpha_s}{\alpha_s + \beta_s} \tag{14}$$

The rate constant, k_s, in equation (13) is found to be

$$k_s = 1/\tau_s = \alpha_s + \beta_s \tag{15}$$

where τ_s is the time constant of the first-order process governing the potassium conductance change; typically τ_s is about 2 sec at V_m between -90 and -70 mV.

The magnitude of g_{K_2} in equation (11) is also governed by a voltage-dependent rectifier function showing inward-going rectification similar to that known to govern instantaneous voltage-dependent membrane potassium conductance, g_{K_1}. Consequently, equation (10) should be expanded to include the rectifier function, giving

$$i_{K_2} = f_2(V_m, V_K) \cdot s \cdot (V_m - V_K) \tag{16}$$

where $f_2(V_m, V_K)$ represents the rectifier function, which has been found to depend on both transmembrane voltage, V_m, and the distribution of potassium ions across the membrane [therefore, V_K—see equation (7)]. Thus, the amplitude of the S-shaped i_{K_2} current–voltage relationship (Figure 8) is dependent in a nonlinear fashion upon the transmembrane voltage at which the holding clamp voltage is set. The i_{K_2} shows strong inward-going rectification with a negative slope conductance which appears at voltages 30 mV or more positive to V_K; owing to the rectifier function, i_{K_2} approaches zero at about 0 mV even though s is 1 at this V_m (Hauswirth et al., 1972).

Even though the cardiac cell membrane rectifier properties are complicated and, as yet, incompletely characterized, the concept of rectification of ionic conductances is useful to explain the nonlinear behavior of observed membrane currents. Together with the more completely understood kinetic behavior, the concept of rectifier properties allows a description of membrane ionic behavior by mathematical expressions; this facilitates our ability to characterize effects of various interventions on ionic behavior, to construct mathematical membrane models, and ultimately to describe possible geometric configurations (on a molecular level) which may be important in membrane ionic conductances.

In terminating this section on potassium pacemaker current analysis, a few words of caution seem appropriate. Elegant mathematical analyses such as those of pacemaker and plateau slow current changes carried out by Hauswirth et al. (1972) are dependent upon selection of Purkinje fiber segments which show current changes in the voltage ranges under study. Although we think such analyses are applicable to repolarization and spontaneous depolarization in *normal* Purkinje fibers, we should nonetheless reserve some degree of circumspection on this point, since experimental fibers do not always generate action potentials with normal plateaus or normal spontaneous phase 4 depolarization. It is encouraging that fibers with normal action potentials have, indeed, been shown to have characteristic i_{K_2} current properties in the voltage range of spontaneous phase 4 depolarization (Vassalle, 1966; Peper and Trautwein, 1969; Weld and Bigger, personal observations).

3. Electrogenic Na^+ Pumping

As mentioned earlier, the intracellular Na^+ concentration is much lower than the extracellular concentration. The intracellular Na^+ concentration in bovine Purkinje fibers is about 25 mM (Bosteels and Carmeliet, 1972a, b). Extrusion of Na^+ from cardiac cells is regarded as an active process, since Na^+ must move against a steep electrochemical gradient. The conditions for coupling of Na^+ extrusion to cellular uptake of K^+ (i.e., sodium transport is electrically neutral) and those for which Na^+ pumping is electrogenic (i.e., Na^+ moves outward without being in 1:1 balance with inward movement of positive charge) are not fully delineated. When cardiac fibers are cooled (0–4°C), they lose K^+ and gain Na^+; this effect is explained by a decrease in cation pumping in the cold (Délèze, 1960). When atrial muscle, ventricular muscle, or Purkinje fibers have been cooled for long periods of time in low K^+ solutions and then rewarmed, hyperpolarization has been observed (Glitsch, 1972; McDonald and MacLeod, 1971; Page and Storm, 1965; Tamai and Kagiyama, 1968; Hiraoka and Hecht, 1973). For instance, after 24 hr at 2–4°C in Tyrode solution with K^+ at 1.0 mmole/liter, the transmembrane voltage of Purkinje fibers is about −20 to −30 mV. When warmed to 37°C in Tyrode containing 5.4 mmol/liter K^+, the V_m polarizes to about −110 mV (Hiraoka and Hecht, 1973), a value 20 mV more negative than that obtained with control fibers. The magnitude of this polarization is proportional to cooling time and is abolished by pretreatment with ouabain or low K^+ solutions (Hiraoka and Hecht, 1973). Large hyperpolarizations, many mV negative to the potassium equilibrium potential were noted by Tamai and Kagiyama (1968) on warming previously cooled cat ventricular muscle. When cooled cardiac muscle is allowed to load with lithium rather than sodium, no hyperpolarization occurs on warming. This is consistent with reports that lithium can utilize sodium channels for entry into the cell but that extrusion of lithium is very slow (Carmeliet, 1964). Thus, it appears that pumping of sodium from cardiac cells can be electrogenic. When electrogenic pumping is activated, it provides outward current which opposes diastolic depolarization. Electrogenic sodium pumping has been proposed to explain such phenomena as hyperpolarization of Purkinje fibers by catecholamines and suppression of phase 4 depolarization in cardiac Purkinje fibers by rapid stimulation (see below).

B.   Inward Currents

Inward current is a prerequisite for diastolic depolarization. Two inward currents will be discussed in this section: the background inward current which participates in slow diastolic depolarization and the rapid, inward sodium current which is responsible for the action potential upstroke.

1.   Background Inward Current

As noted earlier, a significant diastolic inward current is apparent from the fact that resting V_m is significantly less negative than the equilibrium potential for potassium. This diastolic inward current depolarizes the membrane as i_{K_2} deactivates. Peper and Trautwein (1969) found a rather large inward current in Purkinje fibers clamped to their estimated V_K. However, the ionic species which carries the current is still in contention. Peper and Trautwein (1969) found that the current is not diminished in Purkinje fibers exposed to low sodium solutions. Also, Purkinje fibers do not usually spontaneously polarize to V_K when superfused with low Na^+ solutions, although V_m may move in a negative direction (Hall et al., 1963). Tracer studies reveal a considerable sodium efflux from quiescent bovine Purkinje fibers (Bosteels and Carmeliet, 1972a); presumably, the passive influx of sodium is equal to this active efflux.

Some of the background current flowing at diastolic values of V_m may be carried by calcium ions, and an electrogenic potassium pump has even been suggested as a candidate for this current (Peper and Trautwein, 1969). We currently assume that most of the background inward current is carried by sodium and that magnitude of the current is a linear function of the driving force on this ion.

2. Regenerative Inward Sodium Current (i_{Na})

In spontaneously automatic Purkinje fibers, phase 4 depolarization is terminated by an action potential upstroke produced by regenerative inward sodium current. This current also contributes significantly to the late portion of diastolic depolarization. The time and voltage dependence of fast inward sodium current was well characterized in squid axon by Hodgkin and Huxley (1952a–d). It has not been possible, however, to define precisely the kinetics of sodium currents in heart muscle because of the series resistance-linked membrane capacitance and technical inadequacies of the voltage clamp techniques used in heart muscle. The steady-state voltage dependence of the sodium channels and the voltage-dependent rate coefficients have been studied in cooled Purkinje fibers and strongly resemble these properties in nerve (Dudel and Rüdel, 1970). In fact, reasonably successful reconstruction of cardiac action potential upstrokes has been accomplished utilizing modified Hodgkin–Huxley equation (Noble, 1962; McAllister, 1970).

There are three important differences between potassium currents and fast inward sodium current in cardiac Purkinje fibers. First, the membrane does not rectify sodium current as it does i_{K_1} and i_{K_2}. Second, two gating variables (instead of one) must be postulated to explain the increase and then decrease of sodium current during a step voltage clamp. Third, the kinetics of these two gating variables, called m and h (Hodgkin and Huxley, 1952a–d; Dudel and Rüdel, 1970), have time constants measured in milliseconds instead of seconds, as is the case for i_{K_2}.

The equation describing sodium conductance is

$$g_{Na} = m^3 h(\bar{g}_{Na}) \tag{17}$$

where m is the activation factor reponsible for the large increase in g_{Na} upon sudden membrane depolarization, h is the inactivation factor responsible for the subsequent decrease in g_{Na} for the depolarized membrane, and $\bar{g}_{Na}$ is the maximum sodium conductance obtainable under any transmembrane voltage conditions. The kinetic behavior of m and h is described by:

$$\frac{dm}{dt} = \alpha_m(1 - m) - \beta_m m \tag{18}$$

$$\frac{dh}{dt} = \alpha_h(1 - h) - \beta_h h \tag{19}$$

A   B

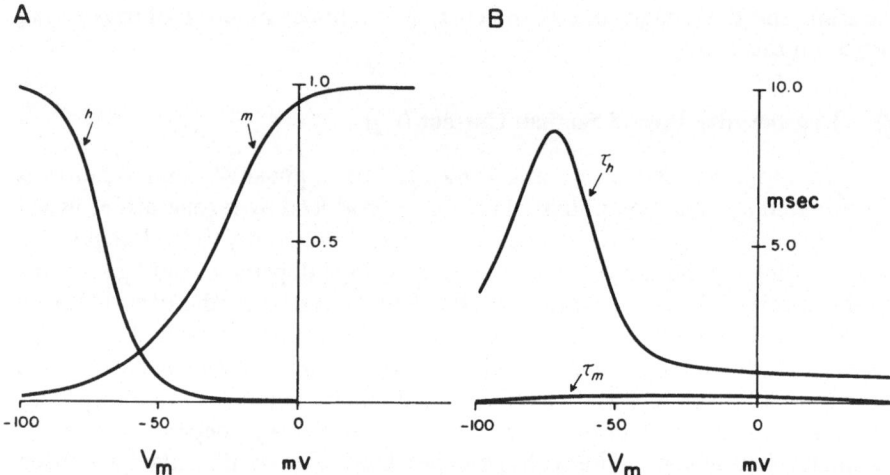

Figure 12A. Steady-state voltage dependence of the kinetic factors, m and h, for fast inward sodium conductance. These curves follow the values of m and h when the transmembrane voltage has been held constant for a long period of time. Note that the value of m^3h, a major determinant of the magnitude of sodium conductance [equation (17)], is always small in the steady state.

Figure 12B. The time constants of m and h [from equations (20) and (21)] are also plotted as functions of voltage. Note the much smaller time constant for m at all transmembrane voltages; this allows m to attain its steady-state value following a transmembrane voltage step far more rapidly than h.

where α_m and α_h represent voltage-dependent rate constants describing conversion of the m and h gates from nonconducting to conducting for sodium ions, and β_m and β_h represent voltage-dependent rate contants describing conversion of the m and h gates from conducting to nonconducting. Both m and h must be open for sodium ions to pass through these specific channels. Note that m allows sodium passage only at depolarized transmembrane voltages in the steady state, whereas h allows sodium passage only at repolarized (near resting) transmembrane voltages in the steady state (Figure 12A). It is only the slower rate of change of h as opposed to m (Figure 12B) which allows a sudden pulse of sodium ions to cross the membrane at the time of a sudden transmembrane voltage change from a repolarized to a depolarized value (Figure 13). This can also be mathematically appreciated from the solutions to equations (18) and (19) for m and h:

$$m = m_\infty - (m_\infty - m_0)e^{-t/\tau_m} \tag{20}$$

$$h = h_\infty - (h_\infty - h_0)e^{-t/\tau_h} \tag{21}$$

where m_0, h_0, and m_∞ and h_∞ represent steady-state values of the kinetic factors at the initial and final transmembrane voltages; t is time following an instantaneous step between the initial and final transmembrane voltage; τ_m and τ_h are the time constants describing the rapidity of change of m and h at a given voltage (see Figure 12B).

A full consideration of excitatory sodium current in cardiac cells is not our main concern in this discussion of diastolic pacemaker currents and can be found elsewhere (Dudel and Rüdel, 1970; Dudel et al., 1967a; Rougier

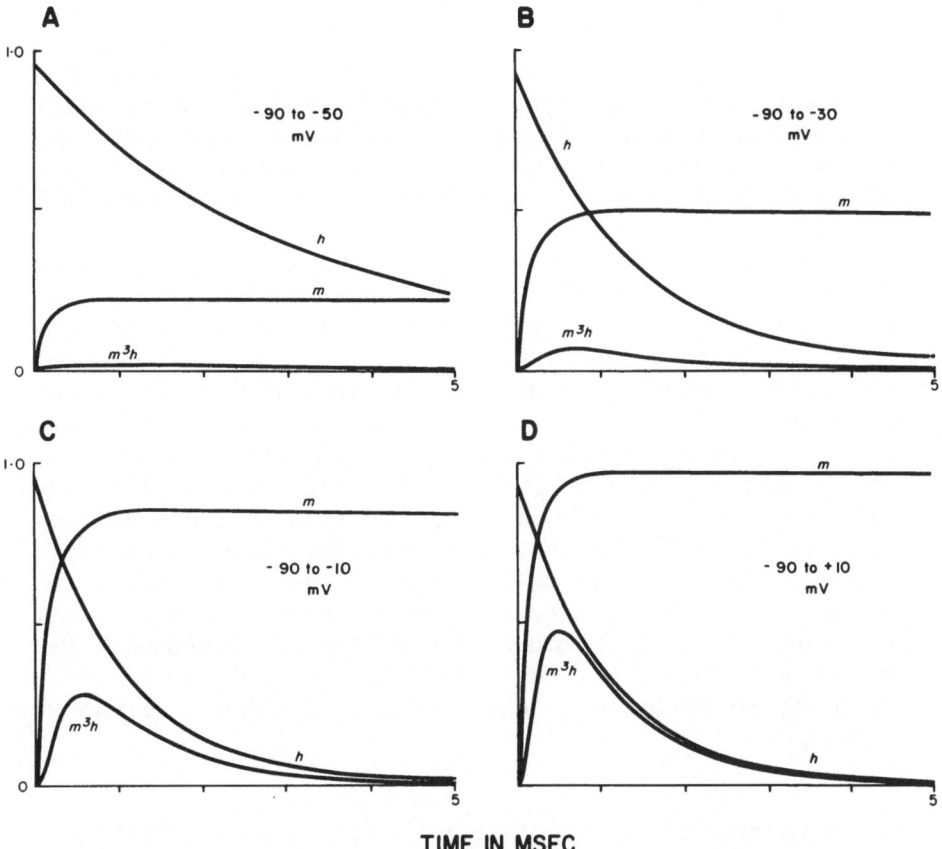

TIME IN MSEC

Figure 13. Time course of change of m, h, and m^3h following "instantaneous" voltage-clamp steps as indicated in each panel. Note that the kinetics of each curve are accounted for by equations (20) and (21), with values for m_∞ and h_∞, τ_m and τ_h taken from Figure 12. Maximum inward sodium conductance, which is proportional to m^3h, is greatest for the voltage step to $+10$ mV.

et al., 1968). However, fast inward sodium current is instrumental in the determination of the membrane's critical firing threshold, which is the transmembrane voltage at which inward current exceeds outward current to initiate the action potential upstroke. Modification of either the voltage dependence or the time dependence of the sodium conductance can alter the threshold voltage. Thus a voltage-dependent decrease in either m or h in the neighborhood of the critical firing voltage will result in less inward sodium current [equation (17) and Figure 12A] and a shift of the critical voltage to more positive values. A direct consequence of this would be the requirement of a greater deactivation of i_{K_2} or a smaller i_{K_1} in order to bring such a membrane to excitation. Significant modification of the time dependence of sodium conductance is probably limited to alteration of the h time constant: phase 4 depolarization is a slow process, making it unlikely that even marked slowing of the rapid m factor kinetics would cause a change in m at any given voltage (Figure 12B). However, there is good evidence in frog atrial cells (Haas *et al.*, 1971) that the kinetics of the fast sodium system's h factor are slow enough to cause a significant deviation of h from h_∞ during repolarization and diastole.

Since h_∞ is larger at more negative transmembrane voltages, a slowing of the rate of change of h during phase 4 depolarization results in a larger value of h than is the case if h can achieve its steady-state value throughout the time–voltage course of phase 4. There are two consequences of an isolated slowing of h inactivation upon phase 4 depolarization: first, since inward sodium current is larger at any transmembrane voltage [equations (8b) and (17); Figures 12A and 13], threshold voltage becomes more negative, enhancing automaticity (Figure 1C). Second, excitation of the fiber (e.g., by a propagating wavefront) results in a larger rate of rise of action potential phase 0 [equation (2)], and thus a faster conduction velocity. The final expression of enhanced automaticity and increased conduction velocity in the intact heart is modified by many other variables. Also, it is clear that shifts in the kinetics of i_{Na} can importantly alter the last portion of diastolic depolarization. The accelerated rate of depolarization during late diastole is importantly contributed to by an increase in i_{Na}, as well as a decrease in i_{K_2} and i_{K_1}.

IV. MODIFICATION OF AUTOMATICITY BY PHYSICAL AND CHEMICAL AGENTS

The preceding section has discussed the changes in membrane ionic conductance which cause spontaneous diastolic depolarization. We relied heavily on data obtained in mammalian cardiac Purkinje fibers using the voltage clamp technique. Unfortunately, such data are absent or sparse for other cardiac cell types, particularly for the sinoatrial and atrioventricular nodes. In this section we will discuss some of the many physical and chemical influences which alter normal automaticity. We will discuss the factors which modify phase 4 depolarization in the framework of three broad categories: (1) normal ionic constituents and neurohumoral agents, (2) physical factors, and (3) exogenous chemical factors.

A. Normal Ionic Constituents and Neurohumors

1. Potassium

Alteration of extracellular potassium ion concentration, $[K]_0$, has profound effects on cardiac pacemaker cells, more so in cells within the ventricular specialized conducting system than within the sinoatrial node. Changes in $[K]_0$ also have profound effects on nonpacemaker electrophysiological properties of heart muscle.

An increase in $[K]_0$ shortens the action potential, depolarizes the cell, and shifts threshold to more positive voltages. When potassium depolarizes the cell sufficiently, the rate of rise and amplitude of phase 0 decrease. These effects on phase 0 are probably not effects of the potassium ion *per se*, but are more likely a result of the more positive transmembrane voltage (Weidmann, 1955a; Trautwein and Schmidt, 1960). Recently, Tritthart *et al.* (1969) have provided evidence to suggest that changes in the extracellular potassium concentration may alter the kinetics of the sodium current, but this is not yet proven. The effects of potassium on resting transmembrane voltage are intimately related to the effects of potassium on cardiac automaticity. Adrian (1956) showed in frog skeletal muscle that the membrane depolarizes approximately as predicted by the Nernst equation [equation (7)] when extracellular potassium is raised above the normal level; this behavior is also seen in cardiac muscle (Weidmann, 1956; Arnsdorf and Bigger, 1972). When extracellular potassium falls to very low concentrations, the membrane also depolarizes. This descending limb on the curve relating transmembrane resting voltage to the extracellular potassium concentration results in a V_m of about -60 mV both when $[K]_0$ is 1.0 mM and when $[K]_0$ is 13.5 mM. The decrease in V_m at low values of $[K]_0$ is the result of a decrease in membrane potassium conductance (g_K) (Carmeliet, 1960; Hall *et al.*, 1963; Arnsdorf and Bigger, 1972). When $[K]_0$ is increased within the physiologic range, changes in electrophysiologic properties are very dependent on the cell type, and the initial and final potassium concentrations. For example, when $[K]_0$ is increased from 2.7 to 5.4 mM in Tyrode solution perfusing isolated Purkinje fibers, V_m does not change significantly but g_K doubles

(Vassalle, 1966). In this instance, the 18-mV decrease in V_K almost precisely offsets the increase in g_K which causes V_m to move closer to V_K—the net result being little or no change in V_m. The increase in g_K resulting from an increase in $[K]_0$ is the result of increases in both g_{K_1} and g_{K_2} (Noble and Tsien, 1968). When $[K]_0$ is increased, the instantaneous potassium current, i_{K1}, increases at any given transmembrane voltage; i_{K1} increases substantially even for increments in $[K]_0$ within the physiological range. Also, the position of the i_{K2} activation curve does not shift on its voltage axis when $[K]_0$ is changed over the range 2.0–6.0 mEq/liter, even though these same changes in $[K]_0$ both increase the amplitude of the i_{K2} activation curve and decrease the rectification of the cardiac membrane for i_{K2} (Noble and Tsien, 1968). The augmentation in potassium conductances induced by increasing the extracellular potassium concentration opposes depolarization of the membrane by inward currents. This action of potassium is a powerful deterrent to phase 4 depolarization and automatic firing.

At $[K]_0$ greater than 6.0 mM, the cell membrane of cardiac Purkinje fibers will depolarize and threshold voltage will shift in a positive direction owing to a voltage-dependent decrease in the i_{Na} gating factor, h (see Figure 12A), and increased membrane potassium conductance. This shift in threshold (Antoni *et al.*, 1963) has a potent antiautomatic action, but is accompanied by the arrhythmogenic potential of slowed conduction and, if $[K]_0$ is increased enough, block.

2. Sodium

It is unlikely that variation in the extracellular sodium concentration within the physiologic range causes large changes in either inward sodium currents or other ionic currents. However, under adverse circumstances, such as digitalis intoxication or hypoxia, sodium may accumulate in cells, causing a signficant decrease in the driving force for sodium across the membrane [see equations (7) and (8b)]; this state would tend to oppose normal automaticity. Outside the physiologic range, reduction of the external sodium concentration may have significant effects on either normal or abnormal automaticity. In sodium-poor or sodium-free solutions, i_{K_2} is greatly reduced in cardiac Purkinje fibers (Deck and Trautwein, 1964; McAllister and Noble, 1966). Preliminary results suggest that removal of sodium from solutions bathing Purkinje fibers does not greatly alter the s kinetics but does reduce the amplitude of i_{K_2} (Noble and Tsien, 1969a). Recently, it has been reported that addition of small concentrations (8 mM) of sodium to Purkinje fibers which exhibit spontaneous calcium-dependent action potentials in sodium-free solution will inhibit this form of automaticity (Wiggins and Cranefield, 1974). Addition of sodium not only diminished spontaneous activity but also caused the cells to hyperpolarize by as much as 20 mV. Addition of lithium to such preparations neither inhibited automatic firing nor caused any hyperpolarization. Wiggins and Cranefield (1974) interpreted their results to mean that the addition of sodium stimulated electrogenic sodium pumping.

3. Calcium

The early studies of the effect of calcium on Purkinje fibers (Weidmann, 1955b) revealed a shift in threshold to more positive values when extracellular calcium concentration, $[Ca]_0$, was increased. The rate of diastolic depolarization was not significantly affected, but the spontaneous firing rate decreased considerably owing to the shift in threshold. When rate is held constant by electrical stimulation, elevation of $[Ca]_0$ enhances the rate of phase 4 depolarization somewhat (Temte and Davis, 1967). Elevation of $[Ca]_0$ also shortens the duration of the Purkinje fiber action potential when drive rate is controlled. The increase in the rate of phase 4 depolarization and the more positive values of threshold voltage at higher $[Ca]_0$ have been ascribed respectively to a shift of the i_{K_2} curve in the depolarizing direction on its voltage axis and to a similar shift in the voltage dependence of the fast inward sodium kinetics (Hauswirth et al., 1969). Although the shift in the i_{K_2} curve alone would promote pacemaker activity, the change in the sodium kinetics would have the opposite effect. Since the later phase of pacemaker depolarization in Purkinje fibers is quite sensitive to changes in sodium current, the net result of increasing $[Ca]_0$ is a reduction of firing rate (Weidmann, 1955b; Temte and Davis, 1967; Colatsky and Hogan, 1964). Increasing $[Ca]_0$ to 7.2 mM augments overdrive suppression of pacemakers (see below) but may induce postoverdrive membrane oscillations and automatic firing; this type of activity has been observed in both canine Purkinje fibers and frog sinus venosus (Colatsky and Hogan, 1964; Gough et al., 1974).

4. Chloride

Studies in cardiac Purkinje fibers show that the chloride ion provides background current at diastolic and plateau values of transmembrane voltage and a brief current transient in the initial portion of the action potential. The distribution of chloride ions in cardiac muscle is thought to be passive and determined by membrane voltage (Carmeliet, 1961; Hutter and Noble, 1961) so that, in fibers which have been at rest for long periods of time, the chloride equilibrium potential, V_{Cl}, should be equal to V_m. In cardiac muscle which is repeatedly activated, V_{Cl} will assume a value between the plateau and diastolic voltages, about -50 mV (Hutter and Noble, 1961). Under these conditions, I_{Cl} will reverse in the course of the cardiac cycle, providing inward current during diastole and outward current during the plateau. Thus, during pacemaker activity a time-independent background inward current carried by chloride will contribute to the pacemaker potential. In addition to this small time-independent chloride current, a larger, outward chloride current contributes to phase 1 of the action potential, i.e., repolarization from the peak of phase 0 to the initial portion of the action potential plateau. This current, which has been called the "initial outward current" and "positive dynamic current," has been studied with voltage-clamp techniques; it was found to activate at about -20 mV and inactivate at plateau voltages with a time constant of about 50 msec. The amplitude of this current is greatly reduced by decreasing the extracellular chloride concentration (Dudel *et al.*, 1967c; Fozzard and Hiraoka, 1973). The recovery from inactivation of this transient chloride current is slow, 0.5–2.0 sec, and dependent on membrane voltage (Peper and Trautwein, 1968; Reuter, 1968; Fozzard and Hiraoka, 1973).

5. Po$_2$

Isolated ventricular muscle and Purkinje fiber preparations exposed to low values of Po$_2$ depolarize and show shortening of the action potential plateau; ultimately, these changes become pronounced and conduction velocity decreases (Trautwein *et al.*, 1954; Coraboeuf *et al.*, 1958). The membrane depolarization in Purkinje fibers is accompanied by an increase in spontaneous phase 4 depolarization, leading to increased automaticity (Trautwein *et al.*, 1954). On the other hand, when Deck (1964a) equilibrated his Tyrode solution with air instead of 95% O_2–5% CO_2. he noted a fall in spontaneous firing rate of rabbit and cat sinus preparations, which he attributed to hypoxia.

The duration of hypoxia tolerated prior to abnormal electrophysiological behavior is shortened by increasing the drive rate of the preparation in both ventricular muscle and Purkinje fibers, and cardiac tissue is more sensitive to each of a series of hypoxic exposures (Trautwein *et al.*, 1954). There is an important difference between ventricular muscle and Purkinje fibers: Although the electrophysiological changes are qualitatively similar in both tissues, Purkinje fibers can withstand far longer periods (hours) of hypoxia prior to showing abnormal changes. Transmembrane ionic gradients are maintained by an ATP-dependent cation pump. When high-energy phosphate stores are consumed under anoxic conditions, anaerobic glycolysis must supply the energy required by the pump. Since cardiac muscle contraction consumes vastly more energy than does electrical excitation, it seems reasonable to assume that the greater energy requirement of ventricular muscle is responsible for its greater intolerance of low oxygen concentrations than Purkinje tissue, which has a lower energy requirement. Unpublished studies from our laboratory in collaboration with Dr. Marianne Legato indicate that Purkinje fiber glycogen stores are depleted at the time of appearance of hypoxia-induced electrophysiological changes.

6. Acid–Base Buffer System

The physiological acid–base buffer system in mammals is primarily determined by the concentrations of carbonic acid and bicarbonate in blood, according to the Henderson–Hasselbalch equation. It is difficult to selectively identify the result of a change in pH, P_{CO_2}, or HCO_3^-, because a change in any one of these determinants produces a change in the other two. Therefore all three of these determinants of acid–base balance are considered together.

Results of studies of acid–base imbalance on spontaneous phase 4 depolarization have been variable. Coraboeuf and Boistel (1953) demonstrated a slowing of spontaneous phase 4 depolarization in Purkinje fibers when the CO_2 in their gassing mixture was raised to 10%, whereas Hoffman and Cranefield (1960) reported an increase in spontaneous phase 4 depolarization, also in Purkinje fibers, when the concentration of sodium bicarbonate in their Tyrode solution was decreased. Each maneuver decreases the pH of the perfusing solution. Hecht and Hutter (1965) studied Purkinje fibers at pH 5.9 and found no significant increase in pacemaker activity; Brown and Noble (1972) studied Purkinje fibers at this same pH and found variable effects on spontaneous automatic rate. Deck (1964a) found that rabbit and cat sinus automaticity was enhanced by alkalinization and depressed by acidification as pH was varied from 7.3 to 8.3 by means of a tris-maleic acid buffer.

Threshold voltage is moved in a positive direction by a decrease in pH (Hecht and Hutter, 1965; Brown and Noble, 1972), and this is perhaps the most consistent electrophysiological effect of lowering pH. In their voltage-clamp analysis, Brown and Noble (1972) found no voltage shift of the i_{K_2} current–voltage relationship by acid, but some decrease in the rectifier function for i_{K_2} (an antiautomatic effect since i_{K_2} will increase). These authors also noted that acid increased inward current at their holding voltage of -70 mV, which is consistent with slightly less negative maximum diastolic voltages which Hecht and Hutter (1965) found in an acid environment. The ionic basis of pH-dependent electrophysiologic changes is unknown, although Hille (1968b) has suggested inactivation of sodium channels through protonation of surface acidic radicals to explain voltage-dependent shifts in sodium conductance factors in frog node of Ranvier at low pH.

An increase of P_{CO_2} to 20% (equilibrated with 14 mM bicarbonate) results in appearance of premature depolarization during phase 3 repolarization, and an increase to 50% can produce partial membrane depolarization and generation of repetitive abnormal action potentials or membrane oscillations (Coraboeuf and Boistel, 1953)—abnormal forms of automaticity. Another interesting point in this paper is that normal action potentials persisted when pure O_2 was bubbled through the perfusate despite the high pH which must exist in such a perfusate. Other action potential changes resulting from acidosis are similar to those caused by hypoxia (see above), except that refractoriness is prolonged or variably affected (Lathrop et al., 1974; Mandel and Obayashi, 1974). These changes in refractoriness may be accounted for by the action potential prolongation seen in Purkinje fibers exposed to solutions with a pH of 5.9 (Hecht and Hutter, 1965).

7. Lactate

Recently, the effects of lactate (lactic acid buffered with sodium bicarbonate to pH 7.35) on cardiac Purkinje fibers have been investigated. Lactate, in clinically encountered concentrations, produced increased spontaneous phase 4 depolarization, a fall in (more positive) resting transmembrane voltage, a decrease in rate of rise of action potential phase 0, and a decrease in action potential duration (Wissner, 1974). This work correctly draws attention to the similarity between the electrophysiological effects of lactate and those of tissue ischemia. The membrane ionic conductance changes responsible for the observed action potential alterations are unknown.

8. Acetylcholine

Acetylcholine is the neurohumoral transmitter for vagal postsynaptic terminals and is thus an important mediator of cardiac control by the central nervous system. The literature on cardiac electrophysiological effects of acetylcholine is extensive, and well reviewed by Hoffman and Cranefield (1960). An increase in conductance of atrial membranes was implicated by the discovery of a shorter length constant and time constant of fiber bundles from frog atria (Trautwein et al., 1956). Since membrane hyperpolarization and decreased phase 4 depolarization accompanied the increase in membrane conductance, the findings were best explained by an acetylcholine-induced increase in membrane conductance to an ion with a negative equilibrium potential—one which could supply more outward current. By showing a corresponding change of the membrane's resting potential toward the calculated equilibrium potential for potassium (at varying potassium concentrations) under the influence of acetylcholine, Trautwein and Dudel (1958a) concluded that an increase in potassium, rather than chloride, conductance was the appropriate explanation for the mechanism of action of acetylcholine. Atropine is a competitive antagonist for acetylcholine and blocks all the effects mentioned above.

Although fibers of the working ventricular myocardium and specialized ventricular conducting system have long been considered unresponsive to vagal action, and thus to acetylcholine (Hoffman and Cranefield, 1960), more recent investigations of isolated specialized conducting cells distal to the atrioventricular junction have shown a significant negative chronotropic response to high concentrations of acetylcholine (Bailey et al., 1972).

9.   Catecholamines

Myocardial cells are regularly exposed to catecholamine under a wide variety of circumstances and from a number of sources. Under normal physiological conditions, cardiac cells are regulated by catecholamines released from atrial and ventricular adrenergic terminals when traffic increases on cardiac sympathetic nerves in response to stress. Under pathological conditions, cardiac fibers are also exposed to adrenal catecholamines released in response to circulatory failure or to catecholamines released from sympathetic nerve terminals by local ischemia. Under abnormal conditions, catecholamines may be important in the genesis of cardiac arrhythmias.

The slope and rate of spontaneous phase 4 depolarization are increased by epinephrine and norepinephrine both in Purkinje and in sinoatrial fibers; high concentrations of catecholamines can also lead to secondary humplike depolarizations during phase 3 repolarization of the action potential (Hoffman and Cranefield, 1960). Trautwein and Schmidt (1960) showed that epinephrine lacked any significant effect on the availability of fast inward sodium current. Kassebaum (1964) showed that an epinephrine concentration of 2.5×10^{-6} g/ml had no effect on the Purkinje fiber current–voltage relationship (current-clamp method) in sodium-free Tyrode, indicating a lack of effect in the instantaneous potassium conductance (i_{K_1}). However, a voltage-clamp analysis within the pacemaker voltage range of Purkinje tissue subjected to epinephrine at 5×10^{-7} g/ml showed a shift in the depolarizing direction in the activation curve for pacemaker current (i_{K_2}) of almost 30 mV (Hauswirth et al., 1968a). By referring to Figure 9, we can appreciate that such a shift of the i_{K_2} curve would produce more depolarization when i_{K_2} deactivates after repolarization. Computer reconstructions indicate that a shift of the i_{K_2} activation curve by 10–20 mV in the depolarizing direction should more than double the rate of spontaneous firing of Purkinje fibers (Hauswirth et al., 1968a), suggesting that the effect of catecholamines on phase 4 depolarization is mediated through the β-adrenergic receptor. Since epinephrine is positively charged, an alternate explanation for its action is that it might act in a manner similar to calcium, i.e., by directly changing the external membrane surface charge and thereby altering the membrane field in the vicinity of the i_{K_2} channel (Tsien, 1973b). Tsien (1973b) then provided evidence that the effect of epinephrine on phase 4 depolarization is not simply mediated by alterations in the surface charge of the cell membrane, but rather through an adenylate cyclase-dependent mechanism. He showed that theophylline, a phosphodiesterase inhibitor (and a neutral molecule at physiological pH), could mimic the action of epinephrine on the i_{K_2} activation curve. Further evidence for a role for cyclic AMP as mediator of adrenergic enhancement of phase 4 depolarization is the demonstration that iontophoresis of cyclic AMP into Purkinje fibers causes changes in phase 4 depolarization similar to extracellular application of catecholamines (Tsien, 1973a).

Catecholamines can also influence phase 4 depolarization in cardiac Purkinje fibers by their effects on membrane ion pumping. Norepinephrine increases ^{42}K influx in Purkinje fibers, an effect attributed to stimulation of a membrane Na^+-K^+ pump (Vassalle and Barnabei, 1971). Trautwein and Schmidt (1960) showed that catecholamines could increase resting trans-membrane voltage in canine atrial or Purkinje fibers which showed partial depolarization. They attributed this effect to activation of electrogenic cation transport on the basis of experiments with 2,4-dinitrophenol, sodium cyanide, and iodoacetic acid. Although catecholamines definitely stimulate cation pumping in cardiac Purkinje fibers and can stimulate electrogenic cation pumping in partially depolarized fibers, it is uncertain to what extent they can induce electrogenic pumping in normally polarized fibers. Vassalle and Carpentier (1972) did show that norepinephrine could enhance the hyper-polarization of rapid stimulation in Purkinje fibers (see Section IV–B–1).

Epinephrine has been shown capable of inducing spontaneous activity in sinoatrial node fibers "paralyzed" by extracellular potassium concentrations as high as 36 mM (Antoni et al., 1963), as has norephinephrine in Purkinje fibers following overdrive at an extracellular potassium concentration of 5.4 mEq/liter, a concentration which usually precludes automatic behavior (Vassalle and Carpentier, 1972). Whether or not this phenomenon is related to a shift of the steady-state i_{K_2} current–voltage relationship to more positive voltages, as suggested by these authors, remains to be proven, since voltage-clamp analysis of these preparations was not undertaken. Catechol-amines have also been shown important in the resistance of the sinoatrial node to high extracellular potassium concentrations (Vassalle et al., 1973). Both sympathetic tone and adequate extracellular calcium supported sinoatrial automaticity, which decreased in their absence. Recently, the epinephrine-induced acceleration of phase 4 depolarization in frog sinus venosus has been shown to depend upon extracellular calcium, and can be blocked by Mn^{2+}, a calcium blocking agent (Gough et al., 1974). The seasonal change in sensitivity of this preparation to epinephrine raises the interesting question of how seasonal change of ionic conductances in the bullfrog sinus venosus are mediated.

B. Physical Factors

1. Frequency of Regenerative Depolarization

Suppression of cardiac automaticity by external electrical stimuli was known to investigators of the previous century (Gaskell, 1884). Clinicians have long recognized that the first heartbeat to follow cessation of a tachyarrhythmia frequently appears after a delay which far exceeds the beat-to-beat interval of the normal cardiac rhythm. Ventricular pacing in dogs either with experimental heart block or with vagally induced sinus suppression and in patients with Stokes–Adams syndrome produced an escape interval which was directly related to the rate and duration of the induced tachycardia (Linenthal et al., 1960; Vassalle et al., 1967a). Lu et al. (1965) also correlated the duration and intensity of a late postoverdrive acceleration in sinoatrial fibers with duration and frequency of drive rate. Lange (1965) and her co-workers showed differential depression of various cardiac tissues by overdrive, with atrioventricular and ectopic atrial pacemakers more prone to overdrive suppression than sinoatrial cells. They felt that the responses of overdrive suppression and of postoverdrive late acceleration to neostigmine, atropine, cocaine, reserpine, and guanethidine were consistent with catecholamine release during overdrive. Using isolated perfused Purkinje fibers, Vassalle (1970) more clearly characterized overdrive suppression: An initial fall of (more positive) maximum diastolic potential during the start of rapid pacing was followed by a later recovery of maximum diastolic voltage to levels more negative than control, during maintained overdrive. After cessation of a 2-min overdrive, the late increase in maximum diastolic voltage returned to control values over 2–5 min. Substitution of lithium (which cannot be actively extruded from the cell) for sodium or exposure to 2,4-dinitrophenol abolished the late overdrive hyperpolarization. At higher external potassium concentrations the effect of overdrive on membrane voltage was less. Additionally, membrane resistance was not altered by rapid driving rates, despite a decreased slope of phase 4 depolarization and a positive shift in threshold voltage. He concluded that overdrive activates electrogenic sodium pumping, and that this is an adequate explanation for overdrive suppression in Purkinje fibers.

2. Stretch

Cat ventricular muscle can be stretched to a tension of 1000 g/cm^2 and dog Purkinje fibers to 150% of resting length with the appearance of an afterpotential but little change in resting and action potentials; only when the muscle is irreversibly damaged by stretch does resting membrane voltage depolarize, duration of phase 0 upstroke prolong, and action potential plateau shorten (Dudel and Trautwein, 1958). These authors note, however, that as little as 10% increase in resting length of dog Purkinje fibers can lead to accelerated phase 4 depolarization and repetitive firing. Deck (1964a), using concentric stretch (about 30% increase in resting length) in rabbit and cat sinoatrial preparations, also notes an increase in spontaneous automatic rate for these cardiac tissues. He feels that the greater amount of atrial tissue surrounding the rabbit sinus accounts for its smaller increase in firing rate compared to cat sinus. Similarly, he attributes a stretch-protective quality to increased sinoatrial "plastic" (elastic–connective) tissue in older cats, which have less stretch-induced enhancement of automaticity than preparations from younger animals. Electrophysiologic changes accompanying the enhanced automaticity are reversible, thereby excluding significant membrane injury as the cause for the stretch-induced increase in firing rate. The most reliable (but by no means invariable) electrophysiologic change resulting from stretch is a more positive maximum diastolic voltage (an automatic effect—Figure 1D); a more positive threshold voltage and altered rate of spontaneous phase 4 depolarization are less frequent (Deck, 1964b).

Contrary to the findings of Dudel and Trautwein (1958), Deck (1964a) has not observed premature or rapid repetitive depolarizations in Purkinje fibers stretched by as much as 80% of their resting length, unless clear signs of physical injury are apparent. Again he notes a stretch-induced reversible change of maximum diastolic voltage to more positive values.

Deck (1964b) notes that Purkinje cells superficially located in relatively thick false tendons are more sensitive to stretch than cells more centrally located in fibers with thick connective tissue coats, implying a protective action of Purkinje fiber connective tissue similar to that of sinoatrial preparations. The ionic basis for stretch-induced automaticity, however, is not clear. The depolarization of resting transmembrane voltage in Purkinje fibers stretched to 140% of resting length (Deck, 1964b) is nearly as large when recorded in sodium-poor as when recorded in normal-sodium Tyrode solution, thus making an increase in sodium conductance an unlikely mechanism. Evaluation of the cable properties of stretched fibers has shown an increase in membrane resistance and length constant (Deck, 1964b), further negating an increased sodium conductance and suggesting a decreased potassium conductance as the etiology of the depolarization. However, even fibers which do not show any stretch-induced resting transmembrane voltage change do show increases in membrane resistance and length constant (Deck, 1964b), thereby making an isolated decrease in g_K unlikely. Arnsdorf and Bigger (1972) have observed that lidocaine repolarizes stretched Purkinje fibers; since lidocaine is known to increase g_{K_1} (Weld and Bigger, 1974), this is further indirect support for the role of a decrease in g_K in the genesis of stretch-induced membrane depolarization and increased membrane resistance.

In view of the impressive degrees of cardiac dilation which may occur in both acute and chronic cardiac diseases, stretch phenomena may play an as yet not fully appreciated role in some cardiac arrhythmias. For instance, an attractive explanation for the clinical "rule of bigeminy" in atrial fibrillation (which predicts that ventricular premature depolarizations will follow QRS complexes terminating the longer R–R intervals) is that antegrade conduction is blocked by virtue of stretching of a portion of the ventricular specialized conducting system with prolonged ventricular filling, thereby setting the stage for a reentrant circuit (Langendorf et al., 1955). The ability of lidocaine to repolarize fibers partially depolarized by stretching, by increasing membrane potassium conductance (Arnsdorf and Bigger, 1972), makes this a theoretically appropriate agent for arrhythmias with this etiology.

3. Temperature

Cooling cardiac Purkinje fibers over the range 40–25°C causes a slight decrease in maximum diastolic transmembrane voltage. All phases of the action potential are slowed by a decrease in temperature, but phases 2 and 4 are the most profoundly affected, the Q_{10} for the plateau being 4.6 and that for phase 4, 6.2 (Coraboeuf and Weidmann, 1954). Noble and Tsien (1968) measured the temperature dependence of i_{K_2} kinetics, i.e., the change in τ_s as a function of temperature, between 28 and 38°C. The Q_{10} for τ_s was about 6, indicating a large temperature dependence of s kinetics and accounting for the marked slowing in spontaneous diastolic depolarization and firing rate when temperature is lowered. Noble and Tsien (1968) also mention that lowering temperature decreased the total amplitude of the i_{K_2} activation curve.

4. Tissue Ischemia

Important differences between anoxia and ischemia for in situ preparations have been described (Bagdonas et al., 1961). Dogs on cardiopulmonary bypass subjected to anoxia for a matter of hours did not develop ventricular arrhythmias, whereas those animals which underwent aortic cross-clamping (with cessation of coronary flow and thus true tissue ischemia) invariably developed multiple ectopic rhythms and then ventricular fibrillation within minutes. After only 10 min of ischemia, electrical activity in ventricular muscle was markedly reduced, whereas electrograms were recorded from the ventricular specialized conduction system for hours. [Note the similarity of these observations to the *in vitro* anoxia-resistance of Purkinje fibers compared to ventricular muscle (Trautwein *et al.*, 1954).] These data suggest that tissue consequences of ischemia are more damaging than hypoxia alone.

Since tissue ischemia is characterized by low pH and high extracellular P_{CO_2}, potassium, catecholamines, and lactic acid, one or more of these components probably causes ischemic rhythm disturbances, which cannot be explained by hypoxia alone. Investigations in experimental acute myocardial infarction, for example, have shown that arteriovenous potassium concentration changes of the order of 1 mEq/liter can be associated with alarming arrhythmias (Regan *et al.*, 1967; Thomas *et al.*, 1970).

The individual metabolic consequences of ischemia (e.g., hypoxia, low pH, high K^+, etc.) produce acute electrophysiological changes in isolated "normal" cardiac fibers which are quite different from the electrophysiological abnormalities of ischemic tissue or tissue surviving experimental myocardial infarction. For instance, the expected effect of ischemia upon action potential duration is an abbreviation, as is seen individually with hypoxia, hyperkalemia, and high lactate levels. However, such is not the case: Friedman *et al.* (1973) report a reproducible prolongation of action potential duration in subendocardial Purkinje cells in infarcted canine ventricle 24 hr after a two-stage ligation of the anterior descending coronary artery. Furthermore, these surviving subendocardial Purkinje fibers show a lidocaine-induced depression of action potential amplitude, phase 0 rate of rise, and conduction velocity at much lower drug concentrations than do Purkinje fibers in adjacent noninfarcted ventricle (Sasyniuk and Kus, 1974). These observations raise questions as to the applicability of acute *in vitro* experiments to chronic myocardial infarction *in vivo* and the accuracy of extrapolation from results obtained in ostensibly normal laboratory animal hearts to ischemic tissue.

C. Exogenous Chemical Factors

1. Blockers of Sodium Conductance

The prototype agent of this group is the puffer fish poison, tetrodotoxin. At very low concentrations (10^{-7} to 5×10^{-9} M) tetrodotoxin selectively blocks the fast sodium channel of nerve membranes, probably by binding at their outer surface in a one-to-one relationship of toxin molecules to sodium channels; there is no significant effect upon either the kinetic behavior or the voltage-dependent inactivation of unblocked fast sodium channels (Narahashi et al., 1964; Takata et al., 1966; Hille, 1968a; Narahashi, 1972). These same studies have failed to show an effect on other ionic conductances in nerve. In cardiac tissues tetrodotoxin has been less extensively studied, but at high concentrations (10^{-5} M) has no effect on spontaneous pacemaker depolarization or on the pacemaker current in Purkinje fibers, while simultaneously blocking the fast inward sodium current (Dudel et al., 1967a). The reason for the higher concentrations of tetrodotoxin required to block fast sodium current in cardiac Purkinje fibers, as opposed to nerve fibers, is unknown, but the lack of effect on the cardiac pacemaker current is consonant with the previously mentioned absence of tetrodotoxin's activity in nerve on ionic conductances other than fast inward sodium. Zipes and Mendez (1973) and Shigenobu and Sperelakis (1972) have shown no effect of fast sodium blockade on phase 4 depolarization and action potential upstrokes of rabbit atrioventricular nodal cells and cultured embryonic chick ventricular cells. These studies emphasize the different ionic basis for the action potential upstroke both in different cell types from the same heart, and also in the same cell type during embryological development.

2. Blockers of Calcium Conductance

The calcium antagonists (e.g., verapamil and D 600) were originally tested for their ability to depress myocardial contraction and thereby decrease myocardial oxygen demand in myocardial ischemia (Fleckenstein et al., 1969a, b, 1972; Fleckenstein, 1970). Verapamil's depression of myocardial contractility can be reversed by increased $[Ca^{2+}]_0$ or catecholamines (Fleckenstein, 1970). Initial studies showed 10^{-5} M verapamil to be relatively free of electrophysiological effects on working ventricular myocardium while causing nearly complete inhibition of contractile force (Fleckenstein et al., 1969b). However, when verapamil at 2×10^{-6} g/ml (less than 5×10^{-6} M) is applied to atrioventricular or sinoatrial nodal cells or Purkinje fibers, it causes a decreased rate of spontaneous phase 4 depolarization and a more positive threshold voltage (Tritthart et al., 1971), suggesting possible antiarrhythmic properties. Further investigation of verapamil in canine Purkinje fibers (at even lower concentrations) has revealed these same findings and also decreased action potential amplitude and lower phase 0 upstroke velocity, enhancement of phase 1, and increased slope of phase 2 (Rosen et al., 1974). Voltage-clamp studies of calcium channel blockers will be important for an ionic clarification of their depression of phase 4 depolarization; however, available data do suggest that verapamil and related compounds may prove to be antiautomatic owing to their depression of membrane calcium conductance.

Manganese ion (2–4 mM), also a blocker of inward calcium current, suppresses spontaneous depolarization and action potentials of rabbit atrioventricular node without interfering with regenerative responses in either atrial muscle or His bundle fibers (Zipes and Mendez, 1973). This differential depression of atrioventricular node by Mn^{2+} (but not by tetrodotoxin) is evidence for excitatory mechanisms involving slow rather than fast ionic conductances.

Carmeliet and Vereecke (1969) and Pappano (1970) have shown that slowly rising action potentials can originate and propagate in Purkinje fibers and atrial muscle depolarized by high $[K]_0$ in the presence of catecholamines. These "slow action potentials" or "slow responses" are elicited at resting transmembrane voltages which cause essentially full inactivation of the fast inward sodium conductance, and can generate reentrant arrhythmias (Wit et al., 1972). Abolition of these slow responses by Mn^{2+} (0.2–2 mM) and enhancement by divalent cations known to pass through calcium channels ($Ba^{2+}, Sr^{2+}, Ca^{2+}$) suggest that an increase in calcium conductance mediates these abnormal potentials (Carmeliet and Vereecke, 1969; Pappano, 1970). Mn^{2+} (1 mM) also blocks the calcium-dependent slow potentials induced by elevated $[K]_0$ and catecholamines in tetrodotoxin-treated embryonic chick heart cells (Shigenobu and Sperelakis, 1972).

Enhanced phase 4 depolarization and delayed after-depolarizations arising from ouabain excess or hypokalemia are suppressed by verapamil at 2×10^{-6} M (Rosen et al., 1974). This depression of abnormal automatic mechanisms is thus at least in part an action on inward calcium current.

3. β-Adrenergic Blocking Agents

The β-adrenergic blocking agents were originally thought to be antiarrhythmic solely owing to their depression of spontaneous phase 4 depolarization, an antiautomatic action resulting from blockade of cardiac β-receptors. However, β-adrenergic blocking agents have subsequently been found to possess electrophysiological actions aside from their β-adrenergic blockade: Reduction of action potential amplitude and upstroke velocity and also striking alteration of action potential duration have been demonstrated, depending on which β-adrenergic blocking agent is studied. It is now clear that the β-adrenergic blocking agents constitute a heterogeneous group with regard to their antiarrhythmic actions on membrane ionic conductances.

a. Pronethalol. Hoffman and Singer (1967) demonstrated that pronethalol (1 mg/liter) decreases spontaneous phase 4 depolarization in Purkinje fibers without diminishing phase 0 rate of rise or action potential amplitude. Using a voltage-clamp technique, Hauswirth et al. (1968b) have shown that pronethalol (1 mg/liter) reverses an adrenaline-induced depolarizing shift of the i_{K_2} current curve along the voltage axis of the i_{K_2} current–voltage relationship. Hence pronethalol's action on the i_{K_2} pacemaker current in Purkinje fibers is probably caused by β-adrenergic blockade.

Pronethalol at 1 mg/liter shifts the membrane responsiveness curve to more negative voltages (Hoffman and Singer, 1967); since phase 0 amplitude and rate of rise are unaffected at 1 mg/liter, this hyperpolarizing shift of the membrane responsiveness curve results from a hyperpolarizing shift of the steady-state voltage dependence of the fast sodium current and/or a slowing of its reactivation kinetics, rather than from a decrease in maximum obtainable I_{Na} (blockage of fast sodium channels). Exposure to higher concentrations of pronethalol causes generalized depolarization and inexcitability of the fiber (Hoffman and Singer, 1967).

b. Propranolol. At 0.1 mg/liter propranolol completely blocks enhancement by epinephrine of spontaneous phase 4 depolarization in Purkinje fibers (Davis and Temte, 1968); this classical β-adrenergic blocking action occurs, as already noted for pronethalol, at a concentration below that required to reduce phase 0 rate of rise and action potential overshoot (actions which reflect reduction of fast sodium current).

Exposure to propranolol at 3.0 mg/liter decreases the ability of both ventricular muscle fibers and Purkinje fibers to respond to high stimulation frequencies (Davis and Temte, 1968), suggesting that h reactivation may be significantly slowed during action potential repolarization. Tritthart *et al.* (1971) have likewise shown that propranolol (1 mg/liter) markedly reduces the maximal upstroke velocity of guinea pig papillary muscle at faster driving rates, again supporting a drug-induced prolongation of fast sodium current recovery time. Contrary to these findings in mammalian Purkinje fibers and ventricular muscle, frog atrial fibers exposed to an even higher concentration of propranolol (10 mg/liter) show only variable prolongation of fast sodium recovery time following either spontaneous repolarization or repolarization with a voltage-clamp technique even when maximum inward sodium current is markedly decreased (Tarr *et al.*, 1973). These authors conclude that the major action of propranolol on inward sodium current in frog atrial fibers is a blockage of the sodium channels, similar to that described earlier for tetrodotoxin in nerve.

Purkinje fiber action potential duration and refractory period are shortened by propranolol (Davis and Temte, 1968), raising the question of earlier or greater activation of outward currents which terminate the action potential plateau or else diminution of inward currents which maintain the plateau. In squid axon, propranolol ($1-3 \times 10^{-5}$ M) increases steady-state potassium conductance (Wu and Narahashi, 1972); if propranolol likewise increases cardiac potassium conductance(s), this effect could explain both propranolol's abbreviation of action potential duration and depression of phase 4 depolarization in Purkinje fibers. Clarification will have to await further voltage-clamp studies.

  c. Sotalol (*MJ 1999*). At a concentration of 10^{-4} M, sotalol fails to significantly decrease spontaneous firing rate of isolated canine Purkinje fibers; sotalol does block the positive chronotropic effect of isoproterenol but only at concentrations much higher than β-blocking concentrations of propranolol (Strauss *et al.*, 1970). This weak β-adrenergic blocking action may account for the ineffectiveness of sotalol in suppressing ouabain-induced phase 4 depolarization in contrast to propranolol at less than one tenth the concentration (Koerpel and Davis, 1972).

  Strauss *et al.* (1970) showed no observable depression of resting voltage or phase 0 amplitude or maximum rate of rise in concentrations as high as 5×10^{-4} M; they did, however, find a significant prolongation of action potential duration and refractory period. This action suggests a mechanism operant in the voltage range of the action potential plateau diametrically opposite to the possibility outlined for propranolol, and actually has led to the suggestion of an additional class of antiarrhythmic action by Singh and Vaughan Williams (1970).

  d. Practolol. At identical concentrations, practolol has less β-adrenergic blocking activity than propranolol and is also relatively free of sodium antagonizing action; it does not, however, prolong action potential duration as sotalol does (Papp and Vaughan Williams, 1969).

  Other β-adrenergic blocking compounds share the characteristics of these four agents to varying degress (Singh, 1972). Thus members of this group act upon the i_{K_2} pacemaker current, the rapid inward sodium current, and also the current(s) involved in action potential repolarization. The degree to which each β-adrenergic blocking agent acts on each of these currents is highly variable and is strongly dependent both upon drug concentration and upon cardiac cell type.

4. Lidocaine

  The spontaneous firing rate of rabbit sinoatrial node shows a modest decrease only at high or toxic concentrations of lidocaine, with a fall of 14% in rate at a 5×10^{-4} M concentration (Mandel and Bigger, 1971). At clinically encountered lidocaine concentrations, neither the rate of phase 4 depolarization nor the spontaneous sinus rate are significantly decreased. This lack of effect on sinoatrial automaticity contrasts with the impressive decrease in phase 4 depolarization and spontaneous firing in canine Purkinje fibers at lower concentrations (10^{-6} to 10^{-5} M) of lidocaine (Bigger and Mandel, 1970). The depression of spontaneous phase 4 depolarization in Purkinje fibers can be explained by an increase in membrane potassium conductance: Lidocaine increases membrane conductance and moves V_m toward V_K, the magnitude of the movement being proportional to the difference between V_m and V_K (Arnsdorf and Bigger, 1972). Specifically, lidocaine increases steady-state outward (potassium) current, i_{K_1}, throughout the voltage range of spontaneous phase 4 depolarization in Purkinje fibers, while concomitantly reducing the magnitude of the i_{K_2} pacemaker current (Weld and Bigger, 1974). This observation raises the intriguing possibility that lidocaine may partially eliminate the time-dependent deactivation of the s gating mechanism which governs the i_{K_2} pacemaker current (Section III–A–2), thereby transforming an i_{K_2} channel into an i_{K_1} channel. This possible mechanism is purely speculative at the present time. Koerpel and Davis (1972) have shown that lidocaine prevents or decreases enhancement by ouabain of spontaneous phase 4 depolarization (which may be mediated through modification of calcium conductance); whether or not this protection is solely a result of the ability of lidocaine to increase g_{K_1} is not yet known.

At low concentrations (1 mg/liter) lidocaine has little effect on the voltage-dependent magnitude of fast inward sodium current, but at higher concentrations (5 mg/liter) does diminish this current, as reflected by a decrease in the maximum rate of action potential phase 0 depolarization elicited at a given voltage (Weld and Bigger, 1973). Since hyperpolarization restores the ability of the membrane to pass a maximal sodium current, the decrease in inward current at a given voltage probably reflects a shift to more negative voltages of the $h_\infty - V_m$ relationship (Figure 12A), rather than a tetrodotoxin-like blockage of sodium channels. By using subthreshold test voltage clamp steps both positive and negative to the holding voltage, Weld and Bigger (1973) have also demonstrated a slowing of both h inactivation and h reactivation in the presence of lidocaine at 5 mg/liter.

Lidocaine causes shortening of Purkinje fiber action potential duration, largely through an abbreviation of the action potential plateau (Bigger and Mandel, 1970). Although an increase in i_{K_1} in the voltage range of action potential phase 2 and phase 3 can explain this effect, an antagonistic action against inward calcium current and/or an enhancement of additional (largely potassium) currents, which are at least in part responsible for action potential repolarization (Hauswirth et al., 1972), have not been excluded.

Like many of the β-adrenergic blocking compounds, then, lidocaine has multiple actions on membrane ionic conductances which are potentially antiarrhythmic.

5. Diphenylhydantoin

Similar to lidocaine, diphenylhydantoin fails to slow spontaneous sino-atrial firing rate or to decrease rate of phase 4 depolarization at low concentrations (10^{-8} to 10^{-6} M), and slows sinus rate by only 16% at a 10^{-4} M concentration (Strauss et al., 1968). Furthermore, diphenylhydantoin (10^{-5} M) fails to decrease enhancement by isoproterenol of sinoatrial spontaneous firing rate (Strauss *et al.*, 1968), although this antagonism is seen in Purkinje fibers (Bigger *et al.*, 1968). In canine Purkinje fibers, diphenylhydantoin decreases spontaneous firing rate owing to a decrease in the rate of phase 4 depolarization (Bigger *et al.*, 1968), an observation consonant with this agent's ability to increase ventricular escape time both during vagal stimulation in intact dogs and also after ventricular overdrive in dogs with heart block (Bigger *et al.*, 1970).

Diphenylhydantoin enhances membrane responsiveness (relationship of phase 0 maximal rate of depolarization to transmembrane voltage during phase 3 repolarization) of ordinary atrial and of specialized Bachmann's bundle fibers at low concentrations (10^{-7} to 10^{-6} M), providing a higher maximal upstroke velocity at a given V_m (Strauss *et al.*, 1968). Although membrane responsiveness is not altered by diphenylhydantoin in normal Purkinje fibers, responsiveness unequivocally improves in Purkinje fibers "depressed" by stretch, cold, hypoxia, or ouabain administration when diphenylhydantoin is administered (Bigger *et al.*, 1968). Such a differential effect in normal vs. depressed Purkinje fibers leads one to suspect that diphenylhydantoin may modify transmembrane ionic gradients (and thus ionic driving forces), perhaps through action on the membrane cation pump, rather than act on the fast inward sodium conductance of Purkinje fibers. With regard to a possible effect on transmembrane ionic gradients, it is interesting that diphenylhydantion (10^{-8} to 10^{-7} M) protects canine Purkinje fibers from hypoxia-induced depolarization and reduced rate of rise of phase 0 (Bassett *et al.*, 1970). However, the mechanism by which diphenylhydantoin does improve membrane responsiveness either in atrial tissues or in depressed Purkinje fibers is not yet established.

Diphenylhydantoin shortens canine Purkinje fiber action potential duration through an abbreviation of all phases of repolarization (Bigger *et al.*, 1968). It is possible that an increase in membrane potassium conductance(s) partially mediates both this effect and also the above-mentioned decrease in Purkinje fiber phase 4 depolarization. The effects of diphenylhydantoin on the voltage–time course of the Purkinje fiber action potential are very reminiscent of the actions of lidocaine. It is quite likely that the same ionic conductances mediate these changes. However, an accurate analysis of membrane ionic conductance changes must await application of a voltage-clamp technique.

6. Quinidine

One of the most prominent electrophysiological effects of quinidine (3–12 mg/liter) on cardiac Purkinje fibers is a reduction of the slope of spontaneous phase 4 depolarization (Weidmann, 1955b; Hoffman, 1957; Hoffman and Cranefield, 1960; Bigger and Jaffe, 1971). Concentrations of quinidine greater than 10 mg/liter are considered potentially toxic and can actually enhance phase 4 depolarization in Purkinje fibers (Hoffman, 1957). An analysis of the phase 4 current change(s) responsible for modification of spontaneous depolarization by quinidine is not yet available.

Quinidine at concentrations less than 10 mg/liter significantly decreases the fast inward sodium current, as reflected by action potential phase 0 amplitude and/or maximum rate of rise from a given V_m, in rabbit atria (Vaughan Williams, 1958) and in canine Purkinje fibers (Hoffman, 1957). Membrane hyperpolarization can largely overcome these actions of quinidine on Purkinje fibers (Weidmann, 1955b) thereby suggesting a quinidine-induced shift of the $h_\infty - V_m$ relationship (Figure 12A) in a hyperpolarizing direction on its voltage axis, rather than actual blockage of sodium channels. Quinidine (less than 10 mg/liter) also increases the effective refractory period of atrial and Purkinje cells (Vaughan Williams, 1958; Hoffman, 1957), thus indicating a probable delay in reactivation of the sodium carrying system for these fiber types. At 10 mg/liter slowing of the sodium reactivation by quinidine in guinea pig ventricular muscle is so marked that normal action potential amplitude and rate of rise can be fully restored by sufficiently slow stimulation rates (Johnson and McKinnon, 1957). This last finding seems at variance with the report of Tritthart et al. (1971) that an unspecified concentration of quinidine causes only slight frequency dependence of the upstroke velocity in guinea pig papillary muscle.

Both the decrease in fast inward sodium current at a given V_m and the delay in reappearance of available inward sodium current following action potential repolarization result in a decrease in inward current. This decrease in inward current can explain quinidine's change of threshold voltage toward zero and may even contribute to quinidine's suppression of phase 4 depolarization.

7. Procaine Amide

The qualitative effects of procaine amide on action potential characteristics are so similar to those of quinidine that all investigators agree that these two pharmacological agents belong in the same electrophysiological classification. The earliest observable electrophysiological action of procaine amide (10 mg/liter) on canine Purkinje fiber action potentials is suppression of spontaneous phase 4 depolarization (Rosen et al., 1972). In fact, these authors report no other consistent electrophysiological changes in Purkinje fibers at procaine amide concentrations less than 30 mg/liter. The mechanism of procaine amide's suppression of spontaneous phase 4 depolarization is not straightforward. Sheep Purkinje fibers exposed to procaine amide (5 and 50 mg/liter) in a sodium-poor physiological solution at $[K]_0 = 1$ mEq/liter fail to show a change of V_m toward V_K, and the current–voltage relationships for shortened Purkinje fiber' segments at $[K]_0 = 4$ mEq/liter remain unaltered throughout the voltage range of phase 4 depolarization (Weld and Bigger, 1972). Both findings indicate that procaine amide, unlike lidocaine, does not exert its antiautomatic action through an increase in membrane potassium conductance. It seems probable, therefore, that procaine amide acts to decrease inward current (sodium and/or calcium) which depolarizes the cell membrane during spontaneous phase 4 depolarization. A final decision must await a voltage-clamp analysis of the effect of procaine amide on pacemaker current(s).

Weidmann (1955b) found that higher concentrations of procaine amide (50 mg/liter) resulted in gradual depolarization of the resting transmembrane voltage, loss of phase 0 amplitude and upstroke velocity, and, finally, inexcitability of sheep Purkinje fibers. As he had found with quinidine, the relationship between upstroke velocity and transmembrane voltage was shifted to more negative voltages. The resulting smaller inward sodium current at any given transmembrane voltage may well prove to be responsible (entirely or in part) for procaine amide's depression of spontaneous phase 4 depolarization.

Although a marked delay in reactivation of inward current following repolarization could theoretically contribute to a slowing of spontaneous phase 4 depolarization, the voltage–time course of phase 4 is far slower than the recovery of the fast sodium current following repolarization. A delay in fast sodium reactivation probably is responsible, however, for the increased effective refractory period of Purkinje fibers exposed to procaine amide (Hoffman, 1957). In guinea pig papillary muscle exposed to procaine amide (50 mg/liter), there is little or no decrease in upstroke velocity with increasing stimulation frequency (up to 240 depolarizations/min), suggesting no drug-induced slowing of fast sodium reactivation in this cardiac cell type (Tritthart et al., 1971). This observation is one of the few demonstrations of a difference between the electrophysiological actions of procaine amide and quinidine, and may be attributable to the fact that the concentrations employed are not comparable.

8. Digitalis

The spontaneous sinus rate of intact animals decreases at low digitalis doses, but may accelerate at higher levels (Hoffman, 1969). Electrophysiological evaluation of digoxin (10^{-7} M) on isolated perfused canine Purkinje fibers has shown enhanced spontaneous phase 4 depolarization (Mandel et al., 1972); ouabain (2×10^{-7} M) induces a similar enhancement of phase 4 depolarization in Pukinje fibers, which is more pronounced at $[K]_0 =$ 2.5 mEq/liter than at 4.0 mEq/liter, and which is further augmented by higher stimulus rates (Davis, 1973; Rosen et al., 1973b). An earlier study (Kassebaum, 1963) failed to show an enhancement of spontaneous phase 4 depolarization of sheep Purkinje fibers exposed to G-strophanthin (1.4×10^{-6} M) in Krebs solution at $[K]_0 = 4.69$ mEq/liter, probably owing to the antiautomatic effect of this relatively high $[K]_0$. No study has demonstrated digitalis-induced spontaneous phase 4 depolarization in either atrial or ventricular muscle cells.

The cause of enhanced phase 4 depolarization by digitalis compounds is still not totally clear. Kassebaum (1963) determined current–voltage relationships for Purkinje fibers exposed to 1.4×10^{-6} M G-strophanthin and found an initial decrease in membrane conductance after 45 min exposure, followed by a large increase in membrane conductance after 60 and 90 min exposure. These current–voltage relationships were performed in sodium-free physiological solutions and therefore support the contention that digitalis compounds at high concentrations initially decrease and later increase membrane potassium conductance of sheep Purkinje fibers. These actions may explain the initial action potential prolongation and subsequent shortening on prolonged exposure to strophanthin or digoxin (Kassebaum, 1963; Mandel et al., 1972), and the former may play a role in the early stages of digitalis-enhanced automaticity. Aronson et al. (1973) have used a voltage-clamp technique to evaluate Purkinje fiber pacemaker current changes on exposure to 2×10^{-7} M ouabain. Paradoxically, these authors have found a progressive (and largely reversible) decrease in the magnitude of the i_{K_2} pacemaker current, without an appreciable shift of the voltage range for i_{K_2} activation—an antiautomatic action. Furthermore, the steady-state current–voltage relationship shows a striking increase in background inward current as i_{K_2} diminishes by less than 40% (20–40 min exposure), but this is followed by a decrease in background inward current as i_{K_2} decreases by more than 80% (60–90 min); theoretically, a decrease in i_{K_2} and the associated net increase in inward current should lead to less spontaneous phase 4 depolarization and a more positive maximum diastolic voltage. Their explanation for the eventual decrease in inward current with prolonged exposure to ouabain is a decrease in the transmembrane cationic gradients [and, therefore, decreased sodium current—see equations (7) and (8b)] resulting from inhibition of the membrane cation pump. Cation pump inhibition can exert two additional actions: electrogenic sodium pumping can decrease, resulting in more rapid phase 4 depolarization; and V_K can move in a positive direction as intracellular potassium concentration decreases, thereby reducing the driving force for repolarizing membrane potassium currents. Both effects potentiate membrane depolarization. The finding by Kassebaum (1963) that strophanthin (1.4×10^{-6} M) shifts the maximum upstroke velocity vs. transmembrane voltage relationship to more negative voltages without decreasing the maximum obtainable upstroke velocity raises the additional possibility that digitalis compounds may act directly on determinants of sodium conductance as well as on the cation pump.

"Toxic" electrophysiological manifestations of digitalis compounds include a more positive resting voltage and diminished action potential amplitude and upstroke velocity (Vassalle et al., 1962). After exposure to digitalis, these changes are seen much sooner in Purkinje fibers than in ventricular muscle (Vassalle et al., 1962; Mandel et al., 1972). Polimeni and Vassale (1971) have attributed the earlier advent of ouabain toxicity in Purkinje fibers to a 7-fold higher rate of potassium exchange in Purkinje fibers compared with ventricular muscle. Since ouabain inhibits the membrane cation pump, the transmembrane potassium gradient in Purkinje fibers declines more rapidly owing to a more rapid loss of intracellular potassium. An increase in stimulation rate increases transmembrane ionic fluxes and probably promotes earlier digitalis toxicity in both ventricular muscle and Purkinje fibers by this same mechanism—overload of an impaired cation pump (Polimeni and Vassalle, 1971).

The ability of digitalis compounds to enhance spontaneous phase 4 depolarization is an augmentation of a "normal" electrophysiological automatic mechanism, despite the various contributing etiologies (outlined above) for this phenomenon on an ionic basis. These agents also promote automaticity through a clearly abnormal electrophysiological automatic mechanism: Both ouabain (2×10^{-7} M) and acetylstrophanthidin (up to 2×10^{-7} g/ml) elicit delayed afterdepolarizations in canine Purkinje fibers (Rosen et al., 1973b; Ferrier et al., 1973). These delayed afterdepolarizations, which follow action potential repolarization, are increased by higher stimulation rates and also higher $[K]_0$ (4.0 mEq/liter vs. 2.5 mEq/liter), contrary to the effect of $[K]_0$ on spontaneous phase 4 depolarization (Rosen et al., 1973b); in fact, delayed afterdepolarizations are actually associated with depression of normal phase 4 depolarization (Ferrier et al., 1973). Verapamil, previously discussed for its role as a calcium blocking agent, effectively suppresses ouabain-induced afterdepolarizations—an effect which can be reversed in part by increasing extracellular calcium concentration (Rosen et al., 1974). Thus digitalis-induced delayed afterdepolarizations may be mediated through an action on membrane calcium conductance. This abnormal automatic mechanism will probably prove to be a major etiology of digitalis-toxic ventricular tachyarrhythmias.

Inhibition of the membrane cation pump with a resultant decrease in intracellular potassium has been correlated both in time-course of effect and magnitude with the positive inotropic action of 10^{-8} to 10^{-6} M ouabain

(Müller, 1965). The protection of his ungulate ventricular fibers from generalized depolarization and inexcitability both by the lower concentrations of ouabain and by $[K]_0 = 4.05$ mEq/liter instead of 2.7 mEq/liter was also accompanied by a less marked loss of intracellular potassium.

The physical site at which digitalis compounds bind to exert their effects must lie deep within the cell membrane, since digoxin and ouabain are unable to reach membrane receptor sites when covalently bound to large protein molecules, even via long flexible polyamide side chains (Smith et al., 1972); these preparations are fully active when tested against a solubilized sodium–potassium ATPase system. Despite the relatively covert receptor site for digoxin, however, digoxin-specific antibody can reverse electrophysiological digoxin toxicity when added to the superfusate within a matter of minutes (Mandel et al., 1972).

V. SUMMARY

The ionic determinants of spontaneous phase 4 depolarization and normal automaticity have been outlined. Although the major current responsible for normal pacemaker depolarization is the i_{K_2} current, we have seen that modification of other outward and also inward currents have important actions on spontaneous automaticity.

The modification of automaticity by physical and chemical agents is accomplished by actions on both the voltage-dependent and kinetic properties of the ionic conductances themselves and by actions on cellular metabolism and transmembrane ionic gradients. The wide spectrum of possible antiautomatic and antiarrhythmic activities at an ionic level which individual agents exhibit should caution us in extrapolating from single laboratory observations to clinical efficacy. In addition, differences between the various cardiac cell types of the heart, between in vivo hearts and isolated, denervated cardiac tissues, between laboratory animals and man, and between normal and ischemic myocardium, all render correlation of electrophysiological observations with clinical arrhythmias somewhat tentative. There is a great need for additional voltage-clamp analysis of both normal and abnormal automaticity, in an effort to further characterize membrane electrical behavior which produces pacemaker depolarization under various environmental conditions. An accurate definition of this ionic behavior will contribute to the eventual identification of the molecular basis of automaticity. Such an understanding will promote the optimal use and development of agents to control automaticity.

REFERENCES

Adrian, R. H., 1956, The effects of internal and external potassium concentration on the membrane potential of frog muscle, *J. Physiol. (London)* **133**:631.

Adrian, R. H., 1969, Rectification in muscle membrane, *Prog. Biophys. Mol. Biol.* **19**:341.

Antoni, H., Herkel, K., and Fleckenstein, A., 1963, Die Restitution der automatischen Erregungsbildung in Kalium-gelähmten Schrittmacher-Geweben durch Adrenalin, *Pfluegers Arch.* **277**:633.

Arnsdorf, M. F., and Bigger, J. T., Jr., 1972, Effect of lidocaine hydrochloride on membrane conductance in mammalian cardiac Purkinje fibers, *J. Clin. Invest.* **51**:2252.

Aronson, R. S., Gelles, J. M., and Hoffman, B. F., 1973, Effect of ouabain on the current underlying spontaneous diastolic depolarization in cardiac Purkinje fibers, *Nature (New Biol.)* **243**:118.

Arvanitaki, A., 1938, *Propriétés rhythmiques de la matière vivante. II. Etude experimentale sur le myocarde d'hélix,* Hermann & Cie., Paris.

Bagdonas, A. A., Stuckey, J. H., Piera, J., Amer, N. S., and Hoffman, B. F., 1961, Effects of ischemia and hypoxia on the specialized conducting system of the canine heart, *Am. Heart J.* **61**:206.

Bailey, J. C., Greenspan, K., Elizari, M. V., Anderson, G. J., and Fisch, C., 1972, Effects of acetylcholine on automaticity and conduction in the proximal portion of the His-Purkinje specialized conduction system of the dog, *Circ. Res.* **30**:210.

Bassett, A. L., Bigger, J. T., Jr., and Hoffman, B. F., 1970, "Protective" action of diphenylhydantoin on canine Purkinje fibers during hypoxia, *J. Pharmacol. Exp. Ther.* **173**:336.

Bassett, A. L., and Wit, A. L., 1973, Recent advances in electrophysiology of antiarrhythmic drugs, *Prog. Drug. Res.* **17**:33.

Bigger, J. T., Jr., 1972a, Antiarrhythmic drugs in ischemic heart disease, *Hosp. Pract.* **7**:69.

Bigger, J. T., Jr., 1972b, Arrhythmias and antiarrhythmic drugs, *Adv. Intern. Med.* **18**:251.

Bigger, J. T., Jr., and Jaffe, C. C., 1971, The effect of bretylium tosylate on the electrophysiological properties of ventricular muscle and Purkinje fibers, *Am. J. Cardiol.* **27**:82.

Bigger, J. T., Jr., and Mandel, W. J., 1970, Effect of lidocaine on the electrophysiological properties of ventricular muscle and Purkinje fibers, *J. Clin. Invest.* **49**:63.

Bigger, J. T., Jr., and Weld, F. M., 1976, Arrhythmias and antiarrhythmic drugs, in *Cardiac Physiology* for the Clinician (M. Vassalle, ed.), Academic Press, New York.

Bigger, J. T., Jr., Bassett, A. L., and Hoffman, B. F., 1968, Electrophysiological effects of diphenylhydantoin on canine Purkinje fibers, *Circ. Res.* **22**:221.

Bigger, J. T., Jr., Weinberg, D. I., Kovalik, A. T. W., Harris, P. D., Cranefield, P. F., and Hoffman, B. F., 1970, Effects of diphenylhydantoin on excitability and automaticity in the canine heart, *Circ. Res.* **26**:1.

Bonke, F. I. M., 1973a, Passive electrical properties of atrial fibers of the rabbit heart, *Pfluegers Arch.* **339**:1.

Bonke, F. I. M., 1973b, Electrotonic spread in the sinoatrial node of the rabbit heart, *Pfluegers Arch.* **339**:16.

Borasio, P. G., and Vassalle, M., 1970, Effects of norepinephrine on active transport and automaticity of cardiac Purkinje fibers, *Physiologist* **13**:152.

Bosteels, S., and Carmeliet, E., 1972a, Estimation of intracellular Na concentration and transmembrane Na flux in cardiac Purkinje fibers, *Pfluegers Arch.* **336**:35.

Bosteels, S., and Carmeliet, E., 1972b, The components of the sodium efflux in cardiac Purkinje fibers, *Pfluegers Arch.* **336**:48.

Bozler, E., 1943, Tonus changes in cardiac muscle and their significance for the initiation of impulses, *Am. J. Physiol.* **139**:477.

Brown, R. H., Jr., and Noble, D., 1972, Effect of pH on ionic currents underlying pacemaker activity in cardiac Purkinje fibers, *J. Physiol (London)* **224**:38P.

Burdon-Sanderson, J. S., and Page, F. J. M., 1880, On the time relations of the excitatory process in the ventricle of the frog, *J. Physiol. (London)* **2**:384.

Burdon-Sanderson, J. S., and Page, F. J. M., 1884, On the electrical phenomena of the excitatory process in the heart of the frog and of the tortoise, as investigated photographically, *J. Physiol. (London)* **4**:327.

Carmeliet, E., 1960, L'influence de la concentration extracellulaire du K sur la perméabilité de la membrane des fibres de Purkinje de mouton pour les ions ^{42}K, *Helv. Physiol. Pharmacol. Acta* **18**:C15.

Carmeliet, E., 1961, Chloride ions and the membrane potential of Purkinje fibres, *J. Physiol. (London)* **156**:375.

Carmeliet, E., 1964, Influence of lithium ions on the transmembrane potential and cation content of cardiac cells, *J. Gen. Physiol.* **47**:501.

Carmeliet, E., and Bosteels, S., 1969, Coupling between Cl flux and Na or K flux in cardiac Purkyne fibers: Influence of pH, *Arch. Int. Physiol. Biochim.* **77**:57

Carmeliet, E., and Vereecke, J., 1969, Adrenaline and the plateau phase of the cardiac action potential: Importance of Ca^{++}, Na^+, and K^+ conductance, *Pfluegers Arch.* **313**:300.

Carmeliet, E., and Willems, J., 1971, The frequency dependent character of the membrane capacity in cardiac Purkyně fibres. *J. Physiol. (London)* **213**:85.

de Carvalho, A. P., Hoffman, B. F., and de Paula Carvalho, M., 1969, Two components of the cardiac action potential. I. Voltage–time course and the effect of acetylcholine on atrial and nodal cells of the rabbit heart, *J. Gen. Physiol.* **54**:607.

Colatsky, T. J., and Hogan, P. M., 1964, Effect of calcium and overdrive on automaticity in spontaneous and driven ventricular pacemaker cells, *Fed. Proc.* **33**:432.

Coraboeuf, E., and Boistel, J., 1953, L'action des taux élevés de gaz carbonique sur le tissu cardiaque, étudiée à l'aide de microélectrodes intracellulaires, *C.R. Soc. Biol. (Paris)* **147**:654.

Coraboeuf, E., and Weidmann, S., 1954, Temperature effects on the electrical activity of Purkinje fibres, *Helv. Physiol. Pharmacol. Acta* **12**:32.

Coraboeuf, E., Gargouil, Y.-M., Lapland, J., and Desplaces, A., 1958, Action de l'anoxie sur les potentiels électriques des cellules cardiaques de mammifères actives et inertes (tissu ventriculaire isolé de cobaye), *C.R. Acad. Sci., Ser.* **246**:3100.

Davis, L. D., 1973, Effect of changes in cycle length on diastolic depolarization produced by ouabain in canine Purkinje fibers, *Circ. Rec.* **32**:206.

Davis, L. D., and Temte, J. V., 1968, Effects of propranolol on the transmembrane potentials of ventricular muscle and Purkinje fibers of the dog, *Circ. Res.* **22**:661.

Deck, K. A., 1964a, Dehnungseffekte am spontanschlagenden, isolierten Sinusknoten, *Pfluegers Arch.* **280**:120.

Deck, K. A., 1964b, Änderungen des Ruhepotentials und der Kabeleigenschaften von Purkinje-Fäden bei der Dehnung, *Pfluegers Arch.* **280**:131.

Deck, K. A., and Trautwein, W., 1964, Ionic currents in cardiac excitation, *Pfluegers Arch.* **280**:63.

Deck, K. A., Kern, R., and Trautwein, W., 1964, Voltage clamp technique in mammalian cardiac fibres, *Pfluegers Arch.* **280**:50.

Délèze, J., 1960, Possible reasons for drop of resting potential of mammalian heart preparations during hypothermia, *Circ. Res.* **82**:553.

Dominguez, G., and Fozzard, H. A., 1970, Influence of extracellular K^+ concentration on cable properties and excitability of sheep cardiac Purkinje fibers, *Circ. Res.* **26**:565.

Draper, M. H., and Weidmann, S., 1951, Cardiac resting and action potentials recorded with an intracellular electrode, *J. Physiol. (London)* **115**:74.

Dudel, J., and Rüdel, R., 1970, Voltage and time dependence of excitatory sodium current in cooled sheep Purkinje fibres, *Pfluegers Arch.* **315**:136.

Dudel, J., and Trautwein, W., 1958, Der Mechanismus der automatischen rhythmischen Impulsbildung der Herzmuskelfaser, *Pfluegers Arch.* **267**:553.

Dudel, J., Peper, K., Rüdel, R., and Trautwein, W., 1967a, The effect of tetrodotoxin on the membrane current in cardiac muscle (Purkinje fibers), *Pfluegers Arch.* **295**:213.

Dudel, J., Peper, K., Rüdel, R., and Trautwein, W., 1967b, The potassium component of membrane current in Purkinje fibers, *Pfluegers Arch.* **296**:308.

Dudel, J., Peper, K., Rüdel, R., and Trautwein, W., 1967c, The dynamic chloride component of membrane current in Purkinje fibers, *Pfluegers Arch.* **295**:197.

Falk, G., and Fatt, P., 1964, Linear electrical properties of striated muscle fibres observed with intracellular electrodes, *Proc. R. Soc. London, Ser. B* **160**:69.

Ferrier, G. R., Saunders, J. H., and Mendez, C., 1973, A cellular mechanism for the generation of ventricular arrhythmias by acetylstrophanthidin. *Circ. Res.* **32**:600.

Fleckenstein, A., 1970, Die Zügelung des Myocardstoffwechsels durch Verapamil: Angriffspunkte und Anwendungsmöglichkeiten, *Arzneim. Forsch.* **20**:1317.

Fleckenstein, A., Tritthart, H., Fleckenstein, B., Herbst, A., and Grün, G., 1969a, Selective inhibition of myocardial contractility by competitive calcium antagonists (Iproveratril, D600, Prenylamine), *Naunyn Schmiedebergs Arch. Pharmakol.* **264**:S227.

Fleckenstein, A., Tritthart, H., Fleckenstein, B., Herbst, A., and Grün, G., 1969b, A new group of competitive calcium antagonists (Iproveratril, D600, Prenylamine) with highly potent inhibitory effects on excitation–contraction coupling in mammalian myocardium, *Pfluegers Arch.* **307**:525.

Fleckenstein, A., Tritthart, H., Döring, H.-J., and Byon, K. Y., 1972, BAY a 1040- ein hochaktiver Ca^{++}-antagonistischer Inhibitor der elektro-mechanischen Koppelungsprozesse im Warmblüter-Myokard, *Arzneim. Forsch.* **22**:22.

Fozzard, H. A., 1966, Membrane capacity of the cardiac Purkinje fibre, *J. Physiol. (London)* **182**:255.

Fozzard, H. A., and Hiraoka, M., 1973, The positive dynamic current and its inactivation properties in cardiac Purkinje fibres, *J. Physiol. (London)* **234**:569.

Fozzard, H. A., and Schoenberg, M., 1972, Strength–duration curves in cardiac Purkinje fibres: Effects of liminal length and charge distribution. *J. Physiol. (London)* **226**:593.

Freygang, W. H., and Trautwein, W., 1970, The structural implications of the linear electrical properties of cardiac Purkinje strands, *J. Gen. Physiol.* **55**:524.

Friedman, P. L., Stewart, J. R., and Wit, A. L., 1973, Spontaneous and induced cardiac arrhythmias in subendocardial Purkinje fibers surviving extensive myocardial infarction in dogs, *Circ. Res.* **33**:612.

Gaskell, W. H., 1884, On the innervation of the heart, with especial reference to the heart of the tortoise, *J. Physiol. (London)* **4**:43.

Glitsch, H. G., 1972, Activation of the electrogenic sodium pump in guinea-pig auricles by internal sodium ions, *J. Physiol. (London)* **220**:565.

Gough, W. B., Dreifus, L. S., and Morad, M., 1974, Dependence of pacemaker potential on catecholamines and Ca^{+2}, *Fed. Proc.* **33**:432.

Haas, H. G., and Kern, R., 1966, Potassium fluxes in voltage clamped Purkinje fibers, *Pfluegers Arch.* **291**:69

Haas, H. G., Kern, R., Einwächter, H. M., and Tarr, M., 1971, Kinetics of Na inactivation in frog atria, *Pfluegers Arch.* **323**:141.

Hall, A. E., Hutter, O. F., and Noble, D., 1963, Current–voltage relations of Purkinje fibres in sodium-deficient solutions, *J. Physiol. (London)* **166**:225.

Hauswirth, O., 1969a, Influence of halothane on the electrical properties of cardiac Purkinje fibres, *J. Physiol. (London)* **201**:42P.

Hauswirth, O., 1969b, Effects of halothane on single atrial, ventricular, and Purkinje fibers, *Circ. Res.* **24**:745.

Hauswirth, O., 1971, Computer Rekonstruktionen der Effekte von Polarisationsströmen und Pharmaka auf Schrittmacher—und Aktionspotentiale von Herzmuskelfasern, Doctoral thesis, Ruprecht-Karl-Universität zu Heidelberg.

Hauswirth, O., and Schaer, H., 1967, Effects of halothane on the sino-atrial node, *J. Pharmacol. Exp. Ther.* **158**:36.

Hauswirth, O., McAllister, R. E., Noble, D., and Tsien, R. W., 1968a, Measurement of voltage clamp currents and reconstruction of electrical activity in Purkinje fibres under normal conditions and under the influence of adrenaline, *J. Physiol. (London)* **198**:8P.

Hauswirth, O., Noble, D., and Tsien, R. W., 1968b, Adrenaline: Mechanism of action on the pacemaker potential in cardiac Purkinje fibers, *Science* **162**:916.

Hauswirth, O., McAllister, R. E., Noble, D., and Tsien, R. W., 1969, Reconstruction of the actions of adrenaline and calcium on cardiac pacemaker potentials, *J. Physiol. (London)* **204**:126P.

Hauswirth, O., Noble, D., and Tsien, R. W., 1972, Separation of the pace-maker and plateau components of delayed rectification in cardiac Purkinje fibres, *J. Physiol. (London)* **225**:211.

Hecht, H. H., and Hutter, O. F., 1965, Action of pH on cardiac Purkinje fibres, in *Electrophysiology of the Heart* (B. Taccardi and J. Marchetti, eds.), pp. 105–123, Pergamon Press, Oxford.

Hille, B., 1968a, Pharmacological modifications of the sodium channels of frog nerve, *J. Gen. Physiol.* **51**:199.

Hille, B., 1968b, Charges and potentials at the nerve surface: Divalent ions and pH, *J. Gen. Physiol.* **58**:221.

Hiraoka, M., and Hecht, H. H., 1973, Recovery from hypothermia in cardiac Purkinje fibers: Considerations for an electrogenic mechanism, *Pfluegers Arch.* **339**:25.

Hodgkin, A. L., and Huxley, A. F., 1952a, Currents carried by sodium and potassium ions through the membrane of the giant axon of *Loligo*, *J. Physiol. (London)* **116**:449.

Hodgkin, A. L., and Huxley, A. F., 1952b, The components of membrane conductance in the giant axon of *Loligo*, *J. Physiol. (London)* **116**:473.

Hodgkin, A. L., and Huxley, A. F., 1952c, The dual effect of membrane potential on sodium conductance in the giant axon of *Loligo*, *J. Physiol. (London)* **116**:497.

Hodgkin, A. L., and Huxley, A. F., 1952d, A quantitative description of membrane current and its application to conduction and excitation in nerve, *J. Physiol. (London)* **117**:500.

Hodgkin, A. L., and Rushton, W. A. H., 1946, The electrical constants of a crustacean nerve fibre, *Proc. R. Soc. London (Biol.)* **133**:444.

Hoffman, B. F., 1957, The action of quinidine and procaine amide on single fibers of dog ventricle and specialized conducting system, *An. Acad. Bras. Cienc.* **29**:365.

Hoffman, B. F., 1969, Effects of digitalis on electrical activity of cardiac fibers, in *Digitalis* (C. Fisch and B. Surawicz, eds.), pp. 93–109, Grune and Stratton, New York.

Hoffman, B. F., and Cranefield, P. F., 1960, *Electrophysiology of the Heart*, McGraw-Hill, New York.

Hoffman, B. F., and Singer, D. H., 1967, Appraisal of the effects of catecholamines on cardiac electrical activity, *Ann. N.Y. Acad. Sci.* **139**:914.

Hutter, O. F., and Noble, D., 1960, Rectifying properties of cardiac muscle, *Nature (London)* **188**:495.

Hutter, O. F., and Noble, D., 1961, Anion conductance of cardiac muscle, *J. Physiol. (London)* **157**:335.

Johnson, E. A., and McKinnon, M. G., 1957, The differential effect of quinidine and pyrilamine on the myocardial action potential at various rates of stimulation, *J. Pharmacol. Exp. Ther.* **120**:460

Juncker, D. F., Lee, P., Greene, E. A., Stish, R., and Lorber, V., 1974, Measurement of tracer influx profiles during the cardiac cycle, *Fed. Proc.* **33**:445

Kabela, E. L., 1973, The effects of lidocaine on potassium efflux from various tissues of dog heart, *J. Pharmacol. Exp. Ther.* **184**:611.

Kamiyama, A., and Matsuda, K., 1966, Electrophysiological properties of the canine ventricular fiber, *Jpn. J. Physiol.* **16**:407.

Kassebaum, D. G., 1963, Electrophysiological effects of strophanthin in the heart, *J. Pharmacol. Exp. Ther.* **140**:329.

Kassebaum, D. G., 1964, Membrane effects of epinephrine in the heart, *Proc. II Int. Pharmacol. Meeting* **5**:95.

Kawamura, K., 1961, Electron microscope studies on the cardiac conduction system of the dog. II. The sinoatrial and atrioventricular nodes, *Jpn. Circ. J.* **25**:973.

Koerpel, B. J., and Davis, L. D., 1972, Effects of lidocaine, propranolol, and sotalol on ouabain-induced changes in transmembrane potential of canine Purkinje fibers, *Circ. Res.* **30**:681.

Kohlhardt, M., Bauer, B., Krause, H., Fleckenstein, A., 1972, New selective inhibitors of the transmembrane Ca conductivity in mammalian myocardial fibers. Studies with the voltage clamp technique, *Experientia* **28**:288.

Lange, G., 1965, Action of driving stimuli from intrinsic and extrinsic sources on *in situ* cardiac pacemaker tissues, *Circ. Res.* **17**:449.

Langendorf, R., Pick, A., and Winternitz, M., 1955, Mechanisms of intermittent ventricular bigeminy. I. Appearance of ectopic beats dependent upon length of the ventricular cycle, the "Rule of Bigeminy," *Circulation* **11**:422.

Lathrop, D., Greenspan, K., and Freeman, A. R., 1974, Electrophysiological effects of hypoxia, hypothermia, acidity, stretch, and K^+ on cardiac tissue, *Fed. Proc.* **33**:445.

Lenfant, J., Mironneau, J., and Aka, J.-K., 1972, Activité répétitive de la fibre sino-auriculaire de grenouille, *J. Physiol. (Paris)* **64**:5.

Lieberman, M., 1973, Electrophysiological studies of a synthetic strand of cardiac muscle, *Physiologist* **16**:551.

Linenthal, A. J., Zoll, P. M., Garabedian, G. H., and Huber, K., 1960, Ventricular slowing and standstill after spontaneous or electrically stimulated runs of rapid ventricular beats in atrioventricular block, *Circulation* **22**:781.

Ling, G., and Gerard, R. W., 1949, The normal membrane potential of frog sartorius fibers, *J. Cell Physiol.* **34**:383

Lu, H.-H., Lange, G., and Brooks, C. McC., 1965, Factors controlling pacemaker action in cells of the sinoatrial node, *Circ. Res.* **17**:460.

Mandel, W. J., and Bigger, J. T., Jr., 1971, Electrophysiologic effects of lidocaine on isolated canine and rabbit atrial tissue, *J. Pharmacol. Exp. Ther.* **178**:81.

Mandel, W. J., and Obayashi, K., 1974, Effects of changes in pH on action potential characteristics of canine Purkinje fibers, *Clin. Res.* **22**:288A.

Mandel, W. J., Bigger, J. T., Jr., and Butler, V. P., 1972, The electrophysiologic effects of low and high digoxin concentrations on isolated mammalian cardiac tissue: reversal by digoxin-specific antibody, *J. Clin. Invest.* **51**:1378.

McAllister, R. E., 1970, Two programs for computation of action potentials, stimulus responses, voltage clamp currents, and current–voltage relations of excitable membranes, *Comput. Programs Biomed.* **1**:146.

McAllister, R. E., and Noble, D., 1966, The time and voltage dependence of the slow outward current in cardiac Purkinje fibres, *J. Physiol. (London)* **186**:632.

McDonald, T. F., and MacLeod, D. P., 1971, Maintenance of resting potential in anoxic guinea pig ventricular muscle; Electrogenic sodium pumping, *Science* **172**:570.

Meek, W. J., and Eyster, J. A. E., 1914, Experiments on the origin and propagation of the impulse in the heart: IV. The effect of vagal stimulation and of cooling on the location of the pacemaker within the sinoauricular node, *Am. J. Physiol.* **34**:368.

Mobley, B. A., and Page, E., 1972, The surface area of sheep cardiac Purkinje fibres, *J. Physiol. (London)* **220**:547.

Müller, P., 1965, Ouabain effects on cardiac contraction, action potential, and cellular potassium, *Circ. Res.* **17**:46.

Narahashi, T., 1972, Mechanism of action of tetrodotoxin and saxitoxin on excitable membranes, *Fed. Proc.* **31**:1124.

Narahashi, T., Moore, J. W., and Scott, W. R., 1964, Tetrodotoxin blockage of sodium conductance increase in lobster giant axons, *J. Gen. Physiol.* **47**:965.

Noble, D., 1962, A modification of the Hodgkin–Huxley equations applicable to Purkinje fibre action and pace-maker potentials, *J. Physiol. (London)* **160**:317.

Noble, D., 1972, Conductance mechanisms in excitable cells, *Biomembranes* **3**:427.

Noble, D., and Tsien, R. W., 1968, The kinetics and rectifier properties of the slow potassium current in cardiac Purkinje fibres, *J. Physiol. (London)* **195**:185.

Noble, D., and Tsien, R. W., 1969a, Outward membrane currents activated in the plateau range of potentials in cardiac Purkinje fibres, *J. Physiol. (London)* **200**:205.

Noble, D., and Tsien, R. W., 1969b, Reconstruction of the repolarization process in cardiac Purkinje fibres based on voltage clamp measurements of membrane current, *J. Physiol. (London)* **200**:233.

Page, E., and Storm, S. R., 1965, Cat heart muscle *in vitro*: VIII. Active transport of sodium in papillary muscles, *J. Gen. Physiol.* **48**:957.

Papp, J. G., and Vaughan Williams, E. M., 1969, A comparison of the effects of I.C.I. 50172 and l-propranolol on intracellular potentials and other features of cardiac function. *Br. J. Pharmacol.* **37**:391.

Pappano, A. J., 1970, Calcium-dependent action potentials produced by catecholamines in guinea pig atrial muscle fibers depolarized by potassium, *Circ. Res.* **27**:379.

Peper, K., and Trautwein, W., 1968, A membrane current related to the plateau of the action potential of Purkinje fibers. *Pfluegers Arch.* **303**:108.

Peper, K., and Trautwein, W., 1969, A note on the pacemaker current in Purkinje fibers, *Pfluegers Arch.* **309**:356.

Polimeni, P. I., and Vassalle, M., 1971, On the mechanism of ouabain toxicity in Purkinje and ventricular muscle fibers at rest and during activity, *Am. J. Cardiol.* **27**:622.

Regan, T. J., Harman, M. A., Leban, P. H., Burke, W. M., and Oldewurtel, H. A., 1967, Ventricular arrhythmias and K^+ transfer during myocardial ischemia and intervention with procaine amide, insulin, or glucose solution, *J. Clin. Invest.* **46**:1657.

Reuter, H., 1967, The dependence of slow inward current in Purkinje fibres on the extracellular calcium concentration, *J. Physiol. (London)* **192**:479.

Reuter, H., 1968, Slow inactivation of currents in cardiac Purkinje fibres, *J. Physiol. (London)* **197**:233.

Rijlant, P., 1936, Méchanisme de l'envahissement de l'oreillette droite du coeur de mammifère par la contraction, *C.R. Soc. Biol. (Paris)* **121**:1361.

Rosen, M. R., Gelband, H., and Hoffman, B. F., 1972, Canine electrocardiographic and cardiac electrophysiologic changes induced by procainamide, *Circulation* **46**:528.

Rosen, M. R., Gelband, H., and Hoffman, B. F., 1973a, Correlation between effects of ouabain on the canine electrocardiogram and transmembrane potentials of isolated Purkinje fibers, *Circulation* **47**:65.

Rosen, M. R., Gelband, H., Merker, C., and Hoffman, B. F., 1973b, Mechanisms of digitalis toxicity. Effects of ouabain on phase four of canine Purkinje fiber transmembrane potentials, *Circulation* **47**:681.

Rosen, M. R., Ilvento, J. P., Gelband, H., and Merker, C., 1974, Effects of verapamil on electrophysiologic properties of canine cardiac Purkinje fibers. *J. Pharmacol. Exp. Ther.* **189**:414.

Rougier, O., Vassort, G., and Stämpfli, R., 1968, Voltage clamp experiments on frog atrial heart muscle fibres with the sucrose gap technique, *Pfluegers Arch.* **301**:91.

Rougier, O., Vassort, G., Garnier, D., Gargouil, Y. M., and Coraboeuf, E., 1969, Existence and role of a slow inward current during the frog atrial action potential, *Pfluegers Arch.* **308**:91.

Sasyniuk, B. I., and Kus, T., 1974, Comparison of the effects of lidocaine on electrophysiological properties of normal Purkinje fibers and those surviving acute myocardial infarction, *Fed. Proc.* **33**:476.

Shigenobu, K., and Sperelakis, N., 1972, Calcium current channels induced by catecholamines in chick embryonic hearts whose fast sodium channels are blocked by tetrodotoxin or elevated potassium, *Circ. Res.* **31**:932.

Singh, B. N., 1972, Anti-arrhythmic actions of β-adrenergic receptor antagonists: review of fundamental aspects, *N.Z. Med. J.* **76**:333.

Singh, B. N., and Vaughan Williams, E. M., 1970, A third class of antiarrhythmic action. Effects on atrial and ventricular intracellular potentials, and other pharmacological actions on cardiac muscle, of MJ 1999 and AH 3474, *Br. J. Pharmacol.* **39**:675.

Smith, T. W., Wagner, H., Jr., Markis, J. E., and Young, M., 1972, Studies on the localization of the cardiac glycoside receptor, *J. Clin. Invest.* **51**:1777.

Strauss, H. C., and Bigger, J. T., Jr., 1972, Electrophysiological properties of the rabbit sinoatrial perinodal fibers, *Circ. Res.* **31**:490

Strauss, H. C., Bigger, J. T., Jr., Bassett, A. L., and Hoffman, B. F., 1968, Actions of diphenylhydantoin on the electrical properties of isolated rabbit and canine atria, *Circ. Res.* **23**:463.

Strauss, H. C., Bigger, J. T., Jr., and Hoffman, B. F., 1970, Electrophysiological and beta-receptor blocking effects of MJ 1999 on dog and rabbit cardiac tissue. *Circ. Res.* **26**:661.

Takata, M., Moore, J. W., Kao, Y., and Fuhrman, F. A., 1966, Blockage of sodium conductance increase in lobster giant axon by tarichatoxin (tetrodotoxin), *J. Gen. Physiol.* **49**:977.

Tamai, T., and Kagiyama, A., 1968, Studies of cat heart muscle during recovery after prolonged hypothermia: Hyperpolarization of cell membranes and its dependence on the sodium pump with electrogenic characteristics, *Circ. Res.* **22**:423.

Tarr, M., Luckstead, E. F., Jurewicz, P. A., and Haas, H. G., 1973, Effect of propranolol on the fast inward sodium current in frog atrial muscle, *J. Pharmacol. Exp. Ther.* **184**:599.

Temte, J. V., and Davis, L. D., 1967, Effect of calcium concentration on the transmembrane potentials of Purkinje fibers, *Circ. Res.* **20**:32.

Thomas, M., Shulman, G., and Opie, L., 1970, Arteriovenous potassium changes and ventricular arrhythmias after coronary artery occlusion, *Cardiovasc. Res.* **4**:327.

Torii, H., 1962, Electron microscope observations on the SA and AV nodes and the Purkinje fibers of the rabbit. *Jpn. Circ. J.* **26**:39.

Trautwein, W., and Dudel, J., 1958a, Zum Mechanismus der Membranwirkung des Acetylcholin an der Herzmuskelfaser, *Pfluegers Arch.* **266**:324.

Trautwein, W., and Dudel, J., 1958b, Hemmende und "erregende" Wirkungen des Acetylcholin am Warmblüterherzen: Zur Frage der spontanen Erregungsbildung, *Pfluegers Arch.* **266**:653.

Trautwein, W., and Kassebaum, D. G., 1961, On the mechanism of spontaneous impulse generation in the pacemaker of the heart, *J. Gen. Physiol.* **45**:317.

Trautwein, W., and Schmidt, R. F., 1960, Zur Membranwirkung des Adrenalins an der Herzmuskelfaser, *Pfluegers Arch.* **271**:715.

Trautwein, W., and Zink, K., 1952, Über Membran- und Aktionspotentiale einzelner Myokardfasern des Kalt- und Warmblüterherzen, *Pfluegers Arch.* **256**:68.

Trautwein, W., Gottstein, U., and Dudel, J., 1954, Der Aktionsstrom der Myokardfaser im Sauerstoffmangel, *Pfluegers Arch.* **260**:40.

Trautwein, W., Kuffler, S. W., and Edwards, C., 1956, Changes in membrane characteristics of heart muscle during inhibition, *J. Gen. Physiol.* **40**:135.

Tritthart, H., Fleckenstein, B., and Lynker, W., 1969, Der Einfluss von Na$^+$, K$^+$, und Ca^{++}-Ionen auf die Aufstrichsgeschwindigkeit des Aktionspotentials und die maximale Reizfolgefrequenz isolierter, elektrisch gereizter Papillarmuskeln von Meerschweinchen, *Pfluegers Arch.* **311**:R27.

Tritthart, H., Fleckenstein, B., and Fleckenstein, A., 1971, Some fundamental actions of antiarrhythmic drugs on the excitability and contractility of single myocardial fibers, *Naunyn Schmiedebergs Arch. Pharmacol.* **269**:212.

Tsien, R. W., 1973a, Adrenaline-like effects of intracellular iontophoresis of cyclic AMP in cardiac Purkinje fibres, *Nature (New Biol.)* **245**:120.

Tsien, R. W., 1973b, Does adrenaline act by directly modifying the external membrane surface charge of cardiac Purkinje fibres? *J. Physiol. (London)* **234**:37P.

Tsien, R. W., Giles, W., and Greengard, P., 1972, Cyclic AMP mediates the effects of adrenaline on cardiac Purkinje fibres, *Nature (New Biol.)* **240**:181.

Vassalle, M., 1966, Analysis of cardiac pacemaker potential using a "voltage clamp" technique, *Am. J. Physiol.* **210**:1335.

Vassalle, M., 1970, Electrogenic suppression of automaticity in sheep and dog Purkinje fibers, *Circ. Res.* **27**:361.

Vassalle, M., and Barnabei, O., 1971, Norepinephrine and potassium fluxes in cardiac Purkinje fibers, *Pfluegers Arch.* **322**:287.

Vassalle, M., and Carpentier, R., 1972, Overdrive excitation: Onset of activity following fast drive in cardiac Purkinje fibers exposed to norepinephrine, *Pfluegers Arch.* **332**:198.

Vassalle, M., and Musso, E., 1974, Cardiac Purkinje fibers, automaticity, and digitalis, *Fed. Proc.* **33**:432.

Vassalle, M., Karis, J., and Hoffman, B. F., 1962, Toxic effects of ouabain on Purkinje fibers and ventricular muscle fibers, *Am. J. Physiol.* **203**:433.

Vassalle, M., Vagnini, F. J., Gourin, A., and Stuckey, J. H., 1967a, Suppression and initiation of idioventricular automaticity during vagal stimulation, *Am. J. Physiol.* **212**:1.

Vassalle, M., Caress, D. L., Slovin, A. J., and Stuckey, J. H., 1967b, On the cause of ventricular asystole during vagal stimulation, *Circ. Res.* **20**:228.

Vassalle, M., Greineder, J. K., and Stuckey, J. H., 1973, Role of the sympathetic nervous system in the sinus node resistance to high potassium, *Circ. Res.* **32**:348.

Vaughan Williams, E. M., 1958, The mode of action of quinidine on isolated rabbit atria interpreted from intracellular potential records, *Br. J. Pharmacol.* **13**:276.

Vaughan Williams, E. M., 1970, Classification of anti-arrhythmic drugs, in *Symposium on cardiac Arrhythmias* (E. Sandøe, E. Flensted-Jensen, and K. H. Olesen, eds.), pp. 449–469, A. B. Astra, Södertälje.

Vick, R. L., 1969, Suppression of latent cardiac pacemaker: Relation to slow diastolic depolarization, *Am. J. Physiol.* **217**:451.

Weidmann, S., 1951, Effect of current flow on the membrane potential of cardiac muscle, *J. Physiol. (London)* **115**:227.

Weidmann, S., 1952, The electrical constants of Purkinje fibres, *J. Physiol. (London)* **118**:348.

Weidmann, S., 1955a, The effect of the cardiac membrane potential on the rapid availability of the sodium-carrying system, *J. Physiol. (London)* **127**:213.

Weidmann, S., 1955b, Effects of calcium ions and local anaesthetics on electrical properties of Purkinje fibres, *J. Physiol. (London)* **129**:568.

Weidmann, S., 1956, *Elektrophysiologie der Herzmuskelfaser*, Huber, Bern.

Weidmann, S., 1970, Electrical constants of trabecular muscle from mammalian heart, *J. Physiol. (London)* **210**:1041.

Weidmann, S., 1974, Heart: Electrophysiology, *Ann. Rev. Physiol.* **36**:155.

Weld, F. M., and Bigger, J. T., Jr., 1972, Effect of procaine amide on membrane conductance of cardiac Purkinje fibers, *Circulation, Suppl. 2* **45**:39.

Weld, F. M., and Bigger, J. T., Jr., 1973, Effect of lidocaine on kinetics of the fast sodium current in cardiac Purkinje fibers, *Circulation, Suppl. 4* **48**:108.

Weld, F. M., and Bigger, J. T., Jr., 1974, Effect of lidocaine on diastolic potassium currents of cardiac Purkinje fibers, *Fed. Proc.* **33**:476.

Wiggins, J. R., and Cranefield, P. F., 1974, Inhibition of Ca-dependent action potentials in canine cardiac Purkinje fibers by low levels of Na, *Fed. Proc.* **33**:446.

Wissner, S. B., 1974, The effect of excess lactate upon the excitability of the sheep Purkinje fiber, *J. Electrocardiol.* **7**:17.

Wit, A. L., Cranefield, P. F., and Hoffman, B. F., 1972, Slow conduction and reentry in the ventricular conducting system. II. Single and sustained circus movement in networks of canine and bovine Purkinje fibers, *Circ. Res.* **30**:11.

Wu, C. H., and Narahashi, T., 1972, Mechanism of action of propranolol on squid axon membranes, *J. Pharmacol. Exp. Ther.* **184**:155.

Zipes, D. P., and Mendez, C., 1973, Action of manganese ions and tetrodotoxin on atrioventricular nodal transmembrane potentials in isolated rabbit hearts, *Circ. Res.* **32**:447.

2

Actions of Opiates and Their Antagonists on Cholinergic Transmission in the Guinea Pig Ileum

SEYMOUR EHRENPREIS

I. INTRODUCTION

Ever since Paton (1957) and Schaumann (1957) developed techniques for electrical or transmural stimulation of the guinea pig ileum, this tissue has become a favorite tool for examining drug effects on parasympathetic [acetylcholine (Ach)] transmission. In particular the use of this preparation has greatly advanced knowledge of the mechanism of action of opiates as analgesics and addictive drugs. This chapter is a detailed discussion of the actions of various opiates and their antagonists on ilea from normal and addicted guinea pigs. Some new concepts for the molecular mechanism of action of opiates, the development of tolerance, and production of withdrawal symptoms will be suggested.

SEYMOUR EHRENPREIS · New York State Research Institute for Neurochemistry and Drug Addiction, Ward's Island, New York, New York 10035.

Although the ileum is comprised mainly of muscle (longitudinal muscle on the external surface, circular muscle in the inner surface), it also contains a well-defined neural network called Auerbach's plexus. Within the plexus the following elements are recognized: numerous ganglia together with pre- and postganglionic fibers. When current of sufficient intensity is passed through the tissue, there is a selective stimulation of the neural elements, i.e., the muscles do not respond to direct electrical stimulation. As a result, ACh is liberated from the nerve network and the muscle contracts. Contraction can be readily recorded by means of appropriate force transducers.

II. MECHANISM OF CONTRACTIONS INDUCED BY ELECTRICAL STIMULATION

Most of the evidence suggests that electrically induced contractions arise from a selective stimulation of postganglionic fibers; preganglionic stimulation appears to be minimal. Thus the potent inhibitors of ganglionic transmission (hexamenthonium, chlorisondamine) fail to significantly affect contraction of the tissue at concentrations which antagonize the action of ganglionic stimulants on the ileum (Ehrenpreis et al., 1972). If a drug affects contraction by a neuronal mechanism (see below for other ways), it is fairly safe to assume that its action is somewhere in the postganglionic neuron, i.e., to alter axonal conduction or influence ACh release in the terminal.

Although the ileum contains large amounts of catecholamines and serotonin, these do not seem to play a major role in transmission between nerve and muscle. Evidence for this is as follows:

1. Electrically induced contractions may be completely abolished by low concentrations of atropine, a drug which has a high specificity for ACh receptors.
2. Large doses of reserpine administered to a guinea pig have no effect on transmission properties of the ileum (S. Ehrenpreis and J. Greenberg, unpublished results).
3. Serotonin is completely absent from the longitudinal muscle– Auerbach's plexus preparation (S. Spector, personal communication).
4. Phentolamine or methysergide at high concentrations have little if any effect on contractions.

Nevertheless exogenous catecholamines may have a profound effect on transmission in the ileum in vitro (Paton and Vizi, 1969) suggesting that this may also occur in vivo.

III. PROCEDURE FOR SETTING UP THE ILEUM

The procedure for setting up the ileum for transmural electrical stimulation is fairly simple. The tissue is removed from the animal, flushed out thoroughly with Tyrode's solution, and immersed in oxygenated Tyrode's buffer until use. A piece of tissue, approximately $1-1\frac{1}{2}$ inches may then be impaled on two electrodes which serve to anchor it in the organ bath. Alternatively, field stimulation may be used in which case the tissue is attached to one electrode, while the other electrode consists of a wire inserted into the bath. In the latter procedure, far more current passes through the solution and this can have a serious effect on data obtained with drugs. The reason for this is that the effectiveness or potency of many drugs is dependent on strength of electrical stimulation: the stronger the stimulation the higher the drug concentration required to affect transmission (Ehrenpreis et al., 1972). This effect probably arises because the number of fibers recruited is stimulus dependent. In view of the above considerations, it is our contention that only relative values for potency of drug effects on transmission can be obtained.

In our laboratory, the conditions for carrying out experiments on the ileum are as follows: Tyrode's solution, at pH 7.8, is gassed with 95% oxygen–5% CO_2; the temperature of the bath of 50-ml capacity is 37°C. The current duration is 0.4 msec, 40–60 V. This gives approximately 75–80% of maximum contraction height. In most reports on drug effects, a single stimulus parameter is used. We have found that a better procedure for evaluating drug effects is to determine complete duration–response curves before and after drug treatment. The current duration is varied in both instances from threshold to maximum. The shift in midpoint of the duration–response curve then affords a measure of the potency of drug action. We have found two different situations to exist with regard to duration–response curves. Most drugs shift the curve to the right and at the same time lower the maximum response. Others simply shift the curve to the right, but the maximum response is still obtained. This procedure is of particular importance in the latter case: if only maximum or supramaximum stimulation is used, it is obvious that an important component of drug action may be missed. Alternatively, if supramaximum stimulation is used, possible stimulatory action of a drug may be missed.

IV. DETERMINATION OF OPIATE POTENCY

In order to determine potency data, dose–response curves must be obtained. This can be done in one of two ways. The discontinuous method involves addition of a single drug concentration, the effect at equilibrium is noted, the drug washed out, and the procedure repeated with a higher concentration of drug following suitable time for recovery of the tissue. In the cumulative method, the drug concentration is increased progressively without washout (Figure 1). The latter procedure has the great advantage of permitting a complete dose–response curve to be determined in a few minutes. ED_{50} values are then calculated from the dose–response curve for comparative purposes.

The cumulative dose–response method has another advantage in that many of the drugs that are examined are extremely difficult to remove from the tissue simply by washout. This was demonstrated quite conclusively for morphine and naloxone both pharmacologically (Ehrenpreis *et al.*, 1972) as well as by means of radioactive drug (Schonbuch and Ehrenpreis, 1972). Once the ileum is exposed to morphine, many hours are required before the drug is totally removed from the tissue. This finding has implications both for the cumulative as well as the discontinuous determination of drug effects.

V. SITE OF BLOCKING ACTION OF DRUGS

Although the ileum is a relatively simple system, a precise determination of the mechanism of action of drugs in affecting transmission may offer some problems. This is due to the fact that several distinct sites of action are possible: postganglionic axon, nerve terminal, ACh receptors, and extrajunctional interacting components.

At the present time, no distinction can be made between inhibition of axonal conduction and an effect limited to nerve terminal block of ACh release. Both would result in inhibition of transmission. However, a neuronal

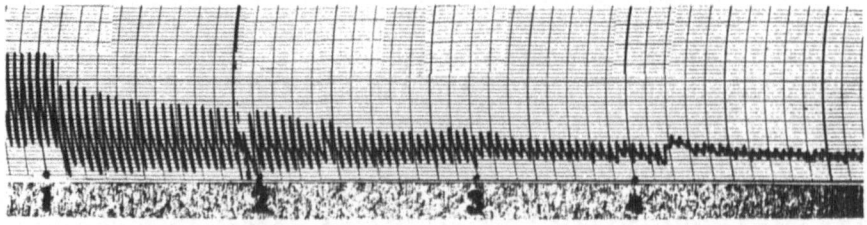

Figure 1. Cumulative dose–response determination for morphine. Current duration, 0.4 msec, 40 V; stimulation rate, 0.2 Hz; bath volume, 50 ml; temperature, 37°C. Morphine concentrations: (1) 4 ng/ml; (2) 8 ng/ml; (3) 16 ng/ml; (4) 32 ng/ml (Ehrenpreis *et al.*, 1972).

site of action can be distinguished from a muscular site simply by determining the effect of exogenous ACh in the presence of the drug. If drug action is confined to neuronal sites, contraction of the tissue by exogenous ACh will be unaffected, i.e., there will be no shift in the dose–response curve to added ACh. If the drug blocks transmission by competitive inhibition of ACh receptors, e.g., atropine, this will be reflected in a shift of the ACh dose–response curve to the right. On the other hand, if the drug blocks by combining with extrajunctional sites, e.g., in muscle membrane or sarcoplasmic reticulum, to inhibit calcium release, etc., this would be reflected in changes in response to potassium ion.

VI. ACTIVITIES OF OPIATES AND ANTAGONISTS ON THE ILEUM

We will now consider the actions of the opiates on cholinergic transmission and the inferences which can be drawn from the studies concerning their effects on cholinergic transmission in a more complex region of the body, namely the central nervous system (CNS). The actions of certain minor analgesics and other drugs which act by a similar mechanism to these, namely, as inhibitors or prostaglandin (PG) synthesis, is also discussed.

All of the opiates depress cholinergic transmission in the ileum. The site of action is exclusively neuronal, since ACh responses are unaffected at the time of block. The fact that at the effective concentration (e.g., 10^{-9}–10^{-7} M for morphine) opiates fail to block conduction in most nerves suggests that their site of action is in the postganglionic nerve terminals. These drugs combine with a specific receptor at this site and inhibit release of ACh as demonstrated by several workers (Paton, 1957; Schaumann, 1957; Lees et al., 1973).

Potency of a series of opiates in effecting transmission is presented in Table 1 along with their analgesic efficacy in mouse and man. A striking correlation exists (correlation coefficient about 0.96) (Harris and Dewey, 1973); the great sensitivity of the preparation together with this correlation suggests that the ileum can serve as a useful tool for understanding opiate action in the CNS. Indeed Pert and Snyder (1973) have obtained evidence on the basis of stereospecific drug binding that the opiate receptor in the ileum and CNS may be quite similar. Quite significantly, the opiate receptor activity was confined to the neuronal elements of the ileum; this is in agreement with pharmacological evidence.

An important point about the opiate receptor of the ileum is its stereospecificity of interaction (Kosterlitz et al., 1973). Thus, whereas dextrorphan

TABLE 1. Potency of a Series of Drugs as Analgesics in Mice and Man and as Inhibitors of Contractions of the Isolated Guinea Pig Ileum[a]

Drug	50% depression of contractions of the ileum: molar potency relative to morphine	Analgesia in mice (hot-plate method): molar potency relative to morphine	Analgesia in man: molar potency relative to morphine
Fentanyl	10,000	250	100
Phenoperidine	2,000	42	10
Oxymorphone	500	13	7.1
Nalorphine	2	0.03	1.1
Diamorphine	1.7	2.8	2.4
Normorphine	1.4	0.05	0.25
Phenazocine	1.2	19	4.0
Morphine	1.0	1.0	1.0
Pentazocine	0.6	0.3	0.42
Codeine	0.15	0.16	0.09
Morphine-N-oxide	0.05	0.10	—
Dextrorphan	inactive		inactive

[a] From Ehrenpreis et al., 1972.

is inert on the ileum, its levo isomer, levorphanol, is even more potent than morphine. The analgesic and binding affinities of these two drugs are in line with the effects on transmission. Similarly, d-methadone is approximately 1/20 as potent as l-methadone on the ileum and in terms of analgesic efficacy. Many other examples of stereospecificity are discussed by Kosterlitz et al., (1973).

It should be noted that the mechanism of action of opiates on the ileum led to similar studies in the CNS with similar results: inhibition of ACh release upon electrical stimulation (Jhamandas et al., 1970). Thus, although it is well recognized that a drug such as morphine has important effects on other CNS transmitters, e.g., serotonin and norepinephrine (Way and Shen, 1971), one possibility is that the primary site of action is on cholinergic transmission, the other transmitter effects being of a secondary nature. The recent results of Harris and Dewey (1973) on effects of various cholinergic drugs in modifying analgesia provide strong support for an important cholinergic component in opiate action.

Two types of narcotic antagonists are known on the basis of animal studies: the pure antagonist, exemplified by naloxone, and the dual-acting or antagonistic agonist, which comprise all the other antagonists. Similar behavior is observed on the ileum (Gyang and Kosterlitz, 1966). Naloxone, levallorphan, and nalorphine all antagonize blockade produced by opiates.

Naloxone acts as a pure antagonist, i.e., has no depressant effect on the ileum when used alone. The other drugs can all cause depression of contractions when used at concentrations somewhat higher than required for reversal of opiate effects. For this reason, we prefer to use naloxone in our studies, since this drug does not offer the additional complexity of agonist action.

Some exceptions to the correlation between ileum and whole animal have been noted. For example, the effect of naloxone can be extremely long lasting (Ehrenpreis *et al.*, 1972) if whole ileum is exposed to fairly high concentrations, e.g., 50–100 ng/ml. This was shown by the fact that even after several washes following naloxone, attenuation of morphine block could be observed. Naloxone reversal of morphine action in whole animal is of short duration. However, Kosterlitz *et al.* (1973) showed a very rapid reversal of naloxone action on longitudinal muscle preparation. It may be noted that they used supermaximum stimulation of the preparation in contrast to our studies on whole ileum where subthreshold conditions were used.

A second exception is that cyclazocine, a fairly potent antagonist of opiates in animals and man, only showed agonistic activity on the ileum (S. Ehrenpreis and J. Greenberg, unpublished results). Naloxone did reverse the cyclazocine block.

Naloxone can produce not only a reversal of opiate block but a contracture of the tissue as well (Ehrenpreis *et al.*, 1972). This phenomenon has been

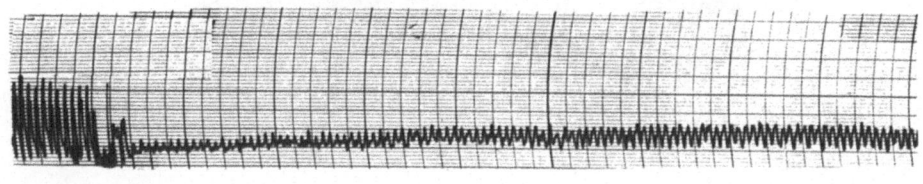

MORPH., 12 ng/ml

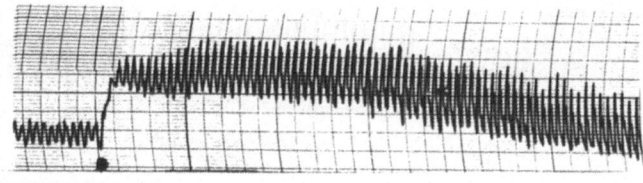

NALOXONE, 16 ng/ml

Figure 2. Naloxone contracture after morphine. A: morphine, 12 ng/ml applied for 10 min; B: naloxone, 16 ng/ml (Ehrenpreis *et al.*, 1972).

discussed in detail elsewhere (Ehrenpreis *et al.*, 1972), but because of its importance some of the factors involved will be summarized here.

1. Contracture is only observed if naloxone is added after morphine, and then only under certain conditions. For example, the degree of contracture depends on the time between exposure to opiate and naloxone. If exposure is less than about 10 min, contracture will be fairly minimal, i.e., only reversal of block will be observed (Figure 3). Furthermore, if the concentration of morphine is sufficient to produce only a minimum block, naloxone will reverse without contracture.

2. Contracture can be dissociated from reversal of block in several ways. If the tissue is exposed to a blocking concentration of opiate and washed, reversal of block can be observed. Addition of naloxone at this time may cause contracture (Figure 4). Naloxone can also cause contracture if added alone to an ileum removed from an addicted guinea pig (Figure 5).

3. Contracture can be rapidly reversed by atropine, suggesting that the phenomenon results from the liberation of ACh within the tissue.

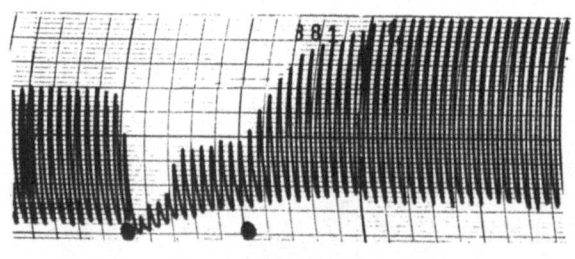

MORPH.   12 ng/ml   NALOXONE, 2 ng/ml

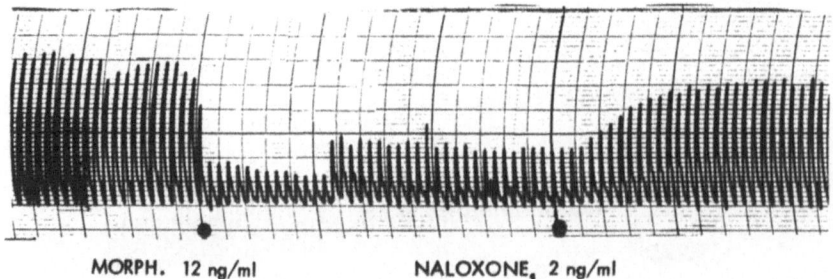

MORPH.   12 ng/ml   NALOXONE, 2 ng/ml

Figure 3. Lack of contracture by naloxone when time interval between naloxone and morphine is reduced to 1 min (upper tracing), 3 min (lower tracing). Concentrations of morphine and naloxone were the same as in Figure 2 (Ehrenpreis *et al.*, 1972).

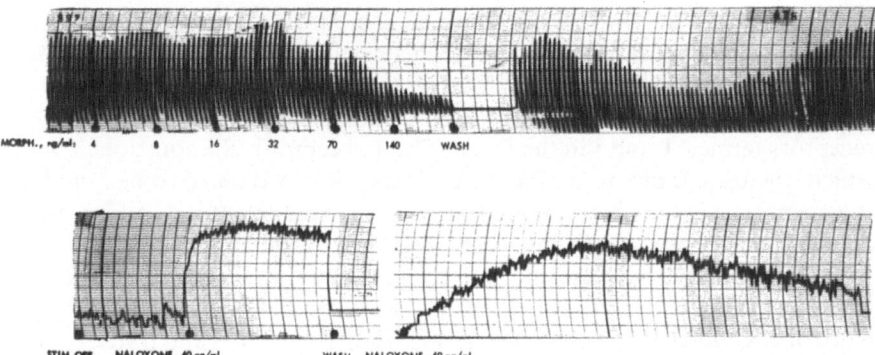

Figure 4. Dissociation of naloxone contracture from improvement of contraction following exposure to morphine. Morphine was first titrated in to give complete block of contractions. Following wash, there is complete recovery of the tissue. Addition of naloxone after the current is shut off results in a marked contracture which can be elicited even after a second wash (Ehrenpreis *et al.*, 1972).

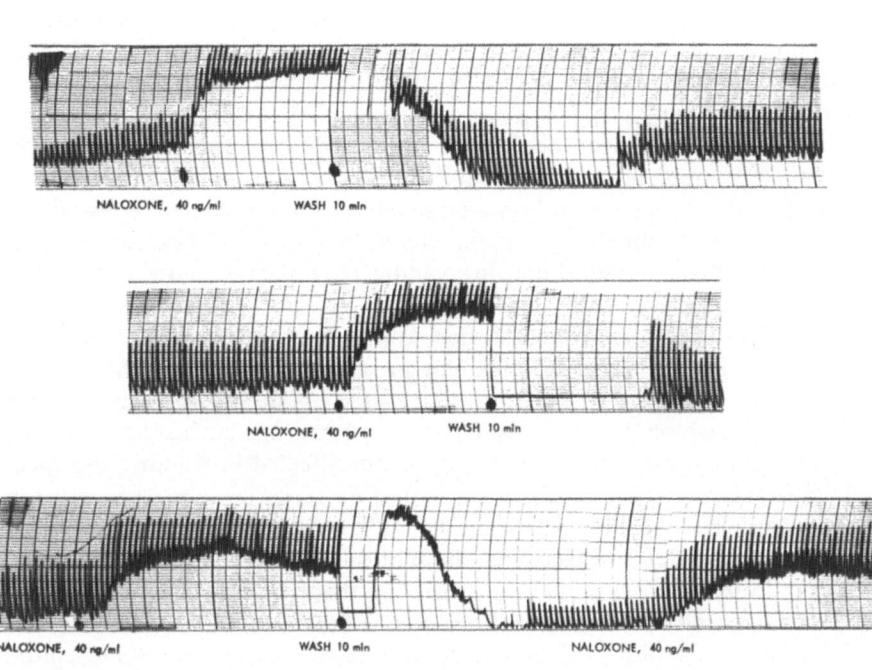

Figure 5. Naloxone contracture of ileum from addicted guinea pig. Note that this contracture can be elicited several times after washout although the height of each contracture diminishes progressively (Ehrenpreis *et al.*, 1972).

Thus at times naloxone may have an excitatory effect on the ileum, but only following exposure to an opiate. This has its exact counterpart in withdrawal precipitated by naloxone or other antagonists in the addicted animal.

These findings have led us to postulate the existence of two opiate receptors termed T and I in the ileum. The T receptor is the constituent with which opiates interact to inhibit ACh release; it is presumed to be found in the membrane of the nerve terminal. The I or internal receptor may be present on synaptic vesicles. When morphine is added to the bath, it first interacts with the T receptors which are more accessible, but also diffuses into the tissue to the I receptors. Binding to I receptors can be extremely tight. When naloxone is added, it first displaces opiate from T receptors and transmission is restored. Naloxone can displace the opiate from the I receptor, this displacement resulting in rupture of vesicles and liberation of ACh. If a significant number of I receptors are occupied, the amount of ACh liberated is sufficient to produce an overt effect, i.e., the contracture. When the tissue is washed following morphine, the drug dissociates first from the T receptor but is still bound to a significant extent to the I receptors. This binding evidently does not influence transmission and is only revealed pharmacologically when naloxone is added. Use of radioactive morphine clearly shows the presence of a component or components in the ileum which retain the drug for many hours (Schonbuch and Ehrenpreis, 1972). In the addicted animal considerable binding to I receptors takes place and thus naloxone alone causes a contracture. The fact that in the ileum from the addicted animal transmission appears to be quite normal (Ehrenpreis et al., 1972) is very significant in view of the fact that there evidently is a large amount of opiate remaining within the tissue. This finding may explain why a drug such as naloxone can precipitate the abstinence syndrome in an addict several days following cessation of intake of opiate.

Prostaglandins and Opiate Action. We have obtained considerable evidence that the T site may be a site for prostaglandins (PG) of the E series (Ehrenpreis at al., 1973). PGE_1 or E_2 reverse opiate block (Figure 6) in a competitive fashion (Figure 7); blockade by other drugs, such as barbiturates, catecholamines, local anesthetics, etc., is not affected thus indicating specificity of the reversal. PGs of the A, B, and $F\alpha$ series are almost inactive in this regard. It is suggested that PGE_1 or E_2 serves as the modulator for coupling ACh release to electrical stimulation. A PG receptor is considered to exist in the nerve terminal for mediating this function. Opiates combine with this receptor and thereby prevent PG from functioning. Other compounds known to block PG by a fairly specific interaction with PG receptors on other tissues [8-oxaprostynoic acid (Fried et al., 1971) and SC 19220 (Sanner, 1971)] also block transmission. This effect is reversed by PGE_1 or E_2.

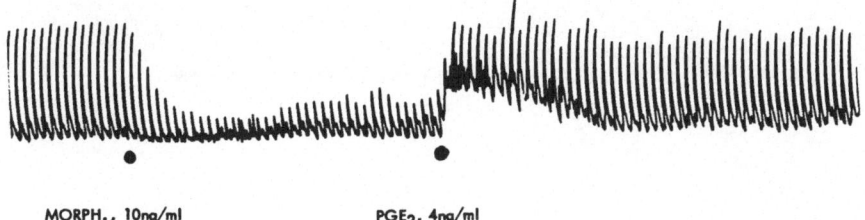

Figure 6. Reversal of morphine block of contractions of ileum by PGE$_2$. The morphine, 10 ng/ml, was applied for 5 min, followed by addition of the PG. Recovery is approximately 80% (Ehrenpreis *et al.*, 1973).

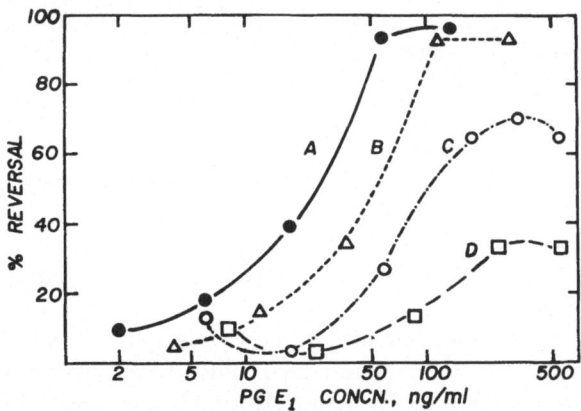

Figure 7. Cumulative dose–response curves for reversal of morphine block by PGE$_1$. Concentrations of morphine were: A, 20 ng/ml; B, 40 ng/ml; C, 80 ng/ml; D, 160 ng/ml. Note that at lower concentrations of morphine reversal is completely surmountable, becoming increasingly unsurmountable as the morphine concentration is increased. A similar series of curves was obtained for the reversal of morphine by naloxone (Ehrenpreis *et al.*, 1973).

VII. ACTIONS OF INHIBITORS OF PROSTAGLANDIN SYNTHESIS

In confirmation of the above hypothesis, we have shown that indomethacin and aspirin also block transmission; this block is reversed specifically by PGs (Figure 8). PGE$_2$ and E$_1$ are far more potent than other PGs. Of considerable interest is the fact that blockade by indomethacin and aspirin is semireversible, i.e., the block is reinstated at least in part when PG is washed

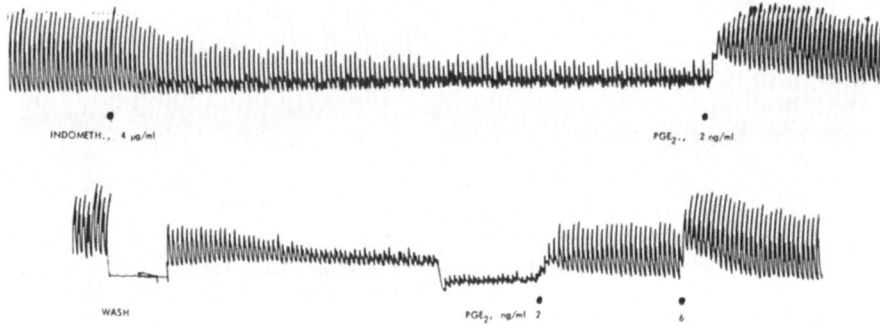

Figure 8. Inhibition of contraction of electrically stimulated guinea pig ileum by indomethacin, 4 µg/ml, acting for 30 min. Note complete reversal of the block by PGE$_2$. Following wash, complete block was reinstated; at this point, transmission was restored by very low concentrations of PG (Ehrenpreis *et al.*, 1973).

out (Figure 8). Transmission is again restored by PGs (Table 2). These drugs are known to inhibit synthesis of PG in an irreversible manner (Smith and Lands, 1971). The fact that inhibition of transmission occurs in the same concentration range as required to inhibit the enzyme and that only a PG restores transmission indicates the essentiality of the PG system for transmission in the ileum.

The recently synthesized inhibitor of prostaglandin synthesis, eicosatetraynoic acid (ETA) (Ahern and Downing, 1970) also proved to be an inhibitor of transmission in the ileum. Although reported to be a reversible inhibitor of prostaglandin synthesis, the effects of this drug were extremely long lasting. In other respects, the drug resembled indomethacin: block of transmission could be reversed by prostaglandin and at time of block there was little effect on exogenous ACh.

TABLE 2. Potency of Various Prostaglandins
in Reversing Indomethacin Block of Electrically
Induced Contractions of Guinea Pig Ileum

Prostaglandin	ED$_{50}$ for complete reversal[a] (ng/ml)[a]
A$_1$	340
B$_1$	70
E$_1$, E$_2$	2
F$_{2\alpha}$	270

[a] These values refer to reversal of block following wash out of the indomethacin (see text for explanation).

In the case of indomethacin, as well as ETA, PGE not only reversed the block under standard conditions of stimulation, but also significantly shifted the entire duration–response curve to the left. Thus PG restores the sensitivity of the tissue close to normal after its depression by inhibitors of PGE synthesis.

We have found an interesting interplay between calcium, magnesium, and PG. It is well known that Mg inhibits release of ACh, and indeed this ion blocks transmission in the ileum. Blockade is of course reversed by adding an equivalent amount of calcium. However, PG at very low concentrations also reverses the block (Figure 9). Interestingly, we have obtained evidence for a synergisim between Ca and PG in this regard.

VIII. MECHANISM OF OPIATE EFFECTS ON CHOLINERGIC TRANSMISSION: RELATION TO THE PROSTAGLANDIN SYSTEM

On the basis of these various findings, we postulate that the active site of the receptor for PG and opiates may bear a negatively charged group, possibly a phosphate. When the nerve is stimulated, an inward movement of calcium takes place (Hubbard *et al.*, 1967). This calcium may complex with the negatively charged group and provide a bridge to link the carboxyl group of PG to the active site. The remaining portion of the PG fixes to the synaptic vesicle and the 2-point attachment serves then to attract the vesicle to the membrane with which it fuses and the contents of ACh are thereby liberated. Opiates would be considered to combine directly with the negative group thereby displacing calcium. Magnesium similarly would combine with the active site preventing binding of calcium at that site. This somehow inhibits complexation with the carboxyl group of the PG, and ACh liberation is inhibited.

The nerve terminal is also the site of synthesis of PG. Inhibition of such synthesis would result in fairly rapid breakdown of PG by various dehydrogenases (Samuelsson *et al.*, 1971). When the level of PG reaches the critical

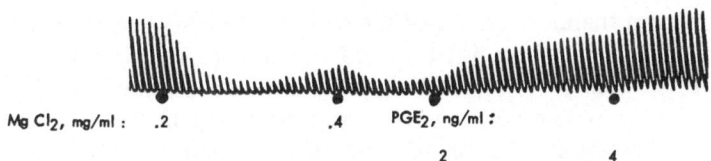

$Mg\ Cl_2$, mg/ml :   .2   .4 PGE_2, ng/ml :

                                                        2   4

Figure 9. Reversal of $MgCl_2$ block by PGE_2. Note that PG is in the ng/ml range, whereas the concentration of MG ion is many orders of magnitude higher.

point, transmission ceases but apparently can be restored simply by adding exogenous PG. At the moment, we have no information concerning the fraction of enzyme which must be inhibited in order to produce the critically low level of PG below which transmission fails. Evidently, very small amounts of PG can maintain transmission, as shown by the fact that only a few nanograms/milliliter in the bath are sufficient for this purpose once synthesis is inhibited. Only a small fraction of what is supplied actually enters into the tissue as shown by uptake studies involving radioactive PGE_2 (S. Ehrenpreis and J. Comaty, unpublished experiments).

Although PG has been shown to alter transmission in vas deferens (Hedqvist and Von Euler, 1972a, b), the conditions for observing this action of PG are somewhat unusual in that brief tetanic stimulation is required. Moreover the action of PG on this tissue is diphasic (Hedqvist and Von Euler, 1972a), i.e., facilitation of transmission at lowest concentrations, inhibition as the concentration of PG is increased. Using the single-shock method, we have been unable to observe significant effects of PGE_1 or E_2 on the vas deferens. Moreover indomethacin *in vitro* or if injected into the animal over a considerable period of time has little effect on transmission. Under similar circumstances of course there is a profound depression of transmission in the ileum which is reversed by PG. Recently Ambache *et al.* (1972) have concluded that in fact the PG system plays little if any role in the transmission mechanism in the vas deferens. In accord with the concept that opiates act via a PG mechanism, morphine has little effect on transmission in the vas deferens of guinea pig or rat even when used in extremely high concentrations. Henderson *et al.* (1972) have recently reported opiate actions on vas deferens of certain strains of mice, the mechanism of action being inhibition of norepinephrine release.

The PG receptor concept as described for the ileum may be important in terms of understanding the selective action of morphine. The reason for this is that the particular PG which is involved in modulating cholinergic transmission may vary from tissue to tissue. For example, $PGF_{2\alpha}$ apparently is the modulator for transmission in the salivary gland (Hahn and Patil, 1972). Apparently the specificity of the receptor for opiates is such that it combines strongly with a receptor for a PG of the E series. Accordingly, the affinity of opiates for the salivary gland receptor would be much less than that of the ileum, and therefore effects of the drug on salivary secretion would be minimal. This kind of specificity could account for the selective action of opiates in various parts of the body, i.e., the lack of generalized effect on cholinergic transmission everywhere. Presumably, in the CNS there are certain select muscarinic synapsis in which transmission is modulated by PG of the E series, e.g., in the periaquaductal gray, where it has been shown conclusively that morphine acts with great specificity (Jacquet and Lajtha,

1973). It is postulated that these are the sites involved with pain perception. Interruption of transmission at these sites either through a PGE receptor mechanism or by inhibition of PGE synthesis could be the basic mechanism for production of analgesia by opiates and nonopiate analgesics.

REFERENCES

Ahern, D. G., and Downing, D. T., 1970, Inhibition of prostaglandin biosynthesis by eicosa-5,8,11,14-tetraynoic acid, *Biochim. Biophys. Acta* **210**:2841.

Ambache, N., Dunk, L. P., Verney, J., and Aboo Zar, M., 1972, Inhibitory nature of the adrenergic innervation of the guinea-pig vas deferens, *Br. J. Pharmacol.* **44**:3598.

Ehrenpreis, S., Light, I., and Schonbuch, G. H., 1972, Use of the electrically stimulated guinea pig ileum to study potent analgesics, in *Drug Addiction: Experimental Pharmacology* (H. Miller and H. Lal, eds.), pp. 319–342. Futura Publishing Co., Mt. Kisco, New York.

Ehrenpreis, S., Greenberg, J., and Belman, S., 1973, Prostaglandins reverse inhibition of electrically induced contractions of guinea pig ileum by morphine, indomethacin and acetylsalicylic acid, *Nature* **245**:280.

Fried, J., Sauthanakrishnan, T. S., Himizu, J., Lin, C. H., Ford, S. H., Rubin, B., and Griggo, E. D., 1971, Prostaglandin antagonists: synthesis and smooth muscle activity, *Nature (London), New Biol.* **231**:232.

Gyang, E. A., and Kosterlitz, H. W., 1966, Agonists and antagonist actions of morphine-like drugs on the guinea pig isolated ileum, *Br. J. Pharmacol. Chemother.* **27**:514.

Hahn, R. A., and Patil, P. N., 1972, Salivation induced by prostaglandin F_{2a} and the modification of the response by atropine and physostigmine, *Br. J. Pharmacol.* **44**:527P.

Harris, L. S., and Dewey, W. L., 1973, Role of cholinergic system in the central action of narcotic agonist and antagonists, in *Agonist and Antagonist Actions of Narcotic Analgesic Drugs* (H. W. Kosterlitz, H. O. J. Collier, and J. E. Villerreal, eds.), pp. 198–206, University Park Press, London.

Hedqvist, P., and Von Euler, U. S., 1972a, Prostaglandin-induced neurotransmission failure in the field-stimulated, isolated vas deferens, *Neuropharmacology* **11**:177.

Hedqvist, P., and Von Euler, U. S., 1972b, Prostaglandin controls neuromuscular transmission in guinea pig vas deferens, *Nature (London), New Biol.* **236**:113.

Henderson, G., Hughes, J., and Kosterlitz, H. W., 1972, A new example of a morphine-sensitive neuro-effector junction: Adrenergic transmission in the mouse vas deferens, *Br. J. Pharmacol.* **46**:764.

Hubbard, J. I., Jones, S. F., and Landau, E. M., 1967, The relationship between the state of nerve-terminal polarization and liberation of acethlcholine, *Ann. N.Y. Acad. Sci.* **144**:459.

Jacquet, Y., and Lajtha, A., 1973, Morphine action at central nervous system sites in rat: analgesia or hyperalgesia depending on site and dose, *Science* **182**:490.

Jhamandas, K., Pinsky, C., and Phillis, J. W., 1970, Effects of morphine and its antagonists on release of cerebral cortical acetylcholine, *Nature*, **228**:176.

Kosterlitz, H. W., Ford, J. A. H., and Watt, A. J., 1973, Morphine receptor in myenteric plexus of the guinea pig ileum, in *Agonist and Antagonist Actions of Narcotic Analgesic Drugs*, (H. W. Kosterlitz, H. O. J. Collier, and J. E. Villerreal, eds.), pp. 45–61, University Park Press, London.

Lees, G. M., Kosterlitz, H. W., and Waterfield, A. A., 1973, Characteristics of morphine-sensitive release of neuro-transmitter substances, in *Agonist and Antagonist Actions of Narcotic Analgesic Drugs* (H. W. Kosterlitz, H. O. J. Collier, and J. E. Villerreal, eds.), pp. 141–152, University Park Press, London.

Paton, W. D. M., 1957, The action of morphine and related substances on contraction and on acetylcholine output of coaxially stimulated guinea pig ileum, *Br. J. Pharmacol. Chemother.* **11**:119.

Paton, W. D. M., and Vizi, F. S., 1969, The inhibitory action of noradrenaline and adrenalin on acetylcholine output by guinea pig ileum longitudinal muscle strips, *Br. J. Pharmacol.* **35**:10.

Pert, C. B., and Snyder, S. H., 1973, Opiate receptor: Demonstration in nervous tissue, *Science* **179**:214.

Samuelsson, B., Granstrom, E., Green, K., and Hamberg, M., 1971, Metabolism of prostaglandins, *Ann. N.Y. Acad. Sci.* **180**:138.

Sanner, J., 1971, Prostaglandin inhibition with a dibenzoxazepine hydrazide derivative and morphine, *Ann. N.Y. Acad. Sci.* **180**:396.

Schaumann, W., 1957, Inhibition by morphine of the release of acetylcholine from the intestine of the guinea pig, *Br. J. Pharmacol. Chemother.* **12**:115.

Schonbuch, G. H., and Ehrenpreis, S., 1972, Uptake of radioactive morphine by isolated guinea pig intestine, *Fed. Proc.* **31**:482.

Smith, W. L., and Lands, W. E. M., 1971, Stimulation and blockade of prostaglandin biosynthesis, *J. Biol. Chem.* **246**:6700.

Way, E. L., and Shen, F., 1971, The effects of narcotic analgesic drugs on specific systems: catecholamines and 5-hydroxytryptamine, in *Narcotic Drugs: Biochemical Pharmacology* (D. H. Clouet, ed.), pp. 229–253, Plenum Press, New York.

3

Pharmacology of Heart Cells During Ontogenesis

ACHILLES J. PAPPANO

I. INTRODUCTION

The reactivity of the embryo heart to drugs has attracted considerable attention. There are several reasons that make cardiac tissue from embryonic and fetal animals advantageous for a systemic investigation of drug action. A study of when and how the heart develops responsiveness to selected chemical probes is an invaluable aid in defining the mechanism of action of drugs and how the mechanism is modified by environmental factors (intra- and extracellular). For example, drug action can be compared in the noninnervated and innervated heart. In this manner, the effects of innervation on receptor sensitivity for transmitter molecules can be examined without the use of surgical or pharmacological techniques to eliminate neural activity. A reasoned examination of the pharmacology of the developing heart necessarily involves a systematic study of the fundamental features of cardiac development itself. The reaction between a drug molecule and a cardiac cell depends upon an interaction with chemical recognition sites (receptors) whose synthesis and assembly have been accomplished at a specified time during ontogenesis. The receptors are associated with electrical (e.g., conductance) and mechanical

ACHILLES J. PAPPANO · Department of Pharmacology, University of Connecticut Health Center, Farmington, Connecticut 06032.

(e.g., myofilament interaction) properties of the cell; therefore, drug action will produce a change in the electrical and mechanical activity of the cell. Heart cells from embryonic and fetal animals also lend themselves easily to study under *in vitro* conditions in cell or organ culture.

A comparative method has been used to discuss drug action on embryo heart cells studied in intact tissues or after disposition in culture. The scope of this discussion is necessarily limited and will deal primarily with selected groups of drugs that have been studied in chick and rodent hearts. A comprehensive review of the mechanical properties of the heart and the changes produced by drugs is given for the fetal lamb heart by Friedman (1972). A comparison of the electrical and chemical properties of intact and cultured heart cells has recently appeared (Sperelakis, 1972a).

II. EXPERIMENTAL METHODS

A. Isolated Cardiac Tissues and Heart Cells in Culture

Many investigators have examined the pulsatile activity of the embryo heart *in situ* having taken suitable precautions to prevent heat loss and evaporation from the tissue. Assessment of drug action on cardiac activity is more conveniently achieved with the organ, or portions of it, isolated and immersed in a superfusing saline solution. Rhythmic spontaneous and evoked electrical and mechanical activity of the isolated tissue can be maintained for reasonable periods of time (e.g., 6–8 hr) during superfusion with a balanced salt solution, such as a modified Tyrode solution, with appropriate control of pH and temperature.

Cardiac cells have been maintained for extended periods of time (several days to weeks) with the application of culture methods. The entire heart has been maintained as a spontaneously contracting organ for three weeks in culture media containing medium 199 (balanced salt solution, glucose, amino acids, fats, vitamins), serum, insulin, and cortisol (Wildenthal, 1971a). Other formulations of synthetic nutrient media have been used (see Waymouth, 1965, for details). Colonies of dispersed heart cells, placed in culture media, have also been used to study the electrical and mechanical properties of the embryo heart. Trypsin and collagenase have served as enzymatic dispersing agents for preparation of cell cultures by many laboratories (see DeHaan, 1967; Sperelakis, 1972a, for details). Two-dimensional monolayer cultures of varying cellular arrangements and three-dimensional aggregates of heart cells have been maintained in culture conditions for weeks with the aid of synthetic media. Recently, heart cells in culture have been grown under experimental conditions that allowed orientation of the cells in prescribed geometric patterns (Lieberman et al., 1972).

B. Measurements of Cellular Activity

Various methods have been used to record the electrical activity of heart cells in isolated tissues and in culture. Electrical stimulation is customarily done with rectangular voltage pulses delivered to the isolated tissue through unipolar or bipolar low-resistance electrodes applied to the surface. Recording of spontaneous and evoked electrical activity from groups of cells can also be accomplished with metal electrodes that lead from the tissue to resistive- or capacitative-coupled amplifiers. The amplified signals, in turn, can be displayed on an oscilloscope or on a pen writer. Membrane resting and action potentials are recorded with the aid of glass capillary microelectrodes filled with 3 M KCl and having tip resistances 10–50 MΩ. The signal from the microelectrode is led through an amplifier with a high input impedance to minimize current leakage from the cell. In addition, an internal feedback capacitance circuit is used to neutralize input capacitance (primarily owing to the microelectrode) and to permit more accurate recording of transient changes in the recorded potentials (e.g., rising phase of the action potential). Again, signals from the amplifier can be displayed on an oscilloscope or pen writer; temporal resolution of the amplitude and time course of intracellularly recorded membrane potentials is more accurate with an oscilloscope because of its greater frequency response capabilities. Differentiation of membrane potentials is a very useful index of cellular electrical activity as exemplified in measurements of the maximum rate of rise of the action potential ($+ \dot{V}_{max}$, see Section IV–D on tetrodotoxin). An operational amplifier can be conveniently used to obtain the derivative of the action potential; alternatively, passive resistance–capacitance networks or recording of a rapid sweep trace can be used to monitor $+ \dot{V}_{max}$. The microelectrode can also be used to lead current into a cell. With a modified Wheatstone bridge circuit, it is possible to use the same microelectrode to pass current and to record voltage from the same cell. This method has been successfully applied to examination of heart cells in culture (see Sperekalis, 1972a). Alternatively, separate microelectrodes can be used to pass current and to record voltage.

Assessment of the mechanical performance of the embryo heart and its constituent tissues has been accomplished by several different techniques.

Force developed by the isolated heart was measured with a photoelectric device by McCarty et al. (1960). Provision was made to adjust resting length of the muscle which was connected to a small deflecting mirror by a thin glass filament attached to a rubber band or metal filament. Heart contractions rotated the filament and the attached mirror; the variations in the amount of incident light reflected by the mirror to the photocell were recorded electronically on an oscilloscope. This apparatus, a modification of that described by Barry (1950) was especially useful in monitoring the mechanical activity (resting and active tension) of very small hearts (4th incubation day). A strain gauge coupled to an oscilloscope or pen writer will provide accurate measurements of cardiac contractions in older hearts that have sufficient mass to allow connections to the recording device. A light source–photocell system has also found usefulness as a recording device to monitor the changes in length of contracting heart cells in culture. With suitable focusing of the reflected light beam, it has been possible to record the displacement of individual cells or portions of cells in culture. The principle of recording is the same as that described above for the intact embryonic heart (see Kaufmann et al., 1969; Boder et al., 1971, for more complete descriptions of the apparatus). Faber (1968) described a recording system that enables the investigator to measure the changes in intracardiac pressure of hearts isolated from animals as early as the 3rd incubation day. Fine-tipped capillaries 100–150 μm tip diameter) were inserted into cardiac chambers, and the pressure changes during the cardiac cycle were recorded on a pen writer through a conventional pressure transducer. The studies of Faber (1968) and McCarty et al. (1960) clearly showed that the young (3–4 day) chick heart operated in accordance with the Frank–Starling mechanism.

The role of Ca^{2+} in the contraction–relaxation cycle of muscle has prompted the development of many techniques for assessing the movement and distribution of this cation across the cell membrane. Recently, measurements of ^{45}Ca exchange have been applied to cultured heart cells grown in monolayers on slides made of glass scintillator material (Langer et al., 1969). Uptake and efflux of ^{45}Ca from spontaneously contracting heart cells were measured directly in an apparatus constructed to provide continuous superfusion of a chamber containing the cells on a slide. Lanthanum quickly displaced the Ca^{2+} in a rapidly exchanging component ($t_{1/2} = 1.15$ min) and reduced the rate of ^{45}Ca efflux from both rapid and slow components (Langer and Frank, 1972). The ability of La^{3+} to uncouple excitation from contraction and to depress ^{45}Ca exchange was attributed to a binding of La^{3+} to the basement membrane of the cell. Extension of studies with this method ought to provide valuable information regarding the role of Ca^{2+} in excitation–contraction coupling in preparations that lack the complicating compartments (e.g., vascular) of intact cardiac muscle.

III. CARDIAC DEVELOPMENT

A. General Morphologic Features

The heart of the chick embryo has been studied by many investigators, and it is helpful to consider some salient features of its development with a view toward achieving an understanding of the changes in structural and functional properties that could determine the actions of drugs.

The chick heart, which appears initially as a tube connecting extraembryonic and intraembryonic vessels (7 somites or 29–33 hr), begins contracting spontaneously within 33–38 hr after fertilization (9 somite stage). Spontaneous electrical activity was detected in cells of the sinoatrial and ventricular regions of the heart at the 8 somite stage, that is, before spontaneous contractions occurred (van Mierop, 1967). Moreover, the pacemaker was located in the sinoatrial region of the heart, since the action potentials recorded from cells in this area preceded those recorded from ventricular cells by a regular interval. Thus, at the inception of action potential generation, the chick embryo heart displays two features of electrical activity that are like those of the adult: sinoatrial pacemaker location and temporal delay between atrial and ventricular excitation (see Lieberman and Paes de Carvalho, 1965).

Enlargement of the tubular heart is accompanied by bending of the structure and the external appearance of definitive cardiac structures including the ventricle (9 somites), atrium (16 somites), and sinus venosus (19 somites). The appearance of these cardiac tissues as clearly delineated regions is sequentially associated with the occurrence of spontaneous contractions. Blood flow through the heart begins at the 16–17 somite stage (45–49 hr). Continued enlargement of the definitive organ is accompanied by appearance of nearly completed septae between the atria (5th incubation day) and the ventricles (6th incubation day), and the external appearance of the heart is like that of the adult by the 8th incubation day (Romanoff, 1960). A useful comparison of the developmental stages of the hearts of various animals, including humans, has been given by Sissman (1970). The ultrastructural changes in cardiac cells, particularly myofilament organization, have been described by Manasek (1968).

B. Innervation and Histochemical Observations

Innervation of the chick embryo heart has been the object of many investigations (see Romanoff, 1960), and it will be treated in some detail. An examination of cardiac innervation patterns provides another landmark in the development of the organ and also has served as a focal point for drug sensitivity studies (see Coraboeuf et al., 1970a). Branches of the vagus nerve appear in the ventricle between 64 and 68 hr and in the atrium at the end of the 4th incubation day (Szepsenwol and Bron, 1936). As development proceeds, vagal neurons are found in the interatrial septum on the 5th incubation day (Kuntz, 1910), in the sinoatrial region on the 6th incubation day, and in the atrial wall at the end of the 7th incubation day (Abel, 1912). The development of the sympathetic cardiac nerves lags somewhat behind that of the parasympathetic. Whereas the primary sympathetic chain appeared between the 4th and 6th incubation days, the secondary sympathetic chain of peripheral adrenergic neurons is not formed before the 6th incubation day (Romanoff, 1960). Indeed, Abel (1912) subscribed to the proposal of His, who reported connections between upper thoracic sympathetic ganglia and the heart on the 10th incubation day. Intrinsic (parasympathetic) cardiac ganglia were reported to appear between the 4th and 6th incubation days (Szantroch, 1929).

Cholinesterase was detected histochemically in the chick embryo heart as early as 68–72 hr (Zachs, 1954). Myocardial cells (atrioventricular wall) displayed a cholinesterase-positive reaction on the 3rd incubation day and cholinesterase staining was quite prominent in atrial and ventricular myocardium on the 7th and 8th incubation days (Gyevai, 1969). Moreover, histochemical demonstration of cholinesterase declined during development for unexplained reasons. It has not been determined whether the enzyme bears a particular relationship to the development of neurons which also appeared about this time. No information is presently available regarding neuronal localization of the enzyme. It can be misleading to view cholinesterase appearance as a sign of cholinergic nerve development because of the widespread distribution of the enzyme (see Karczmar et al., 1973). Histochemical localization of choline acetyltransferase would be a most helpful adjunct in the study of the appearance and development of the functional cholinergic nerves (see Section IV–A on cholinergic transmission and cholinergic drugs).

The Falck paraformaldehyde method has been applied to the embryo heart for histochemical fluorescent studies of adrenergic structures (Enemar et al., 1965). Fluorescence was initially observed in round cells of the bulbus on the 6th incubation day; such cells could be found on the 7th and 8th incubation days. On the 10th incubation day, a plexus of multipolar cells with short processes appeared to replace the small round cells seen earlier; the plexus was believed to correspond to the bulbar plexus of His. It is important to note that the fluorescence observed in cells from the 6th through the 10th incubation days had a yellow color like that characteristic of certain tryptamine derivatives. Fluorescent structures that had a nervelike appearance were first observed on the 16th incubation day as varicose fibers in ventricular musculature. The green color of the fluorescent material observed on the 16th incubation day supported the view that adrenergic nerves were present at this time since green fluorescence is characteristic of catecholamines. The implications of the delay between ingrowth of sympathetic nerves to the heart and the appearance of fluorescent adrenergic nerves will be considered later (see Section IV–B on adrenergic agonists and antagonists).

C. Ion Content and Distribution

The marked changes in cell growth and functional capabilities during development suggest that the ionic environment of the cardiac cell is also subject to change. Early analysis indicated that the Na^+ content of heart was high, whereas that of K^+ was low at the 2nd incubation day (Klein, 1960). The Na^+ content declined markedly from 650 mM (2nd day) to 81 mM (7th day) and to 31 mM (21st day). Potassium content rose from 65–70 mM (2nd–3rd day) to reach peak values of about 75–85 mM (13th day) and then declined to 70–80 mM on the day of hatching. The detection of a large Na^+ content was puzzling, and it was concluded that only a small portion (5–8% at the 7th day) was osmotically and electrochemically active. In fact, subsequent analysis strongly supported the conclusion that the high Na^+ content of the early embryonic heart was a result of binding of Na^+ to mucopolysaccharide cardiac jelly and that the amount of Na^+ bound decreased as the cardiac jelly diminished during ontogenesis (Klein, 1963a). Subsequent analysis of cation distribution between ventricular cells and extracellular environment showed that both Na^+ and K^+ content diminished from the 5th incubation day through the 21st incubation day (Harsch and Green, 1963). Moreover, K^+ content was always greater than Na^+ content at any age, and the inulin (extracellular space) declined with age. Estimates of intracellular ion concentrations (mM) from the data of Harsch and Green yield values on the 8th, 11th, and 18th incubation days as follows: $[Na^+]_i = 23$, 37, and 39; $[K^+]_i = 144$, 115, and 92. Since there was little change in the extracellular concentrations of these cations ($[Na^+]_0$ and $[K^+]_0$), it can be concluded on the basis of ion concentrations that a reduction in the equilibrium potentials (E_{Na} and E_K) occurred during ontogenesis. More recently, ion content, ion concentrations, and inulin space in chick ventricular tissue have been reexamined and the observations of Harsch and Green have been confirmed (McDonald and DeHaan, 1973). Calculations of E_K showed that it decreased slightly during ontogenesis from -94 mV on the 3rd incubation day to -86 mV on the 18th incubation day. No significant differences were estimated in E_{Na} since $[Na^+]_i$ did not vary by more than 10 mM during ontogenesis and the changes were variable and not specifically related to age.

Measurements of ion content in chick atria showed that K^+ content tended to decrease during ontogenesis (Table 1), as in chick ventricle (Pappano, unpublished observations). By contrast, there was no consistent change in Na^+ content during development; the highest value of Na^+ was recorded on the 12th incubation day. The ratio of Na^+ to K^+ was >1 in atria on the 6th, 12th, and 18th incubation days. This pattern is decidedly different from that observed in the chick ventricle where Na^+/K^+ is <1 (Harsch and Green, 1963). It is commonly found that the ratio (Na^+/K^+) exceeds 1 in tissues containing pacemaker cells and the chick atrial preparations included the sinoatrial pacemaker. The relationship between equilibrium potentials and membrane resting and action potentials will be considered in the next section.

D. Electrical Properties of Cardiac Cells

Several studies have been made of the electrical activity of embryo heart cells during ontogenesis with particular reference to the ionic basis of the resting and action potentials. The resting and action potentials of chick ventricular cells (Shimizu and Tasaki, 1966) and of rat atrial and ventricular cells (Couch et al., 1969) increased during maturation. In the chick heart the resting potential (E_m) of ventricular cells increased steadily from about -40 mV at the 3rd incubation day to -65 mV at the 7th–9th incubation days; no further change was noted after this time (Sperelakis and Shigenobu, 1972). Action potential amplitude and the overshoot potential (E_{ov}) underwent a similar increase between the 3rd and 8th incubation days and then did not change through the rest of the chicken life *in ovo*. These findings were confirmed by McDonald and DeHaan (1973). However, they obtained resting E_m values slightly greater (more negative) than did Sperelakis and Shigenobu and also noted that the resting E_m and E_{ov} increased until the 14th incubation day. Atrial cells displayed an increase in resting E_m and amplitude during ontogenesis that appeared to reach a constant value at the 5th–6th incubation days (Table 2). Examination of the K-electrode properties with electro-

TABLE 1. Ion and Water Content of Chick Embryo Atria

Incubation age (days)	Ion (mM/kg wet wt)			H_2O (ml/100 g wet wt)
	Na^+	K^+	Ca^{2+}	
6	63.3 ± 4.7	64.8 ± 6.1	2.8 ± 0.3	87.1 ± 0.8
12	74.9 ± 3.8	57.8 ± 1.4	$2.6 + 0.2$	87.8 ± 1.1
18	69.7 ± 2.5	55.3 ± 1.5	2.4 ± 0.2	86.7 ± 0.6

TABLE 2. Membrane Resting and Action Potentials in
Chick Atria

Incubation age (days)	N^a	E_m (mV)	Amplitude (mV)
3	11	-47 ± 3	57 ± 3
4	9	-56 ± 4	68 ± 5
5	12	-63 ± 2	81 ± 3
6	19	-62 ± 2	82 ± 2

^{a} N refers to number of impalements.

physiological techniques suggested that membrane conductance of K^+ (g_K) increased during ontogenesis (Pappano, 1972a). The slope of the line relating E_m to $[K^+]_0$ increased from 46 mV per 10-fold change in $[K^+]_0$ on the 4th incubation day to reach a value of 59 mV per 10-fold change in $[K^+]_0$ at the 18th incubation day (see Table 5). Estimated $[K^+]_i$ ranged from 125 to 145 mM from the 4th to the 18th incubation days. In addition, suppression of automaticity required only 5–10 mM $[K^+]_0$ on the 18th incubation day as compared to 20–30 mM $[K^+]_0$ on the 4th–6th incubation day. This observation provided an independent measure of g_K since increased g_K is known to inhibit automaticity (Trautwein, 1963). These observations strongly supported the conclusion that g_K increased during ontogenesis. Similar findings were reported by Sperelakis and Shigenobu (1972) using electrophysiologic techniques. These investigators also noted that input resistance of ventricular cells decreased rapidly up to the 8th incubation day and attributed this to an increased P_K. Moreover, it was concluded that the increased resting E_m observed during development was primarily the result of a reduction in the ratio of permeabilities (P_{Na}/P_K) from about 0.2 in young hearts to a value of about 0.05 in older hearts. Estimates of the permeability ratio from ion concentrations and observed resting E_m also suggested that P_{Na}/P_K decreased during maturation (McDonald and DeHaan, 1973). Thus, there is general agreement that the selectivity of the cardiac membrane for K^+ increased with developmental age in the chick heart.

The rising phase of the action potential in chick atrial (Pappano, 1972b) and ventricular cells (Yeh and Hoffman, 1968; Sperelakis and Shigenobu, 1972; McDonald and DeHaan, 1973) depends upon an increased g_{Na}. In ventricular cells, the ratio of g_{Na}/g_K during the overshoot is thought to remain unchanged during ontogenesis because E_{ov} had a slope of about 60 mV/10-fold change in $[Na^+]_0$ (Yeh and Hoffman, 1968; Sperelakis and Shigenobu, 1972). Atrial cells displayed a Ca^{2+} current sufficient to allow excitation in the presence of tetrodotoxin (TTX) in young but not old preparations. Although an inward Na^+ current determined the rising phase of the ventricular action potential, there is some evidence that Ca^{2+} can participate in action potential generation in the presence of TTX alone (McDonald *et al.*, 1973) or in the presence of TTX and catecholamines (Shigenobu and Sperelakis, 1972). A more complete description of the ionic current carriers during excitation in embryo heart cells and in cultured heart cells is given later when the actions of tetrodotoxin are considered. The ionic basis of action potential generation in the embryo heart has many features in common with those of the adult heart (Trautwein, 1973).

E. Changes in Heart Rate During Development

Sinoatrial impulse frequency changed considerably during development, and the pattern of heart rate changes observed *in vitro* has been compared with that obtained *in vivo* (Löffelholz and Pappano, 1974a). This comparison is helpful because changes in spontaneous impulse frequency of the isolated heart often serve as an index of drug action described later. As shown in Table 3, sinoatrial impulse frequency increased during ontogenesis to reach a maximum between the 11th and 15th incubation days. Pacemaker firing rate decreased after the 15th incubation day, reached a minimum around the 21st incubation day and then increased again by the end of the first week after hatching (Table 3). Studies of changes in the rate of spontaneous cardiac contractions done under *in vivo* conditions (Romanoff, 1960) have shown a pattern similar to that observed *in vitro*, and it can be concluded that the variations in spontaneous impulse frequency arose from alterations of activity intrinsic to the pacemaking mechanism. The decline in impulse

TABLE 3. Sinoatrial Impulse Frequency in Isolated
Preparations[a]

Incubation age (days)	Spontaneous impulse frequency (AP/min)[b]
6	101 ± 3
9	112 ± 2
11	116 ± 4
13	115 ± 5
15	116 ± 6
18	89 ± 4
21 (hatching)	71 ± 7
28	90 ± 7

[a] Measurements made in isolated sinoatrial preparations bathed in modified Tyrode solution (5.4 mM K^+) at 30°C.
[b] Spontaneous impulse frequency given as action potentials per min (AP/min); measurements are mean ± SEM.

frequency during the third incubation week was associated with a reduction in the rate of slow diastolic depolarization of pacemaker cells. This observation can be explained, in part, by an ontogenetic increase in membrane conductance to K^+ (g_K) in sinoatrial cells (Pappano, 1972a). The fact that spontaneous rate decreased to a minimum on the day of hatching was attributed to interruption of cardioaccelerator sympathetic reflex activity that could operate on the 21st incubation day (see Section IV–B). This proposal is in accordance with the findings of Bogue (1932), who concluded that sympathetic cardioaccelerator fibers could be reflexively activated in the newly hatched chick by acoustic and optic stimuli. More recently, it has been reported that the reflex sympathetic component of homeothermic regulation develops within the first 5 days after the chick hatches (Wekstein and Zolman, 1968).

IV. MODIFICATION OF ELECTRICAL AND MECHANICAL ACTIVITY OF EMBRYO HEARTS PRODUCED BY DRUGS

A. Cholinergic Transmission and Cholinergic Drugs

The responsiveness of the chick embryo heart to acetylcholine (ACh) and to cholinomimetic substances has been studied by many investigators. In an early report of cholinomimetic action, Pickering (1893) reported that muscarine had no specific effect on the rate of spontaneous contractions in the young chick heart (72nd–100th incubation hour). He later concluded that the appearance of cardioinhibition by muscarine around the 8th incubation day could be related to the development of inhibitory nerves within the heart (Pickering, 1896). By contrast, Plattner and Hou (1931) concluded that ACh-mediated cardioinhibition did not require innervation, since responsiveness to the drug could be demonstrated in the noninnervated chick heart (72–94 hr incubation age). It was subsequently shown that ACh produced atropine-sensitive inhibition of spontaneous cardiac beating in the 10 somite (33–38 hr incubation age) embryo (Hsu, 1933; Cullis and Lucas, 1936). Thus, the cardioinhibitory action of ACh is manifest shortly after initiation of spontaneous contractions (Patten and Kramer, 1933), and the atropine-sensitive cholinergic receptor appears before the ingrowth of cardiac autonomic neurons (see Section III–B). Considerable attention has been given to the possibility that vagal innervation was associated with an increased sensitivity of the heart to cholinergic agonists (reviewed by Coraboeuf et al., 1970a). Although morphologic innervation of the heart had been studied in detail, functional innervation by vagal neurons was not known.

1. Development of Cholinergic Neuroeffector Transmission

Field stimuli were delivered to chick embryo hearts to determine when efferent vagal innervation of the heart began to transmit information to pacemaker cells. Neurotransmitters can be released from intracardiac autonomic neurons by application of high-frequency impulse trains (see Vincenzi and West, 1963; Blinks, 1966, for details). Neurally mediated cardioinhibition appeared for the first time in ontogenesis on the 12th incubation day; this is illustrated in Figure 1 (Pappano and Löffelholz, 1974). Pharmacological analysis suggested that field stimulation evoked release of inhibitory transmitter (presumably ACh) by initiating propagated impulses in postganglionic cholinergic nerves. Both membrane hyperpolarization and the duration of inhibition increased in proportion to the frequency of applied stimuli (Figure 2). These findings were consistent with the possibility that increasing the frequency of stimulation augmented the amount of ACh released from intracardiac nerves. Membrane hyperpolarization and inhibition of pacemaker

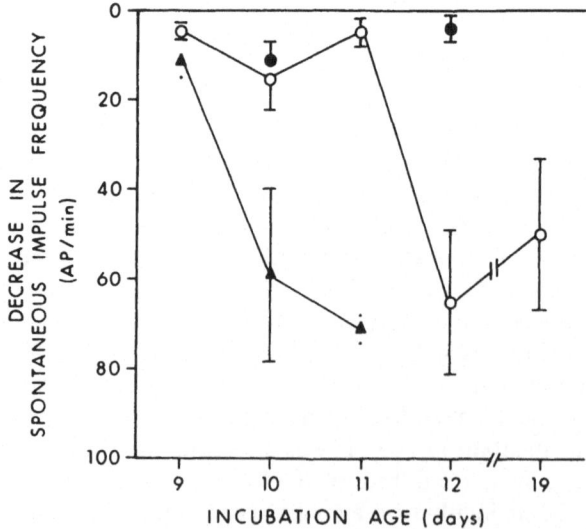

Figure 1. Ontogenetic appearance of atropine-sensitive cardioinhibitory nerve transmission. Ordinate: decrease in sinoatrial pacemaker impulse frequency in action potentials (AP/min); abscissa: incubation age of chick embryo from which heart was isolated. The nonfilled and filled circles show the pacemaker response to field stimulation in the absence and presence, respectively, of 2.8×10^{-7} M atropine. Filled triangles indicate responses obtained in physostigmine (3.6×10^{-6} M). Each symbol is the mean ± SEM of 4–8 measurements except those for physostigmine on the 9th and 11th incubation days. (From Pappano and Löffelholz, 1974; reproduced with permission of the *Journal of Pharmacology and Experimental Therapeutics.*)

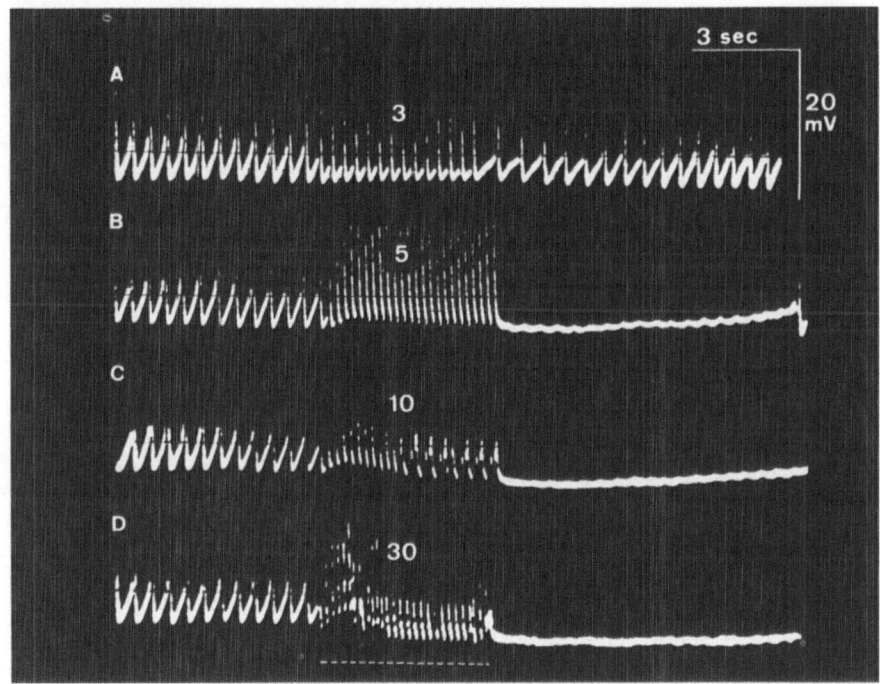

Figure 2. Frequency-dependent effects of field stimulation on membrane of pacemaker cell (12th incubation day). The records were obtained from a single cell and show only the lower portions of the action potential. Trains of stimuli at 3 Hz (A), 5 Hz (B), 10 Hz (C), and 30 Hz (D) were applied to the sinoatrial region during the period indicated by discontinuous line below trace D.

activity caused by field stimulation were prevented by tetrodotoxin TTX which blocks impulse initiation and conduction and by atropine which competitively occludes the postsynaptic cholinergic receptor (Figure 1). The failure of hexamethonium to block field stimulation-dependent cardioinhibition strengthened the argument that the stimulation procedure effected transmitter release from postganglionic cholinergic neurons. Stimulation of the extracardiac (cervical) vagus trunk elicited hexamethonium-sensitive cardioinhibition on the 12th incubation day lending credence to the proposal that efferent vagal innervation of the chick heart was structurally and functionally similar to that described in adult amphibia and mammals.

The ontogenetic appearance of cholinergically mediated cardioinhibition could be shifted two days earlier (10th incubation day) by treating the preparations with physostigmine, a reversible cholinesterase inhibitor (Pappano and Löffelholz, 1974). However, field stimulation did not elicit cardioinhibition on the 9th incubation day, even in the presence of physostigmine

(Figure 1). This finding suggested that the onset of inhibitory transmission to cardiac pacemaker cells was limited, at least in part, by the amount of ACh available for release by cholinergic nerves. The specific activity of choline acetyltransferase (ChAc), the enzyme catalyzing the synthesis of ACh from choline and acetyl CoA, increased for the first time in ontogenesis on the 10th incubation day and continued to rise throughout the remainder of embryogenesis (Gifford *et al.*, 1973). Assuming that the amount of transmitter available for release increased when enzyme activity rose, this observation strongly supports the hypothesis that the onset of inhibitory neuroeffector transmission depended upon availability of transmitter.

Pickering (1896) observed that application of interrupted currents for 3–4 min evoked cardioinhibition in chick hearts after 8.5 days. He concluded that the inhibitory effects of electrical stimuli were a result of activation of intracardiac nerves. However, it is possible that the inhibition was the result of overdrive suppression caused by direct effects of prolonged electrical stimulation on the membrane (see Vassalle, 1970). As mentioned previously, antagonism by atropine of the cardioinhibitory effects of field stimulation is consistent with the neural basis of the phenomenon and will distinguish cholinergically mediated inhibition from that owing to direct suppression of the membrane. Coraboeuf *et al.*, (1970*b*) reported that electrical stimulation of noninnervated chick heart (72-hr incubation age) produced atropine-sensitive inhibition of automaticity. The inhibition was attributed to release of an ACh-like substance from either "connective cells" or myocardial cells; a bioassay system was used to detect the material released from the hearts. In connection with this observation, it has been suggested that the ChAc found in the 72-hr chick heart is extraneuronal in origin. The fact that the chick heart contained an ACh-like material on the 3rd incubation day had been noted by Lissák *et al.* (1942). However, the material was thought to be within intracardiac nerves on the basis of histological examination of the tissues and organ culture experiments. Experiments in our laboratory did not reveal atropine-sensitive postdrive inhibition until the 12th incubation day, but this phenomenon was neurally dependent. Failure to observe inhibition by field stimulation from the 6th through the 11th incubation days does not preclude the possibility that the release of an ACh-like material from nonneural sources is restricted to the earliest stages of ontogenesis. The hypothesis of Coraboeuf and his colleagues certainly requires further examination.

2. Sensitivity to Cholinergic Drugs and Innervation

The onset of cholinergic neuroeffector transmission was also influenced by cardiac sensitivity to applied ACh (Löffelholz and Pappano, 1974*b*). Sensitivity of the sinoatrial pacemaker to ACh was consistently low between the

6th and 9th incubation days, increased significantly between the 9th and 11th incubation days, and remained consistently high between the 11th and 18th incubation days (Table 4). Accordingly, the increase in ACh sensitivity that occurred just prior to the onset of cholinergic neuroeffector transmission must be included as a factor involved in the onset of functional vagal innervation of the pacemaker. Reconstruction of the roles of pre- and postjunctional elements in the ontogenetic appearance of cholinergic neuroeffector transmission suggests the following pattern: (1) Both transmitter availability and postjunctional sensitivity were too low through the 9th incubation day to allow inhibition by field stimulation. (2) Physostigmine allowed neurally-mediated inhibition on the 10th incubation day because it preserved small amounts of released transmitter from hydrolysis and it sensitized postjunctional receptors to ACh. (3) The availability of transmitter for release delayed the appearance of neurally mediated inhibition until the 12th incubation day (absence of physostigmine) since postjunctional sensitivity to ACh was the same on the 11th and 12th incubation days. The inability of field stimulation to evoke inhibition on the 9th incubation day was probably not due to a lack of impulse propagation for the cervical vagus conducted action potentials at this time.

The increased sensitivity of the chick embryo heart to ACh just prior to functional cholinergic innervation was also associated with a marked change in the duration of inhibition by choline esters (Pappano and Skowronek, 1974). Pacemaker inhibition by ACh, carbamycholine (Carb), and acetyl-β-methylcholine (MCh) was sustained in hearts taken from animals after the 11th incubation day in contrast to the briefer duration of inhibition observed prior to this time (see Figure 3 for details of experiments with ACh). Sinoatrial

TABLE 4. ACh Sensitivity in Chick Sinoatrial
Preparations

Incubation age (days)	ED_{50} ($\times 10^{-7}$ M)
6 (3)[a]	16.0 ± 1.2
9 (3)	22.3 ± 0.8
10 (6)	6.2 ± 2.5[b]
11 (3)	4.1 ± 2.9[c]
18 (6)	2.1 ± 0.5[c]

[a] Number of experiments given in parentheses.
[b] $0.05 < P < 0.02$ when compared to ED_{50} (mean ± SEM) on 9th incubation day.
[c] $P < 0.01$ when compared to ED_{50} on 9th incubation day.

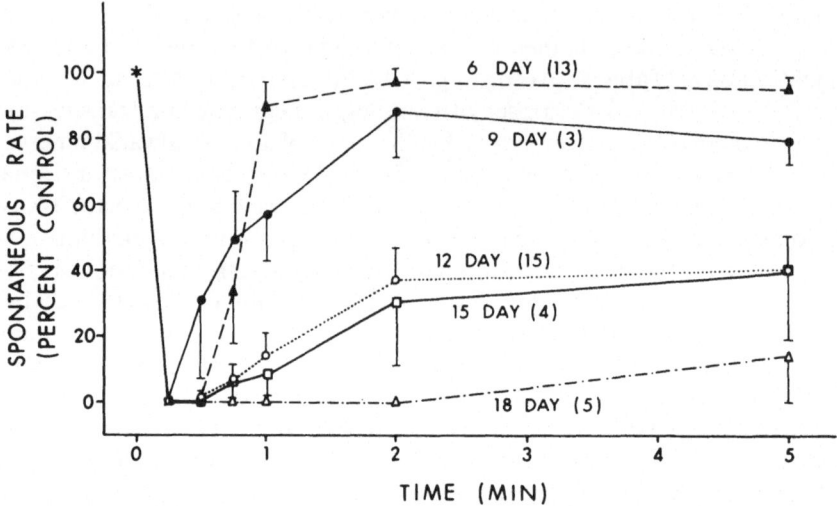

Figure 3. Duration of cardioinhibition by ACh (5.5 × 10⁻⁶ M) in sinoatrial pacemaker during ontogenesis. Ordinate: spontaneous impulse frequency of sinoatrial pacemaker as percent of control; abscissa; time in minutes. Symbols give mean ± SEM of measurements obtained from preparations isolated from chick embryos at incubation age specified. The number of preparations is given in parentheses.

impulse frequency returned to 85–90% of control values within 2 min after application of ACh on the 6th and 9th incubation days, whereas recovery ranged from 0–40% in preparations from the 12th, 15th, and 18th incubation days. These findings are consistent with the possibility that desensitization limited the duration of pacemaker inhibition in hearts from animals prior to functional cholinergic innervation. For example, a second application of drugs did not evoke inhibition at a time when the pacemaker had recovered from the inhibitory effects of a first application. Desensitization was most prominent with Carb for a conditioning application (5.1 × 10⁻⁶ M) completely prevented the effects of a 10-fold greater concentration. This pattern is comparable to that described at the neuromuscular junction (Nastuk *et al.*, 1966). Superfusion with drug-free saline for 10–20 min was needed to restore completely the inhibitory effects of choline esters. Hydrolysis by acetylcholinesterase was not involved in limiting drug action because physostigmine did not prolong the duration of inhibition, and the inhibitory effects of cholinesterase-resistant Carb were as brief as those of ACh on the 6th incubation day. In addition, drug-evoked release of catecholamines from cardiac stores (Lee *et al.*, 1960) in the chick embryo heart did not explain the brevity of inhibition. Propranolol, which blocked cardiac adrenergic receptors, did not prolong the duration of drug action. For these reasons, it can be concluded that the recovery of automaticity in the presence of drug resulted from desensitization of the receptor and/or ionophore so that the drug–receptor interaction was less capable of evoking the conductance change (increased K^+ conductance) responsible for cardioinhibition (see next section). The reduction of action potential duration by ACh, like the negative chronotropic effect, endured for a longer time in atrial cells from preparations older than the 11th incubation day. Recovery of contractions in the presence of ACh had been observed in 33–35-hr embryo hearts (Cullis and Lucas, 1936) and "adaptation" to the inhibitory effect of ACh was seen as late as the 10th incubation day (Dufour and Posternak, 1960). Moreover, physostigmine did not prolong the negative chronotropic effect of ACh nor did it restore the effects of a second application of the drug (Obrecht-Coutris and Coraboeuf, 1967). The fetal rat heart also displayed more persistent effects of ACh on rate and action potential duration on the 20th day than on the 16th day (Pager et al., 1965). These authors concluded that the increased sensitivity of the rat heart to ACh may be related to cholinergic innervation which occurs around the 16th day. Although there are no data available on the onset of cholinergic neuroeffector transmission in the fetal rat heart, this finding bears some similarity to that described in the chick embryo heart. The results obtained with fetal mouse hearts are similar to those described in the chick embryo (Wildenthal, 1973). Sensitivity of the fetal mouse heart to the negative chronotropic effects of ACh increased progressively from the 13th–14th gestational day through the 21st–22nd day (term). The response of the murine heart to ACh continued to increase after ingrowth of cholinergic nerves, an observation similar to that described by Pager et al. (1965) in the fetal rat heart. It would be of interest to know when cholinergic neuroeffector transmission began in the mouse and rat. The temporal relationships between responsiveness to cholinergic drugs, on the one hand, and morphologic and functional innervation by the vagus, on the other hand, would facilitate comparative studies of neural development and receptor mechanisms between the avian and mammalian animals commonly used for study.

The mechanism involved in desensitization to cholinergic agonists is not known. However, the desensitization is rather specific since it does not extend to the cardioinhibitory effects of K^+. Elevation of the external concentration of K^+ ($[K^+]_0$) to 20 mM produced a sustained (up to 1 hr) reduction of the pacemaker firing rate, presumably by increasing membrane conductance to K^+ (g_K). In the presence of elevated $[K^+]_0$, addition of ACh or Carb arrested pacemaker impulse generation for 1–2 min after which time the firing rate returned to the level established by $[K^+]_0$. The desensitization observed in the chick heart may be related to inactivation of the cholinergic receptor as proposed in the model obtained from the neuromuscular junction

(Rang and Ritter, 1970). However, it has been noted that desensitization at the neuromuscular junction may involve a change in the ionic conductances activated by the drug–receptor interaction (Waud, 1968; Magazanik and Vsykočil, 1970).

3. Ionic Determinants of Cholinergic Drug Action

The ionic determinants of the membrane actions of ACh in the chick embryo heart change during ontogenesis. An increase in g_K is responsible for the reduction in rate of slow diastolic depolarization and in atrial action potential duration caused by ACh (Pappano, 1972a). The ability of ACh to increase g_K may increase during development, since the reduction in action potential duration produced by the drug became greater as maturation occurred (see Table 5). This augmentation of the effects of ACh was paralleled by an increase in the sensitivity of atrial cells to K^+. The slope of the relationship between $[K^+]_0$ and the membrane potential (E_m) increased steadily during ontogenesis to attain a value on the 18th incubation day that is near the ideal value for a K-sensitive electrode (Table 5). Another indication that membrane sensitivity to $[K^+]_0$ increased during development was obtained independently from a study of the suppression of automaticity by K^+. Cardiac automaticity depends upon a time- and voltage-sensitive reduction in g_K (Trautwein, 1963; Vassalle, 1966; Noble and Tsien, 1968), and this can be inhibited by elevating $[K^+]_0$. Suppression of automaticity required $[K^+]_0$ of 20–30 mM on the 4th and 6th incubation days, 10–20 mM on the 12th incubation day, and 5–10 mM on the 18th incubation day. Qualitatively similar findings have been reported by Sperelakis and Shigenobu (1972). These investigators also found that membrane resistance of ventricular muscle decreased during ontogenesis, another indication that g_K increased with embryonic age in chick cardiac cells. Suppression of spontaneous contractions in isolated chick heart cells also required less K^+ when the cells were isolated from older hearts (DeHaan, 1970). Thus, the increased sensitivity of embryo heart cells to K^+ observed during development of the organ can be maintained in culture. Accordingly, the progressive increase in membrane g_K and in membrane sensitivity to K^+ per se, tends to support the view that the increase in the sensitivity of sinoatrial cells to cholinergic agonists may arise from ontogenetic changes in membrane conductance.

Additional evidence that the ionic mechanism of ACh action changed during development was obtained from a study of pacemaker cell activity during inhibition. In hearts from the 6th incubation day and afterward, ACh hyperpolarized the membrane. This effect, like the reduction in action potential duration, depended upon an increase in g_K that allowed the membrane potential to approach the potassium equilibrium potential (E_K). Prior to the

TABLE 5. Changes in Effects of ACH and $[K^+]_0$ on Membrane
Potentials of Chick Embryo Atria During Ontogenesis

Incubation age (days)	Change in action potential duration by ACh[a] (msec)	E_m vs. $[K^+]_0^a$ (mV/decade)
4	$+2 \pm 4 (8)^b$	$46 \pm 2 (3)^b$
6	$-15 \pm 3 (11)$	$50 \pm 2 (3)$
12	$-39 \pm 7 (5)$	$53 \pm 1 (3)$
18	$-62 \pm 9 (5)$	$59 \pm 1 (2)$

[a] Measurements given as mean $\pm$ SEM.
[b] Number of experiments given in parentheses.

6th incubation day, ACh did not hyperpolarize the membrane during pacemaker inhibition even though E_K was more negative than the maximum diastolic potential (MDP). This observation confirmed that made by others who had reported that ACh reduced the MDP in chick heart cells (Fingl et al., 1952; Coraboeuf et al., 1970a, b). Coraboeuf and his colleagues had also noted that ACh had no effect on atrial action potential duration in hearts from the 4th incubation day. Thus, ACh increased MDP on the 6th incubation day but decreased MDP on the 4th incubation day when arrest had occurred (Table 6). The apparent depolarizing effect of ACh in a pacemaker cell from the 4th incubation day is shown in Figure 4 taken from a preparation treated with TTX (which had no effect on the membrane actions of ACh). It will be noted that automaticity recovered more rapidly from the inhibitory effects of ACh than did the membrane potential, an observation consistent with separate actions of the drug. This hypothesis was supported by the finding that removal of Na^+ (Tris$^+$ replacement) not only prevented the decrease in membrane potential but also allowed for an increase (hyperpolarization) as shown in Figure 5. The reduction in MDP in the presence of Na^+ was attributed to an increase in g_{Na}, and the inhibition of pacemaker

TABLE 6. Effects of ACh on MDP[a] of Sinoatrial Pacemaker Cells

Incubation age (days)	MDP		Change in MDP by ACh[c]	P
	Control	+ACh[b]		
4 (6)[d]	-62 ± 2	-55 ± 3	-7 ± 1	<0.01
6 (4)	-66 ± 4	-76 ± 5	$+10 \pm 1$	<0.01

[a] MDP is maximum diastolic potential (mV $\pm$ SEM).
[b] 5.5×10^{-6} M ACh arrested all preparations.
[c] Positive sign indicates hyperpolarization; negative sign indicates depolarization.
[d] Number of cells given in parentheses.

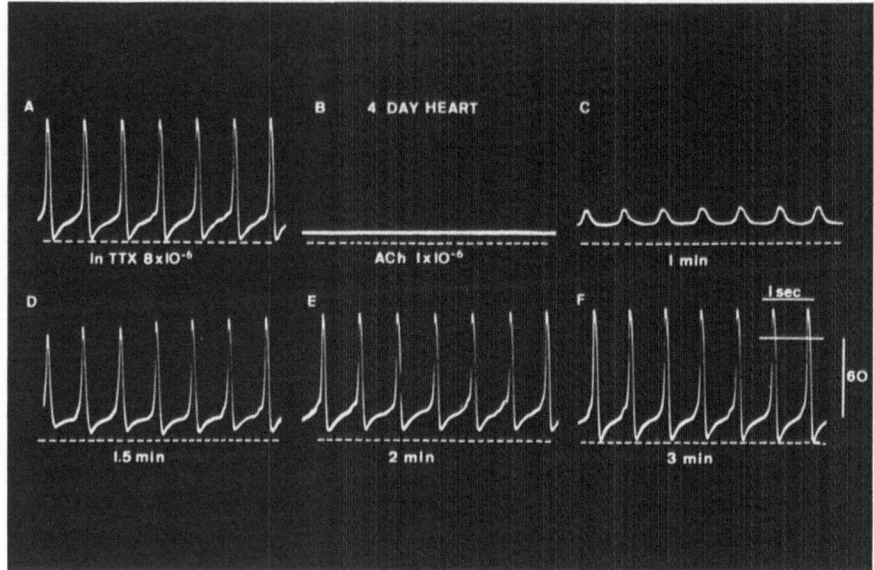

Figure 4. Membrane effect of ACh in pacemaker cell of heart isolated on the 4th incubation day.
The records are from a single impalement in a preparation treated with TTX (8×10^{-6} g/ml =
2.5×10^{-7} M). The discontinuous horizontal line in each record marks the maximum diastolic
potential before addition of ACh shown in the control record (A). ACh (1×10^{-6} g/ml =
5.5×10^{-6} M), given 15 sec before record B, arrested pacemaker potential generation (B)
that recovered within 1 min (C) and initiated action potentials within 1.5 min (D). Membrane
potential declined in ACh as shown in B and did not return to control values for 2–3 min (E–F).
TTX had no effect on membrane actions and pacemaker inhibition caused by ACh. Horizontal
line through action potentials in F marks zero potential; vertical calibration is 60 mV; calibrations apply to all records.

activity to an increase in g_K (Pappano, 1972a). In the absence of a readily
permeable substitute for Na^+, it would be anticipated that the increase in
g_K would dominate and permit ACh to hyperpolarize, The ability of ACh
to increase g_{Na} seemed to decline during ontogenesis, whereas its capacity to
increase g_K increased (see above). The possibility that neurally released ACh
increased g_{Na} as well as g_K had been advanced by Toda and West (1967), who
found that membrane hyperpolarization caused by vagal stimulation increased as $[Na^+]_0$ was reduced.

The decline in desensitization and the increase in sensitivity to cholinergic agonists (Table 4) during ontogenesis are particularly noteworthy
against the background of cholinergic innervation of the pacemaker. Before
functional innervation, the cholinergic receptor has a low sensitivity to ACh

and is rapidly desensitized. At and after cholinergic innervation, the cholinergic receptor has a high sensitivity to ACh and is slowly desensitized. The ontogenetic transition in the properties of the cholinergic receptor, a change associated with functional cholinergic innervation of the sinoatrial region, can be compared with the properties of the cholinergic receptor at the neuromuscular junction. The curare-sensitive receptor at the amphibian neuromuscular junction was differentiated into two types on the basis of morphologic and functional criteria (Feltz and Mallart, 1971a). Junctional

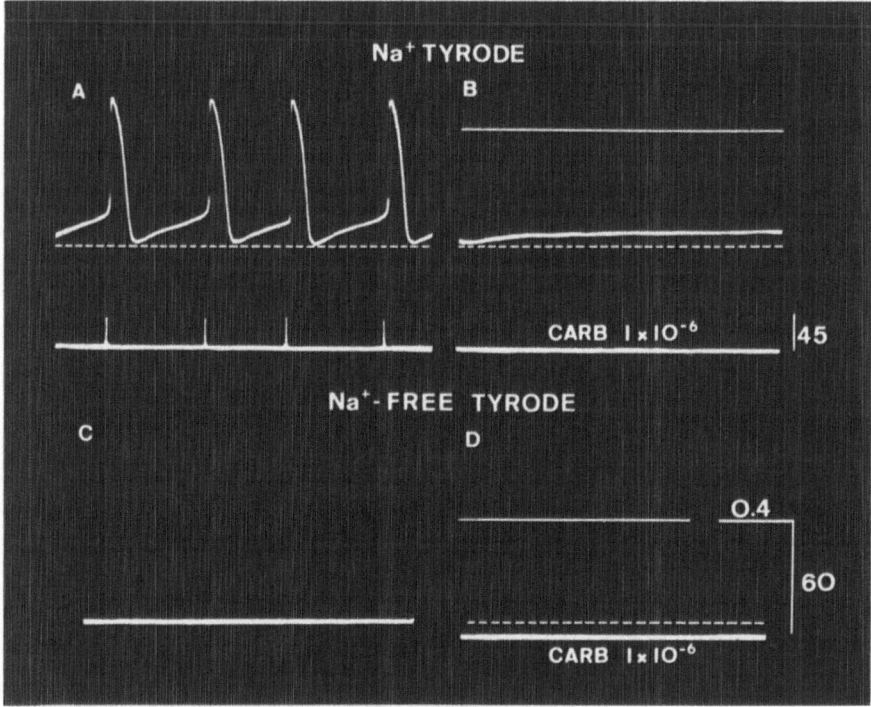

Figure 5. Reversal of Carb-induced depolarization by removal of external Na⁺. Records A and B were taken from a single impalement of sinoatrial cell in a preparation bathed in Tyrode solution containing normal Na⁺. A: Control showing spontaneous action potentials (uppermost trace), maximum diastolic potential level (discontinuous horizontal line), and maximum rate of rise ($+ \dot{V}_{max}$, lowermost trace). B: Carb (1×10^{-6} g/ml = 5.4×10^{-6}M) arrested pacemaker activity and depolarized membrane within 20 sec. Records C and D were taken from a single cell within 15 min after tris⁺ replaced Na⁺ in bathing medium. C: Control, spontaneous action potentials abolished in Na⁺-free saline. D: Carb (1×10^{-6} g/ml) hyperpolarized membrane within 20 sec after addition. Uppermost horizontal lines in B and D are zero potential. Calibrations for voltage (60 mV) and time (0.4 sec) apply to all records; $+ \dot{V}_{max}$ calibration is 45 V/sec. (From Pappano, 1972a; reproduced with permission of the *Journal of Pharmacology and Experimental Therapeutics.*)

receptors, located at the end-plate region, had a high sensitivity to applied ACh and depolarized rapidly when activated. Extrajunctional receptors, located at regions away from the end plate, had a low sensitivity to applied ACh and depolarized slowly when activated. Furthermore, the reversal potential was -16 mV at junctional receptors and -42 mV at extrajunctional receptors indicating a different degree of g_{Na}/g_K activation (Feltz and Mallart, 1971b). In chronically denervated preparations, the cholinergic receptor displayed the functional properties of the extrajunctional type, even at former junctional regions. It should also be noted that the action potentials in chick atria are susceptible to blockade by TTX on the 12th incubation day (functional innervation) but not on the sixth incubation day (Pappano, 1972b). Noninnervated skeletal muscle also is more resistant than innervated muscle to TTX (Harris and Marshall, 1973; see Section IV–D on tetrodotoxin). Interpretation of the observations regarding drug sensitivity and cholinergic innervation demands cautious appraisal. Although the findings in the embryo heart are suggestive, it has not been established that the changes in intensity and duration of cholinergic drug action are causally related to the onset of cholinergic neuroeffector transmission.

4. Heart Cells in Culture

The use of culture techniques has been suggested as a means to study drug effects on heart cells without the complications introduced by the presence of nerve cells (see Sperelakis, 1972a; Wildenthal, 1971b). However, the use of cell culture techniques has often been associated with a lack of responsiveness to ACh and to other drugs (Sperelakis, 1972a; Johnson and Lieberman, 1971). For example, neither ACh nor Carb had any effect on the resting and action potentials, pacemaker firing rate, and spontaneous contractions of chick ventricular cells in culture (Sperelakis and Lehmkuhl, 1965; Sperelakis and Pappano, 1969a). Cultured chick ventricular cells are depolarized by lipidsoluble noracetylcholine dodeciodide (Sperelakis and Pappano, 1969a). The Na-dependent depolarization produced by this lipid soluble ACh analog may not be related to activation of cholinergic receptors since the available evidence (see below) argues against their presence. Failure to observe effects of cholinergic agonists on cultured cells has been attributed to the fact that they are taken from ventricular tissues (Johnson and Lieberman, 1971). For example, trypsin-dissociated ventricular cell cultures were rarely sensitive to 10^{-4} g/ml ACh (Fänge et al., 1956) and 10^{-5} g/ml ACh (Nakanishi and Takeda, 1969), yet these concentrations of the drug reduced spontaneous impulse frequency, hyperpolarized the membrane, and reduced action potential duration in cultures of atrial cells. It has also been suggested that the earlier innervation by the vagus of atrial muscle allows atrial cells to become more sensitive to ACh than ventricular cells (Fänge *et al.*, 1956). The fact that ACh reduced the pulsation rate of isolated heart cells in culture may have been caused by the presence of atrial cells (Harary and Farley, 1960; Ertel *et al.*, 1971). It should be noted that chick ventricular muscle is innervated by cholinergic nerves (Bolton, 1967) and that activation of intracardiac branches of these nerves and addition of ACh evoked atropine-sensitive decrements in developed tension in ventricles isolated from 3-week-old chicks. Therefore, it may be an oversimplification to assume that the inability of ACh to effect contractile force and developed tension in chick ventricular cells in culture stemmed from a lack of innervation. Rather, it can be suggested that the cells may not yet have developed cholinergic receptors during life *in ovo* for there is general agreement that intact ventricular muscle cells from the chick do not respond to ACh before hatching (Pappano, 1972*a*; Sperelakis and Shigenobu, 1972). In addition to a lack of receptor development at the time of culturing, it also appears that the disaggregation procedure inactivates or removes drug receptors (see Section IV–B–4.) For example, atrial and ventricular cells (chick embryo and neonatal mouse) in culture displayed negative chronotropic reactions to ACh that could be reproduced up to 6 months after culture (Boder and Johnson, 1972). The maintenance of reactivity to drugs, including ACh, was attributed to the use of collagenase rather than trypsin as a cell-dispersing agent.

Wildenthal (1971*a*) has described conditions that promote survival of organ cultures of mouse heart. The negative chronotropic effects of ACh are maintained for some time in these preparations that are not subjected to enzymatic disaggregation procedure (Wildenthal, 1971*b*). Furthermore, hearts in organ culture have been considered to be free of functional adrenergic nerves (see Section IV–B–4). Experimental verification of functional innervation or the lack of it by cholinergic nerves in organ culture is lacking. Conceivably, organ culture procedures may provide a ready source of cardiac muscle cells with distinct pharmacologic receptors and lacking autonomic innervation.

B. Adrenergic Transmission and Adrenergic Drugs

Reactivity of the developing heart to sympathetic transmitter and to sympathomimetic drugs, like responsiveness to ACh and cogeners, has been studied by many investigators. Markowitz (1931) concluded that isolated chick embryo hearts did not respond to epinephrine (EPI) on the 2nd incubation day (4 positive results in 16 hearts). Thereafter, the number of hearts displaying positive chronotropic effects to EPI increased gradually (6/22— 3rd incubation day, $>50\%$—4th incubation day, $>60\%$—5th incubation day, 100%—6th incubation day). She concluded that the chick embryo heart on the 2nd incubation day lacked some intermediary substance (receptor) that allowed the organ to respond to EPI and also suggested that the intermediary substance was not a ganglion cell. Acceleration of the chick embryo heart by EPI (10^{-8}–10^{-7} g/ml) was detected as early as the 37th incubation hour by Hsu (1933) who, like Markowitz, posited that drug action was independent of nerve elements. It is generally agreed that the early appearance of responsiveness to EPI preceded sympathetic innervation of the chick embryo heart (Barry, 1950; Fingl *et al.*, 1952). Shideman's laboratory (McCarty *et al.*, 1960) first described the adrenergic cardiac receptor as belonging to the β type because dichloroisoproterenol (DCI) antagonized the increases in rate and displacement caused by EPI and norepinephrine (NE). The possibility that sympathetic innervation changed cardiac sensitivity to catecholamines was advanced by some and denied by others (see McCarty *et al.*, 1960). Furthermore, the onset of sympathetic innervation was equated with the morphologic ingrowth of sympathetic nerve elements.

1. Development of Adrenergic Neuroeffector Transmission

Recent experiments in our laboratory have shown that transmission between adrenergic nerves and sinoatrial pacemaker cells could be detected for the first time on the 21st incubation day, that is, the day of hatching (Pappano and Löffelholz, 1974). The ontogenetic appearance of propranolol-sensitive acceleration of the sinoatrial pacemaker is depicted in Figure 6. Acceleration evoked by 30-Hz stimulus trains was essentially the same on the day of hatching and one week later; the maximum effect observed on the 21st incubation day was the same in the presence and absence of atropine. Acceleration of pacemaker firing was evoked by field stimulation applied in the same manner used when studying the onset of cholinergic neuroeffector transmission. Because cholinergic transmission had begun on the 12th incubation day, field stimulation elicited a biphasic chronotropic effect in hearts taken from animals on the 21st incubation day and thereafter. This is illustrated in the records of Figure 7. Membrane hyperpolarization and a reduction in spontaneous impulse frequency occurred during the period of stimulation and for about 3–4 sec afterward. Pacemaker firing frequency then increased and exceeded the control values for up to 60 sec after stimulation with maximum acceleration occurring at 20–30 sec after the end of the stimulation period. Acceleration of pacemaker activity by field stimulation was associated with an increased rate of slow diastolic depolarization (Figure 7) as expected (see Trautwein, 1963). Attempts to detect neurally-mediated acceleration prior to the day of hatching were unsuccessful. Thus, pretreatment with atropine to prevent cardioinhibition that could mask acceleration was not accompanied by the appearance of any acceleratory effects of field

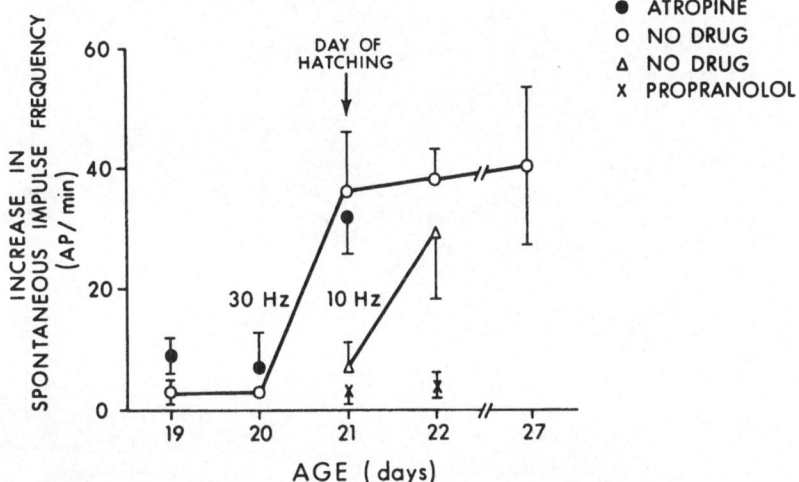

Figure 6. Ontogenetic appearance of propranolol-sensitive cardioaccelerator nerve transmission. Ordinate: increase in spontaneous impulse frequency of sinoatrial preparations; abscissa: incubation age of chick from which heart was isolated. The nonfilled circles and the triangles show the pacemaker response to impulse trains (30 V, 0.5 msec) of 30 Hz and 10 Hz, respectively, in untreated preparations. The responses to 30-Hz impulse trains in the presence of 3.4×10^{-6} M propranolol are given by the "x" and those evoked in the presence of 2.8×10^{-7} M atropine are given by the filled circles. The symbols are the mean $\pm$ SEM of 3–8 measurements. (From Pappano and Löffelholz, 1974; reproduced with the permission of the *Journal of Pharmacology and Experimental Therapeutics.*)

stimulation on the 18th through the 20th incubation days (see Figure 6). Bathing the preparations in EPI-containing saline solution did not reveal acceleration by field stimulation during or after exposure to the catecholamine.

The stimulus frequency range over which acceleration could be evoked (≥ 10–60 Hz) was more restricted than that observed with pacemaker inhibition caused by field stimulation (≥ 3–60 Hz). However, the optimal stimulus frequency needed to evoke inhibition and acceleration was the same, namely 30 Hz. Stimulation of extracardiac sympathetic nerves increased the rate of spontaneous impulse generation; this effect was blocked by propranolol but not by hexamethonium. These data suggest that the pattern of cardiac sympathetic innervation in the chicken is similar to that described in adult mammalian species. Accordingly, the chick heart is innervated by postganglionic sympathetic axons whose cell bodies are situated in extracardiac sympathetic ganglia, thoracic sympathetic ganglion number 1 (Tummons and Sturkie, 1968). In chickens, stimulation of cardiac sympathetic fibers elicited both inhibitory and accelerator effects (Tummons and Sturkie, 1970). In contrast, stimulation of cardiac sympathetic fibers to the heart in

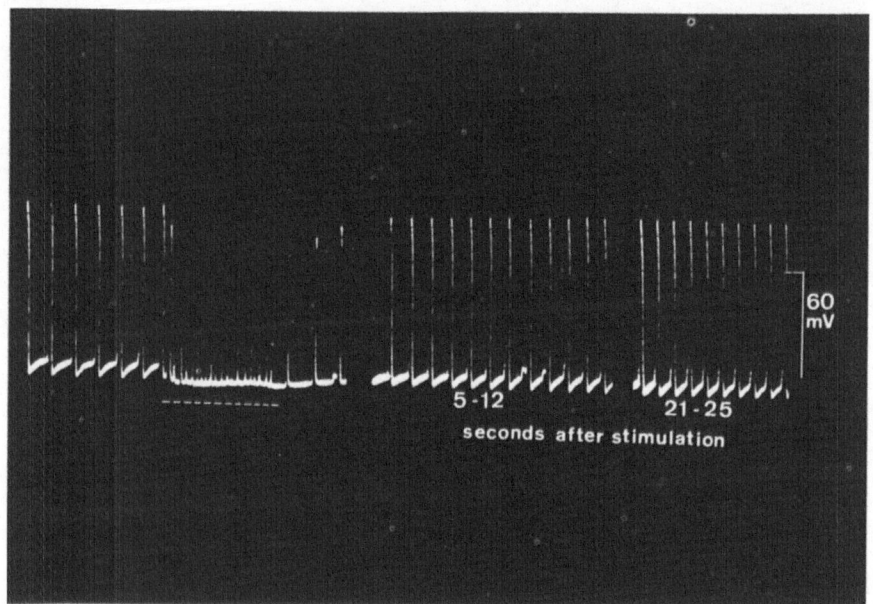

Figure 7. Cardioinhibitor and cardioaccelerator nerve transmission to sinoatrial pacemaker cell in preparation from the 21st incubation day (hatching). Field stimulation (30 V, 0.5 msec, 30 Hz) was applied to the sinoatrial region for 3 sec as indicated by discontinuous horizontal line. The membrane hyperpolarization and inhibition evoked during field stimulation (left-hand panel) dissipated within 5 sec after stimulation. Acceleration became evident during 5–12-sec period (middle panel) after the end of stimulation and reached a maximum during the 21–25-sec period (right-hand panel). The horizontal line in the right-hand panel marks zero potential.

chicks, 5–8 days after hatching, caused only acceleration (Pappano and Löffelholz, 1974). The reason for the discrepancy between our findings and those of Tummons and Sturkie is not known; perhaps it is related to ingrowth of inhibitory fibers within the sympathetic trunk during growth after hatching. It is not known when adrenergic neuroeffector transmission to ventricular cells appears in the chick heart. Bolton (1967) found that application of field stimuli to ventricular muscle of the 3-week-old chick evoked positive inotropic effects sensitive to blockade by β-adrenergic antagonists (DCI, pronetholol, and propranolol) and by adrenergic neuron blocking agents (bretylium, guanethidine, and guanochlor) but not by α-adrenergic antagonists. It is readily apparent that cholinergic transmission to heart cells preceded adrenergic transmission, a pattern that is rooted in phylogenesis as well (Burnstock, 1969).

It was previously noted that ingrowth of sympathetic nerve fibers to the heart occurred early in ontogenesis of the chick (see Section III–B). The appearance of functional cardioaccelerator innervation on the 21st incubation day may be a result of inadequate synthesis and/or release of adrenergic transmitter and to a low sensitivity to the adrenergic transmitter before the 21st incubation day.

The cardiac content of EPI and NE increased continuously from the 21st through the 28th incubation days (Ignarro and Shideman, 1968a; Manukhin et al., 1969). Since these increases occurred after fluorescent nerves were detected (Enemar et al., 1965), it seemed reasonable to assume that they reflected the development of synthetic and uptake capacity of adrenergic nerves for catecholamines as described in other tissues. For example, the capacity of the developing rat heart to accumulate [^{3}H]NE increased in parallel with increments in endogenous NE content, an index of adrenergic innervation (Iversen et al., 1965). However, it is difficult to relate development of adrenergic neurons to endogenous catecholamine content in the chick embryo heart because the content of catecholamines in the organ varies considerably during ontogenesis. Epinephrine content in the chick embryo heart was (in ng/mg protein): 1–2 on the 6th incubation day, 7–8 on the 10th incubation day, 1–2 on the 12th incubation day, about 33 on the 17th incubation day, and 5–6 on the 21st incubation day (Ignarro and Shideman, 1968a). Concomitantly, similar variations occurred in the NE content although the ratio of NE to EPI was >1 on the 10th, 12th, and 21st incubation days, and <1 on the 6th and 17th incubation days. The appearance of the catecholamines in high concentrations (10th and 17th incubation days) was not associated with adrenergic neuroeffector transmission and the variable ratio of NE/EPI does not allow a reasonable prediction of what the transmitter might be. It has been suggested that EPI may be the adrenergic transmitter in the chick heart since this substance comprised a large fraction of total catecholamine in the organ shortly after hatching (Callingham and Cass, 1966) and guanethidine depleted more EPI than NE from the heart. This hypothesis is not supported by the findings of Sturkie and Poorvin (1973), who found that large quantities of EPI were lost from the isolated, perfused adult cock heart in the absence of nerve stimulation whereas large amounts of NE were recovered from the perfusion fluid during accelerator nerve stimulation. The possibility that the adrenergic transmitter could change from EPI to NE during growth and development after hatching has not been explored.

Shideman's laboratory has also studied the ability of cocaine to prevent [^{3}H]NE uptake by the chick embryo heart, an effect attributed to blockade of active transport of the catecholamine by sympathetic nerves (Ignarro and Shideman, 1968b). It is possible that these findings are related to amine uptake capacity of adrenergic nerves at a time when the nerves do not release transmitter in response to electrical stimuli. Alternatively, catecholamine uptake may be associated with the activity of chromaffin cells at the early stage examined (5th–10th incubation day). Dail and Palmer (1973) concluded that catecholamine-containing cells in or near the human fetal heart (8–18 weeks) were probably chromaffin cells and not adrenergic neurons since fluorescent fibers were not detected. It is noteworthy that the fluorescent structures observed in the chick embryo heart did not have a fiber-like appearance until the 16th incubation day; prior to this time the fluorescent structures had a round appearance (Enemar *et al.*, 1965). In this context, it is helpful to consider the relationship between the appearance of fluorescent adrenergic fibers and of transmission in the mouse vas deferens (Furness *et al.*, 1970). Fluorescent nerve fibers were detected in the circular and longitudinal muscle layers at 5 and 9 days after birth, respectively. However, adrenergic neuroeffector transmission, signaled by evoked excitatory junction potentials, did not appear until the 18th postnatal day. It was concluded that the presence of fluorescent nerve fibers need not indicate that transmission will occur when these fibers are stimulated. The gap between morphologic and functional innervation was attributed to the amount of transmitter available for release.

2. Sensitivity to Catecholamines During Ontogenesis

Sensitivity of the chick heart to catecholamines and sympathomimetic substances is advantageously considered against the ontogenetic background described previously. Recent investigations of the adrenergic receptor showed that propranolol antagonized the positive chronotropic effect of isoproterenol (ISO) (Jaffee, 1972; Löffelholz and Pappano, 1974*b*) and of EPI (Löffelholz and Pappano, 1974*b*). These findings confirm the report of McCarty *et al.* (1960) who found the cardiac adrenergic receptor in the chick to be of the β-adrenergic variety. In addition, the early appearance of the adrenergic receptor described by Hsu, who used EPI, has been substantiated by Michal *et al.*, (1967) with NE (2nd incubation day) and by Jaffee (1972) with ISO (50th–55th incubation hour). Early detection of adrenergic responsiveness is not a unanimous observation, for Paff and Glander (1968) contend that the propranolol-sensitive adrenergic receptor did not function until the 4th incubation day. However, it is generally agreed that the adrenergic receptor is functional in the chick heart before the ingrowth of sympathetic nerves and before NE and EPI can be measured (4th incubation day; Ignarro and Shideman, 1968*a*).

Pacemaker sensitivity to EPI and NE has been studied during development (Löffelholz and Pappano, 1974*b*). Estimation of the ED_{50} from the concentration–effect relationships provided a reliable index of pacemaker reactivity to the catecholamines. The results of these experiments are given in Table 8. The sinoatrial pacemaker was more sensitive to ISO than to EPI at each time examined before and after hatching; this finding is consistent with the properties of a β-adrenergic receptor. Moreover, the pacemaker responded in a qualitatively similar fashion to both amines through the time of hatching. For example, sensitivity to EPI was unchanged between the 12th and 18th incubation days. A marked reduction in sensitivity to EPI and ISO occurred on the 19th and 20th incubation days; this was followed by an increase in sensitivity on the 21st incubation day to the values observed on the 18th incubation day. The increased sensitivity on the 21st incubation day coincided with the onset of adrenergic neuroeffector transmission (Löffelholz and Pappano, 1974b).

The parallel shifts in pacemaker reactivity to EPI and ISO could be viewed as indicating some participation of adrenergic neuroeffector transmission in resetting catecholamine sensitivity to high levels. Alternatively, it is possible that the shift in catecholamine sensitivity was related to the removal of a depressant mechanism associated with the terminal stages of ontogenesis. Avid uptake of EPI by the operation of an adrenergic nerve membrane transport system would not satisfactorily explain the reduction in pacemaker sensitivity just before hatching because the sensitivity to ISO, which is not transported by this system (Hertting, 1964), also decreased significantly at the same time. Development of an amine transport system in adrenergic nerves after hatching could explain the finding that sensitivity to EPI was apparently unchanged whereas that of ISO increased (Table 7). Girard (1973) reported that the sensitivity of the chick to the vasopressor

TABLE 7. Responsiveness of Sinoatrial Pacemaker to
Epinephrine and Isoproterenol

Incubation age (days)	Epinephrine ED_{50} ($\times$ 10^{-7} M)	P^a
12 (8)[b]	3.0 $\pm$ 0.6	<0.2
18 (4)	1.7 $\pm$ 0.4	—
19 (6)	15.0 $\pm$ 9.0	<0.3
20 (3)	42.7 $\pm$ 16.6	<0.05
21 (5)	2.6 $\pm$ 1.2	<0.6
28 (3)	3.4 $\pm$ 2.3	<0.5

Incubation age (days)	Isoproterenol ED_{50} ($\times$ 10^{-8} M)	P^a
18 (4)[b]	3.2 $\pm$ 0.5	—
19 (4)	9.6 $\pm$ 0.9	<0.01
20 (3)	10.4 $\pm$ 2.4	<0.02
21 (4)	3.2 $\pm$ 1.5	<0.9
28 (4)	0.5 $\pm$ 0.2	<0.01

[a] Compared to ED_{50} value obtained on 18th incubation day.
[b] Number of experiments.

effects of NE changed during ontogenesis, and the variations are similar to those observed with respect to the positive chronotropic effects of EPI and ISO. Thus, sensitivity of the chick to the pressor effects of NE increased progressively from the 7th through the 17th incubation days, decreased significantly on the 19th and 20th incubation days, and then increased after hatching to attain a sensitivity at 2 days after hatching that was equal to that observed at 3 months. The decline in adrenergic sensitivity on the two days prior to hatching was attributed to the respiratory acidosis that occurs at this time (Girard, 1973). The simultaneous involution of the chorioallantoic circulation and the appearance of thoracic respiratory movements (Romanoff, 1960) on the 18th incubation day are associated with reductions in O_2 consumption, O_2 tensions, and arteriovenous O_2 differences that are maximal on the 20th incubation day (Girard and Muffat-Joly, 1971). The marked increase in adrenergic sensitivity after hatching was referable to the elimination of hypercapnic acidosis and hypoxia (Girard, 1973). It has been shown that hypoxia reduced the sensitivity of isolated papillary muscle to NE (Kent et al., 1972) and that acidosis decreased the affinity of cardiac adrenergic receptors for ISO (Schümann et al., 1972). Because the chronotropic effects of EPI and ISO were studied on isolated preparations that were exposed to the same pH, temperature, and O_2 tension, the reduction in sinoatrial sensitivity to catecholamines could be the result of respiratory acidosis only if this disturbance in vivo produced a change in the heart that persisted in vitro. For example, the hypoxia and metabolic demands of the hatching process could evoke a marked increase in circulating catecholamines released from the adrenal medulla. Sun (1932) noted that the EPI content of chick adrenals decreased abruptly on the 17th and 18th incubation days and then returned to normal levels immediately after hatching. Assuming that the reduced adrenal content of EPI was owing to increased release of this substance into the circulation, it can be speculated that the subsensitivity of the cardiac adrenergic receptor (19th and 20th incubation days) was caused by intense exposure to catecholamines. The β-adrenergic receptor of rat pineal gland displayed an increased sensitivity to ISO in animals after chronic denervation (or reserpine treatment); this "supersensitivity" was manifested as a shift to the left of the concentration–effect relationship describing the increased levels of serotonin-N-acetyltransferase and cyclic AMP caused by ISO (Deguchi and Axelrod, 1973). Moreover, repeated administration of ISO to animals with denervated pineal glands (or reserpine treated) not only prevented the supersensitivity but also revealed a subsensitivity to ISO. Increased catecholamine levels in the circulation of the chick just before hatching, a reflection of sympathetic activity, could reduced the sensitivity of the cardiac adrenergic receptor. This speculative proposal would be materially assisted if catecholamine concentrations in the blood rose during late ontogenesis.

Increased catabolism of applied EPI and ISO may also be involved in the subsensitivity observed just before hatching for the activities of monoamine oxidase (MAO) and catechol-O-methyltransferase (COMT) reached maximum levels on the 19th incubation day and then decreased markedly within 1–2 days after hatching (Ignarro and Shideman, 1968c). The variations in adrenergic sensitivity just before and after hatching could be the result of increased catabolism, provided that extracellularly located COMT was active (this enzyme degrades EPI and ISO). Clearly, the changes in adrenergic receptor sensitivity during late ontogenesis and after hatching are consistent with several possible mechanisms. Although the mechanism remains unclear, the subsensitivity of the adrenergic receptor could interfere with detection of the onset of adrenergic neuroeffector transmission on the 19th and 20th incubation days.

Attention has also been given to the actions of catecholamines in the fetal rat heart. Wildenthal (1973) observed that the maximum positive chronotropic effects of NE increased in two stages during maturation. Norepinephrine produced a small but significant increase at 13–14 days, a greater increase at 15–16, 17–18, and 19–20 days, and a most pronounced increase in atrial rate at 21–22 days (term). A similar pattern of responsiveness was observed with ISO. Although the data suggested that atrial responsiveness in the fetal rat heart increased with age, it is not known whether sensitivity to NE follows the same pattern. It would be instructive to know the ED_{50} values for NE action, i.e., the concentration of NE required to produce a half-maximal effect. The fact that the maximum increase in rate produced by NE increased with age is not, by itself, a sufficient condition for assigning an increased sensitivity to the adrenergic receptor. For example, variations in control heart rate could obscure the fact that sensitivity is unchanged. Another aspect of adrenergic receptor reactivity in the fetal rat heart has been considered by Bernard and Gargouïl (1967). These investigators found that NE (10^{-5} g/ml), but not EPI (10^{-5} g/ml), had a positive chronotropic effect on the 13th day. This pattern was reversed on the 19th and 21st days with EPI but not NE, having a positive chronotropic effect. These observations have been interpreted as indicative of two configurations of β-adrenergic receptor sensitive to either NE or EPI but not to both (Bernard and Gargouïl, 1967). The possibility that reactivity to these catecholamines reversed because of a change in the configuration (? sensitivity) of the β-adrenergic receptor is intriguing, but experimental evidence obtained from concentration–effect relationships and the effect of antagonists is clearly necessary to substantiate this hypothesis.

3. Membrane Effects of Catecholamines: Ionic Mechanisms and Adenyl Cyclase

The ionic mechanism responsible for the positive chronotropic effect of the catecholamines in the embryonic heart is not known; it is not unreasonable to assume that it may be similar to that described in mammalian Purkinje fibers in which EPI shifted the activation curve of the pacemaker current (i_{K_2}) to less negative values of the membrane potential (Hauswirth et al., 1968). The positive inotropic effect appears to be related to an increased Ca^{2+} conductance (g_{Ca}) for the catecholamines restored action potentials and contractions to chick ventricular cells in the presence of TTX or depolarized by elevated $[K^+]_0$ (Shigenobu and Sperelakis, 1972). This mechanism of action is in agreement with the findings made previously in adult vertebrate hearts (Reuter, 1966; Vassort et al., 1969; Carmeliet and Vereecke, 1969; Pappano, 1970). Although Sr^{2+} could replace Ca^{2+} as a current carrier in the chick ventricle, the possibility that Na^+ current flowed through a slow conductance system could not be ruled out.

Cyclic 3',5'-adenosine monophosphate (cAMP), its dibutyryl derivative (dibutyryl cAMP), and the methylxanthines (caffeine and theophylline) restored action potentials to chick ventricular cells poisoned with TTX (Shigenobu and Sperelakis, 1972). Although the effects of these agents resembled those of EPI and ISO, no link between the catecholamines and the adenyl cyclase–cAMP has been substantiated. Isoproterenol (7×10^{-6} M) increased developed tension and cAMP levels of chick embryo hearts on the 7th–9th incubation days, but ISO had no effect on either force of contraction or on cyclic nucleotide levels on the 4th incubation day (Hollman and Green, 1973). In contrast to this pattern, cAMP levels did not increase up to 60 sec after addition of ISO in chick hearts isolated from animals 1–7 days after hatching, yet the catecholamine increased the force of contraction in hearts from this age group. In connection with these findings, it was also reported that the specific activity of cAMP (pM/mg protein) in untreated hearts was 60, 46, and 18 on the 4th incubation day, the 7th–9th incubation days, and 1–7 days after hatching, respectively. It appears that the positive inotropic effect of the catecholamines is not related directly to an increase in cAMP levels in the chick heart. Studies of human fetal heart yielded no evidence in support of a role for adenyl cyclase–cAMP in mediating the cellular actions of the catecholamines. Epinephrine (10^{-7} g/ml) had a positive inotropic effect in ventricular strips and a positive chronotropic effect in hearts taken from human fetuses in the 9th and 10th weeks of gestation (Gennser and Nilsson, 1970). Thus, the human embryo heart has an adrenergic receptor whose activation can initiate characteristic effects of the catecholamines on the rate and force of contractions as early as the 9th–10th week. Interestingly,

NE, EPI, and ISO ($10^{-6}-10^{-3}$ M) did not stimulate adenyl cyclase activity in broken cell preparations of human hearts (6–17 weeks gestation) although the adrenergic receptor is operative at this time (Dail and Palmer, 1973). The adenyl cyclase was capable of activation by fluoride at the 8th week; the specific activity of the enzyme decreased from the 8th to the 17th week. In the case of the human embryo heart, it can be argued that the β-adrenergic receptor and its link to the contractile proteins were present at a time (9–10 weeks) when the catecholamines did not activate adenyl cyclase. Rigorous demonstration that there is no relationship between catecholamine effects and adenyl cyclase stimulation in the human fetal heart would require confirmation that the preparative procedure did not destroy or inactivate the adrenergic receptor moiety. The experiments done on the chick heart were conducted in a manner that precluded the possibility of inactivation of the adrenergic receptor during preparation (Hollman and Green, 1973). Coltart *et al.* (1972) observed that adenyl cyclase activity in human fetal hearts increased between the 12th and 22nd weeks of gestation as did the positive inotropic effect of NE, but the relationship between NE and adenyl cyclase was not reported. The increase in adenyl cyclase during gestation observed by these investigators is contrary to the findings reported by Hollman and Green (chick) and by Dail and Palmer (human).

4. Heart Cells in Culture

The reactivity of heart cells in culture to catecholamines varies considerably. Positive chronotropic effects of EPI, ISO, and NE have been observed in cultured chick heart cells (Wollenberger, 1964; Krause *et al.*, 1970; Ertel *et al.*, 1971; Boder and Johnson, 1972). Insensitivity of cultured heart cells (chick) to EPI, ISO, and NE has been reported by several groups (Sperelakis and Lehmkuhl, 1965; Sperelakis and Pappano, 1969a; Kaufmann *et al.*, 1969). The different results obtained regarding the sensitivity of cells in culture to catecholamines suggest that the techniques used in the culture procedure may be responsible for the loss of reactivity to the catecholamines. Treatment with trypsin, which is used to separate cells, may cause inactivation or digestion of drug receptors (Kaufmann *et al.*, 1969). This view is supported by the findings of Boder and Johnson (1972), who reported that the use of collagenase provided cell cultures with responsiveness to a variety of drugs, including catecholamines. Unsatisfactory cell cultures obtained with collagenase treatment were attributed to high trypsin and clostridiopeptidase β levels in the crude collagenase samples (Boder and Johnson, 1972).

In those preparations that reacted to the catecholamines, the positive chronotropic effects of EPI, NE, and ISO were antagonized by DCI, pronetholol, and propranolol (Wollenberger, 1964; Ertel *et al.*, 1971; Boder and

Johnson, 1972). The role of cAMP in the mechanism of catecholamine action on cultured heart cells has been considered. Dibutyryl cAMP, but not cAMP, had a positive chronotropic effect on heart cell cultures from young rats 10^{-6} M threshold; Krause et al., 1970) and from 2–7-day-old mice (0.2–4 × 10^{-6} M; Boder and Johnson, 1972). Since the effects of dibutyryl cAMP were potentiated by caffeine (Krause et al., 1970) and were not blocked by propranolol (Boder and Johnson, 1972), it appears that the compound is acting in a fashion similar to that proposed for cAMP. However, no measurements have been made of cAMP levels in heart cell cultures displaying positive effects of the catecholamines, so it is not possible to answer whether the cyclic nucleotide may have mediated the actions of the drugs.

Chick heart cells in culture have been used to study the binding of [^{3}H]NE to the myoblasts (Lefkowitz et al., 1973). The binding of [^{3}H]NE to cultured myoblasts attained equilibrium in 30 min and 65–85% of the labeled compound could be displaced from the cells by unlabeled NE, ISO, EPI, and dopamine (5 × 10^{-6} M). Half-maximal inhibition of [^{3}H]NE binding required 40 μg/ml NE; this concentration produced about 50% of the maximum positive chronotropic effect in cultured heart cells (Ertel et al., 1971). These observations are viewed as consistent with the proposal that the bound [^{3}H]NE was associated with the β-adrenergic receptor, although this conclusion is not easily reconciled with the finding that 3 × 10^{-4} M propranolol displaced only 40% of [^{3}H]NE from the cells. Cautious interpretation of the relationship between binding properties and receptor identification has been expressed by Cuatrecasas et al. (1974). These investigators reported that binding of [^{3}H]NE to cells and microsomes represented an interaction of the catecholamine with a membrane-binding protein related to COMT. Furthermore, it was proposed the actual number of receptor binding sites may be very low and therefore not easily detected in the presence of an excess of nonspecific recognition sites for the catecholamines.

C. Nicotine and Tyramine

These agents will be considered together because they are thought to act indirectly in the heart. That is, nicotine and tyramine depend upon the presence of autonomic nerves from which they can release transmitters. It is well known that the mechanism by which nicotine effects transmitter release is different from that of tyramine. A comparison of the effects of these substances on cardiac activity can be helpful in determining the transmitter release capability of developing autonomic nerves.

Low doses of nicotine increased and high doses decreased the rate of spontaneous beating of chick embryo hearts at the 80th incubation hour (Pickering, 1893). The accelerating and decelerating effects of nicotine were attributed to an action on the myoplasm, since the heart was considered to be aneural at this time. More recently, Shideman's laboratory presented evidence that nicotine, as well as ACh and tetramethylammonium (TMA), had a biphasic effect on the rate and developed tension in hearts taken from chick embryos on the 4th incubation day (Lee *et al.*, 1960). Concentrations of nicotine $\geq 2 \times 10^{-5}$ g/ml increased and then decreased the rate of spontaneous beating; the deceleration was more pronounced at higher concentrations of the drug. Atropine prevented the inhibitory actions of nicotine on rate and developed tension and allowed the drug to evoke only positive effects on these parameters. Similar findings were made with ACh and TMA. Because the chick embryo heart was not innervated until the 5th incubation day, it was concluded that the stimulant effects of nicotine (as well as TMA and ACh) were the result of release of endogenous catecholamines from nonneural sites within the heart. Blockade of the stimulant effect of nicotine by reserpine and DCI supported the proposal that the effects are mediated through an action on adrenergic receptors. The ability of nicotine to increase developed tension in the atropinized heart was the same on the 4th and 9th incubation days, that is, before and after sympathetic nerves appeared in the myocardium. This observation is consistent with the possibility that nicotine-induced release of catecholamines may be independent of adrenergic nerves, even in the sympathetically innervated heart. As mentioned previously, neural stores of catecholamines may not appear until the 16th incubation day. The atropine-sensitive negative chronotropic action of nicotine on the 4th incubation day merited little attention, and the possibility of a direct action of nicotine was not considered.

Experiments have been conducted in our laboratory to determine the relationship between functional autonomic innervation of the sinoatrial pacemaker and the chronotropic effects of nicotine (Pappano, unpublished observations). In contrast to results obtained by Lee *et al.* (1960), nicotine ($\leq 10^{-4}$ M) had a negligible effect on spontaneous impulse frequency up to the 10th incubation day. After this time, nicotine (10^{-5} M) progressively reduced sinoatrial impulse frequency through the 13th incubation day (Table 8). The cardioinhibitory actions of nicotine appeared to develop in parallel with the pattern described for cholinergically mediated inhibition of the pacemaker. The earliest evidence for significant inhibition by nicotine was the 11th incubation day, about the time when the activity of choline acetyltransferase within the heart increased for the first time (Gifford *et al.*, 1973) and when atropine-sensitive cardioinhibition produced by field stimulation was observed in the presence of physostigmine (Pappano and Löffelholz, 1974). Maximum inhibition by nicotine occurred on the 12th–13th incubation days. It will be noted that on the 12th incubation day, the cholinergically mediated inhibition of the pacemaker was detected for the first time in the

TABLE 8. Effects of Nicotine on Sinoatrial Impulse Frequency during
Development

Incubation age (days)	Sinoatrial impulse frequency (fraction of control)[a]	
	10^{-5} M nicotine	10^{-5} M nicotine + 2.9×10^{-7} M atropine
6	0.96 ± 0.01 (4)[b]	—
7	0.92 ± 0.02 (4)[b]	—
9	0.85 ± 0.07 (4)[b]	1.00 ± 0.04 (4)
10	0.84 (2)	—
11	0.70 ± 0.12 (5)	—
12 (cholinergic transmission)	0.34 ± 0.12 (3)[c]	0.97 (2)
13	0.27 ± 0.15 (5)[c]	1.01 ± 0.05 (4)
17	0.56 ± 0.08 (3)[c]	—
19	0.83 ± 0.05 (4)[c]	0.95 ± 0.04 (4)
21–22 (adrenergic transmission)	0.45 ± 0.21 (4)[c]	0.93 (2)

[a] Measurements usually given as mean $\pm$ SEM with number of experiments shown in parentheses.
[b] $P > 0.1$ when compared to control rate before addition of nicotine to effect observed in presence of atropine.
[c] $P \leq 0.05$ when compared to control rate before addition of nicotine and to effect observed in presence of atropine.

absence of physostigmine. Nicotine did not evoke cardioinhibition in the presence of 2.9×10^{-7} M atropine (Table 8). In hexamethonium-treated $(3.2 \times 10^{-4}$ M) preparations from the 12th incubation day, nicotine $(10^{-5}$ M) reduced spontaneous impulse frequency to 0.84 ± 0.14 (3 experiments) of control values. This change was significantly less ($P < 0.05$) than the reduction produced by nicotine in the absence of hexamethonium on this day (Table 8). These observations suggest that the inhibitory effects of nicotine, like those caused by nerve stimulation, depended in large part upon the amount of ACh available for release from cholinergic nerves. The release mechanism involved activation of hexamethonium-sensitive (nicotinic) receptors on cholinergic nerves. The advantage of effecting transmitter release by chemical means is tempered by the observation that the inhibitory effects of nicotine $(10^{-5}$ M) decreased after the 13th incubation day, reached a minimum on the 19th incubation day, and then increased by the 21st–22nd incubation days (Table 8). The complex pattern of sinoatrial pacemaker reactivity to nicotine during the last week of the incubation period could be explained by a diminution in the inhibitory effects and/or an increase in the acceleratory effects of the compound. It is known that inhibition produced by field stimulation is as marked on the 19th and 21st incubation days as it is on the 12th incubation day (Pappano and Löffelholz, 1974). In addition, sinoatrial pacemaker sensitivity to ACh does not change between the 11th and 18th incubation days (see Table 4). However, it is possible that the amount of ACh released by nicotine decreases over the last week of ontogenesis in contrast to the apparently stable release caused by nerve stimulation. In addition, sensitivity to applied ACh may decrease just before hatching, as described for the catecholamines. It could be argued that nicotine released catecholamines that accelerate the heart and overcome the inhibitory effects of the drug, but this appears unlikely for the drug did not have a positive inotropic effect even in the presence of atropine (Table 8). It is particularly puzzling to note that nicotine did not evoke acceleration on the 21st–22nd incubation days when adrenergic neuroeffector transmission appeared. Resolution of this problem will be of considerable help in determining the development of function in cardiac autonomic nerves, as well as in understanding the mechanism of action of nicotine during ontogenesis.

Nicotine had no acute effect on the rate of spontaneous contractions or on the electrical properties of the membrane of chick heart cells in culture (Sperelakis and Pappano, 1969a; Ertel et al., 1971). The fact that catecholamines and ACh had direct chronotropic effects (Ertel et al., 1971) on the rate of spontaneous contractions strongly supports the contention that the effects of nicotine in the embryo heart, like those in adult vertebrate hearts, are the result of release of neurotransmitters. It should be noted that chronic effects of nicotine have been observed in rat heart cell cultures (Wenzel et al., 1970). Concentrations of nicotine greater than 3×10^{-6} M prolonged the time during which spontaneous contractions occurred in secondary cell cultures by 10 days. Although the ability to prolong beating activity was not increased by elevation of the nicotine concentration, the rate of spontaneous contractions did increase with concentration (Wenzel et al., 1970). Perhaps these chronic effects of nicotine are related to a direct action on cardiac muscle cells for neural elements are lacking in culture. Vacuole formation was especially prominent with higher concentrations of nicotine, and their appearance was taken as a sign of toxicity. An effect of nicotine on lactic dehydrogenase (LDH) was considered as a possible mechanism to allow longer beating periods in nicotine-treated cultures. This study illustrates the experimental possibilities inherent in use of cell cultures for the study of drugs under controlled environmental conditions for extended periods of time.

Tyramine, an indirectly acting sympathomimetic amine, has been used as a chemical means of evoking catecholamine release from adrenergic structures in adult animals. The release of NE from adrenergic nerves by tyramine differs in several respects from the mechanism utilized by the nerve impulse and by nicotine, the latter two stimuli apparently acting in a similar fashion. Accordingly, the use of tyramine provides an index of the availability of catecholamines for release from cardiac adrenergic stores.

Tyramine (2×10^{-6} g/ml) had a positive effect on the rate and force of contractions when applied to isolated chick atria after the 14th incubation day (Michal et al., 1967). Prior to this time, tyramine (1×10^{-6}–5×10^{-5} g/ml) had no stimulant effect on the atria; however, the drug reduced the rate and force of spontaneous contractions when given in high concentrations (1×10^{-5}–5×10^{-5} g/ml). Thus, the presence of large catecholamine stores prior to the 15th incubation day does not ensure that the catecholamines are available for release by an indirectly acting sympathomimetic amine (see Section IV–B). The cardiostimulant action of tyramine increased after its initial appearance; this effect was attributed to an increase in the catecholamine stores available for release (Michal et al., 1967). Experiments summarized in Table 9 (Pappano, unpublished observations) indicated that tyramine (2.9×10^{-5} M) had a modest positive chronotropic effect that was significant on the 19th incubation day but not on the 11th and 15th incubation days. These observations essentially agreed with those of Michal et al. (1967). A marked increment in the positive chronotropic action of tyramine appeared around the time of hatching. It had been mentioned that adrenergic neuroeffector transmission appeared for the first time in ontogenesis at the time of hatching and that the gap between morphologic and functional adrenergic innervation of the sinoatrial pacemaker was owing to insufficient amounts of transmitter available for release (see Section IV–B). In this connection, the finding that the positive chronotropic effect of tyramine increased significantly at the time of hatching suggests that release of adrenergic transmitter by tyramine, like that evoked by nerve stimulation, depended upon adequate amounts of transmitter available for release. Tyramine-induced acceleration also occurred before adrenergic transmission appeared as pointed out by Michal et al. (1967) and by the results obtained on the 19th incubation day (Table 9). Reserpine, an agent that depletes catecholamines from the chick heart (Lee et al., 1960), prevented the increments in rate and tension caused by tyramine but not those caused by NE (Michal et al., 1967). The dependence of tyramine on catecholamine stores within the heart is also supported by

TABLE 9. Effects of Tyramine on Impulse Frequency in Chick Sinoatrial Pacemaker

Incubation age (days)	Impulse frequency (AP/min)[a]		P
	Control	$+2.9 \times 10^{-5}$ M tyramine	
11	114.5 ± 5.9 (4)[b]	131.0 ± 7.6	<0.1
15	89.0 ± 9.3 (4)	111.0 ± 1.7	<0.1
19	96.4 ± 12.5 (7)	117.7 ± 13.1	<0.02
21–22	63.3 ± 5.9 (3)	138.0 ± 9.2	<0.01

[a] Impulse frequency given in action potentials/min (AP/min).
[b] Figures in parentheses refer to number of experiments.

the observation that significant cardiostimulation by the drug occurred around the time that fluorescent neuron-like structures appeared within the organ (Enemar et al., 1965). Assuming that the appearance of fluorescent nerves signalled the presence of stores of adrenergic transmitter available for release, it can be argued that the initial disposition of the catecholamines permitted their release by tyramine but not by electrical stimulation of the nerves. The possibility that tyramine released catecholamines from non-neural stores (e.g., chromaffin cells) before and after the onset of adrenergic transmission, as well as from adrenergic nerves, must also be considered.

The positive chronotropic effect of tyramine in the fetal mouse heart was attributed to an indirect action mediated by release of catecholamines from adrenergic neurons, since responsiveness to the drug did not appear until the 21st–22nd gestational day, about 6 days after sympathetic nerves appeared in the heart (Wildenthal, 1973). Support for the neural origin of catecholamines involved in the cardiostimulant actions of tyramine has been given by studies on heart cells in organ and cell cultures. Tyramine had no effect on the rate and displacement of spontaneous contractions in cultured heart cells from neonatal mice (Boder and Johnson, 1972) and from chick embryos (Ertel et al., 1971). Tyramine accelerated spontaneous contractions of fetal mouse hearts during the first two days after the organs were placed in culture but not after this time although the positive chronotropic effects of NE persisted for at least two weeks (Wildenthal, 1971b). The failure of tyramine to exert positive effects on the rate and force of contractions was attributed to the absence of adrenergic nerves in heart cell cultures.

Establishment of functional interrelationships among cardiac catecholamine stores, the developing adrenergic neuron, and the effects of chemical releasing agents like tyramine requires further exploration. Studies of the development of function in the adrenergic neuron and receptor ought to include the phenomenon of denervation supersensitivity (see review by Fleming et al., 1973). For example, how soon after the appearance of adrenergic transmission is it possible to induce denervation supersensitivity? Can the sensitivity of the adrenergic receptor be changed by reserpine-induced depletion of catecholamine stores before fluorescent nerves appear in the heart? Studies of the pharmacology of the developing heart have to consider the properties of cardiac nerves as well as those of muscle cells.

D. Tetrodotoxin

Tetrodotoxin (TTX) has been a very useful probe of membrane excitation mechanisms because its pharmacologic properties seem to be restricted to blockade of the early transient conductance (customarily g_{Na}) that allows inward current flow for action potential generation (Kao, 1966; Moore and

Narahashi, 1967; Hille, 1970). This compound has been particularly helpful in studying the ionic mechanisms of excitation in developing cardiac membranes during ontogenesis.

The initial studies of the action of TTX on excitation in developing cardiac cell membranes were done in ventricular cells of the chick (Ishima, 1968) and the rat (Bernard and Gargouïl, 1968, 1970). Tetrodotoxin (10^{-6} g/ml $\simeq 3.1 \times 10^{-6}$ M) reduced the amplitude and the maximum rate of rise ($+ \dot{V}_{max}$) but did not prevent excitation in any of the 50 ventricular preparations isolated from chicks before the 6th incubation day (Ishima, 1968). Thereafter, TTX prevented excitation in some preparations between the 6th and 10th incubation days and in all preparations on the 11th incubation day. Ishima suggested that the susceptibility of the action potential to blockade by TTX increased as the action potential became more dependent upon Na^+. Bernard and Gargouïl (1970) confirmed this finding in the fetal rat heart in which TTX (10^{-5} M) reduced the rapid rising phase of the action potential in ventricular preparations isolated from rats on the 13th and 20th days after fertilization but had no effect on action potentials on the 10th day. They proposed that action potentials in 10-day-old hearts depended upon an increased permeability of a slow channel (conductance for late inward current) system that was not sensitive to TTX but was sensitive to blockade by Mn^{2+}. The appearance of action potential blockade by TTX at the 13th day was attributed to the development of a rapid channel (conductance for early inward current) system that normally carried Na^+ (see Trautwein, 1973, for discussion of rapid and slow inward current systems). Like Ishima, Bernard and Gargouïl suggested that embryonic muscle cells have properties in common with pacemaker cells.

A description of the actions of TTX on ventricular cells during ontogenesis of the chick was provided by Shigenobu and Sperelakis (1971). It was reported that the action potentials recorded from chick hearts before the 5th incubation day were insensitive to TTX (2×10^{-5} g/ml). After the 8th incubation day, TTX ($1-4 \times 10^{-6}$ g/ml) rapidly reduced the $+ \dot{V}_{max}$ and overshoot (E_{ov}) of the action potential and blocked excitation. The toxin had either no effect or completely blocked excitation between the 5th and 8th incubation days; it was during this time that $+ \dot{V}_{max}$ increased from values less than 20 V/sec to more than 60 V/sec. Thus, action potentials with a low $+ \dot{V}_{max}$ were not affected by TTX, whereas those with a high $+ \dot{V}_{max}$ were depressed by the drug. Since the action potentials resistant to TTX (prior to 5th incubation day) were abolished by removal of Na^+ but unaffected by 1 mM La^{3+}, it was concluded that the TTX-insensitive conductance was of the "slow channel" type that carried Na^+ current but not Ca^{2+} current. The possibility that the lower resting E_m of ventricular cells inactivated the early conductance and thus prevented any sign of TTX action from being observed was unlikely; membrane hyperpolarization did not permit any evidence of an effect of TTX on $+\dot{V}_{max}$. Accordingly, it was concluded that chick ventricular cells did not have TTX receptors prior to the 5th incubation day (Shigenobu and Sperelakis, 1971). A marked increase in the ability of TTX to depress the percentage of beating hearts occurred between the 4th and 7th incubation days (McDonald *et al.*, 1972); this effect was also attributed to the appearance of receptors for TTX. It should be noted that measurement of $+\dot{V}_{max}$ is a more precise index of determining whether TTX receptors are present for contraction may be uncoupled from excitation and thereby give misleading results.

The evidence obtained from a study of chick atrial muscle showed that the susceptibility of the action potential to blockade by TTX increased during ontogenesis (Pappano, 1972*b*). Intracellularly recorded action potentials in atria from the 12th and 18th incubation days were blocked by 1.6×10^{-7} M TTX, whereas those recorded in cells from the 6th incubation day were not abolished, even in the presence of 10^{-5} M TTX. The records in Figure 8

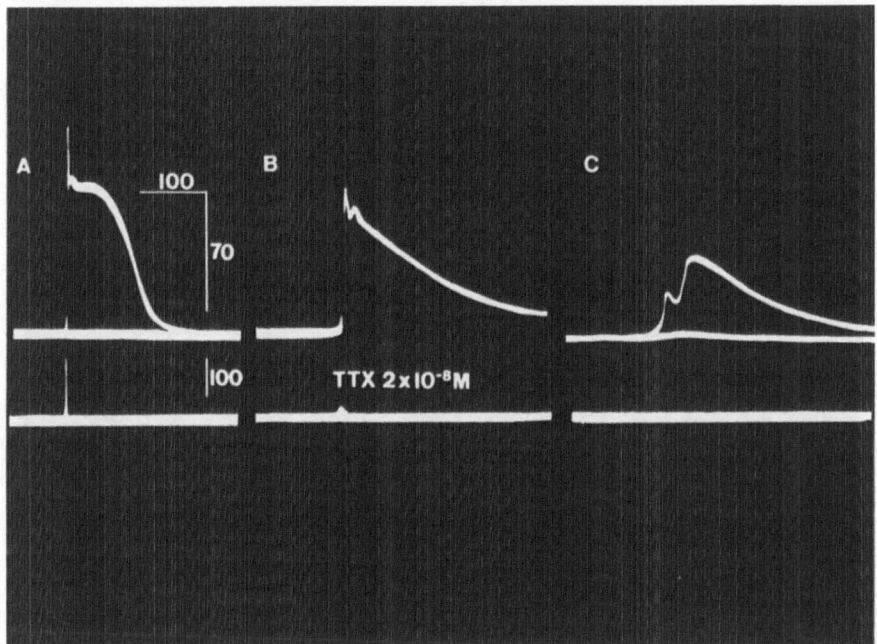

Figure 8. Blockade of excitation by TTX in atrial cell from heart isolated on the 19th incubation day. Calibrations for time (100 msec), voltage (70 mV), and $+\dot{V}_{max}$ (100 V/sec) apply to all records; the time calibration also serves as zero potential mark. A: Control, evoked (10 V, 0.5 msec) action potential recorded from cell in left sinoatrial valve had characteristic appearance of Purkinje fiber. B: Amplitude and $+\dot{V}_{max}$ of action potential reduced at 5 min after addition of 2×10^{-8} M TTX (used 20 V, 0.5-msec stimuli because TTX had reduced excitability). C: Blockade of excitation evoked by stimuli (150 V, 5 msec) at 20 min after TTX.

illustrate the characteristic action of TTX in a Purkinje-like cell from the left sinoatrial valve of a heart isolated on the 19th incubation day. It is noteworthy that both the E_{ov} and $+\dot{V}_{max}$ were diminished in parallel by TTX and complete blockade (Figure 8C) occurred within 20 min. Tetrodotoxin also markedly reduced $+\dot{V}_{max}$ in cells from the 6th incubation day. However, E_{ov} was only slightly reduced as shown in Figure 9, and action potentials persisted in the presence of 10^{-5} M TTX. The effects of TTX on the amplitude and $+\dot{V}_{max}$ of atrial cells on the 6th, 12th, and 18th incubation days are graphically depicted in Figure 10. The maximum rate of rise of atrial action potentials increased during ontogenesis, a finding also noted in ventricular muscle (Bernard and Gargouïl, 1970; Shigenobu and Sperelakis, 1971). The increase in $+\dot{V}_{max}$, an index of the early conductance, was not associated with an increase in resting E_m (at least in the age range examined) suggesting that voltage-dependent inactivation was not an important factor in preventing TTX from blocking the early conductance (see Table 10). In addition, the increase in absolute value of $+\dot{V}_{max}$ during ontogenesis suggested that the density of early (Na^+) conductance channels had also increased (alternatively,

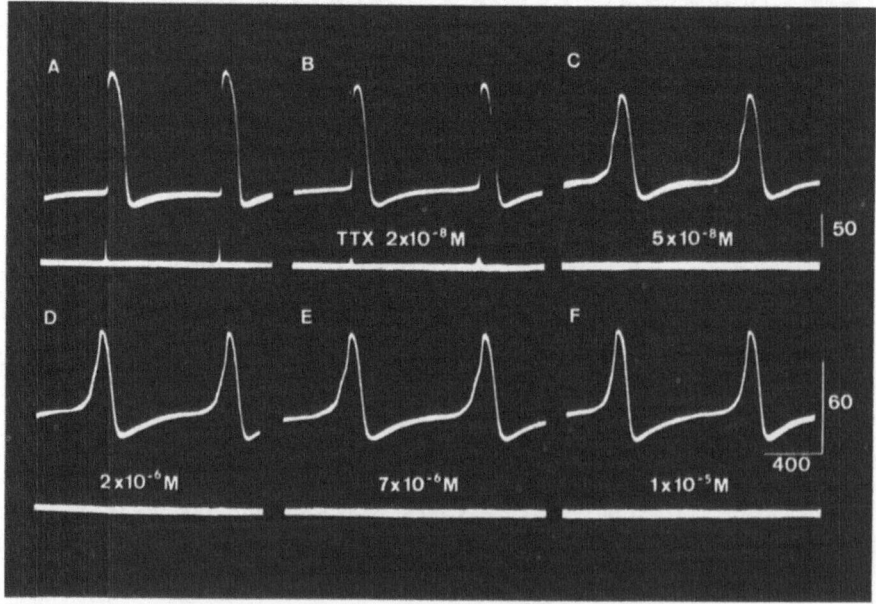

Figure 9. Effects of TTX on action potentials of an atrial cell in a heart isolated on the 6th incubation day. Calibrations are given as in Figure 8. All records are taken from a single cell. A, control; B, 10 min after addition of 2×10^{-8} M TTX; C, 7 min after 5×10^{-8} M TTX; D, 5 min after 2×10^{-6} M TTX; E, 10 min after 7×10^{-6} M TTX; F, 10 min after 1×10^{-5} M TTX. (From Pappano, 1972b; reproduced with permission of *Circulation Research*.)

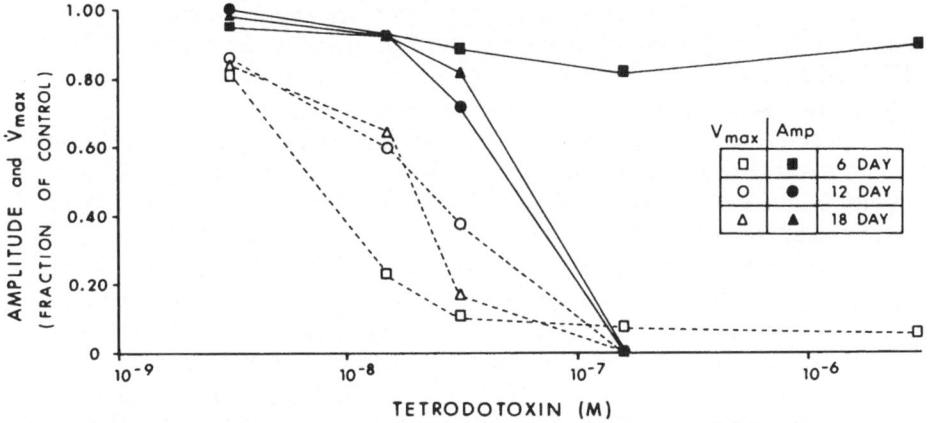

Figure 10. Summary of the effects of TTX on action potential in atrial cells of chick heart. Ordinate: amplitude (Amp) and maximum rate of rise ($+\dot{V}_{max}$) of action potentials in atrial cells from the 6th, 12th, and 18th incubation days. Abscissa: TTX concentration (molar). The symbols are the mean values of 15–30 impalements. (Modified from Pappano, 1972*b*.)

the conductance/channel could have increased to bring about the change observed), a conclusion also reached by Sperelakis and Shigenobu (1972). This proposal was consistent with the observation that the Na-electrode properties of E_{ov} increased in parallel with that found for $+\dot{V}_{max}$. When $[Na^+]_0$ changed by a factor of 10, E_{ov} varied about 10–20 mV for a 10-fold change in $[Na^+]_0$ in atrial cells from the 6th incubation day (when $[Na^+]_0$ ranged from 30–100 mM) and about 60 mV in cells from the 18th incubation day. The 60 mV/10-fold change in $[Na^+]_0$ indicated that the Na-electrode properties had increased considerably, in association with the increased $+\dot{V}_{max}$. Reductions in $[Na^+]_0$ produced proportional reductions in $+\dot{V}_{max}$ of the action potential on the 6th, 12th, and 18th incubation days. This datum showed that the early conductance was Na-dependent and also corresponded to the finding that TTX caused a proportional reduction in $+\dot{V}_{max}$ at each age

TABLE 10. Membrane Potentials in Chick Atria

Incubation age (days)	E_m (mV)	Amplitude (mV)	V_{max} (V/sec)
6 (60)[a]	−66 ± 1	89 ± 1	64 ± 3
12 (63)	−69 ± 1	90 ± 1	78 ± 2[b]
18 (55)	−67 ± 1	91 ± 1	94 ± 3[b]

[a] Number of impalements given in parentheses.
[b] $P < 0.01$ when compared to value in younger heart.

examined (Figure 10). The inability of TTX to block action potentials on the 6th incubation day was not owing to a lack of receptors for the toxin since TTX reduced $+\dot{V}_{max}$ to the same extent as it did in atria from older animals. The concentrations of TTX needed to reduce $+\dot{V}_{max}$ by 50% were 0.9 × 10^{-8} M and 2 × 10^{-8} M on the 6th and 18th days, respectively, an indication of comparable receptor sensitivity to TTX. As shown in Table 11, the sensitivity of chick atrial cells to TTX is about 0.1 of that observed in the frog node of Ranvier and in the squid giant axon. The failure of TTX to eliminate action potentials on the 6th incubation day was a result of the fact that action potential generation was effected by an increased membrane conductance to Ca^{2+} when the early g_{Na} component had been eliminated by the toxin. Overshoot potential depended upon $[Ca^{2+}]_0$ in atrial cells (6th incubation day) bathed in 3.1 × 10^{-6} M TTX as shown in Figure 11. An ideal Ca electrode would have a slope of 30 mV/10-fold change in $[Ca^{2+}]_0$. The relationship between E_{ov} and $[Ca^{2+}]_0$ (0.5–1.7 mM) had a slope of 24 mV/decade; action potentials were abolished when $[Ca^{2+}]_0$ was less than 0.45 mM. At $[Ca^{2+}]_0$ greater than 1.7 mM (Figure 11), the slope became less than 24 mV/decade, perhaps a result of the ability of Ca^{2+} to stabilize excitable membranes. Atrial membranes on the 6th incubation day displayed substantial Ca-electrode properties and thus were able to generate action potentials when TTX had blocked the early g_{Na} system. It appears that the g_{Ca} system involved in the generation of atrial action potentials is representative of a "slow channel" system (see Bernard and Gargouïl, 1970; Trautwein, 1973).

The results obtained in ventricular cells (Ishima, 1968) and in atrial cells (Pappano, 1972b) demonstrated that receptors for TTX are present in the very young heart in contrast to the conclusion reached by others (Sperelakis, 1972a; McDonald et al., 1972). Additional evidence has been obtained in support of the conclusion that TTX receptors appear early in ontogenesis. It has been shown that chick ventricular cell membranes possess TTX receptors as early as the 21–30 somite stage (50–60-hr incubation age; Renaud and LeDouarin, 1972). Tetrodotoxin (5 × 10^{-7} g/ml) depressed the rising

TABLE 11. Comparative Sensitivity of Excitable Membrane to TTX

Preparation	ID_{50} (M)[a]	Reference
Frog—node of Ranvier	1.2 × 10^{-9}	Hille (1970)
Squid giant axon	3.3 × 10^{-9}	Cuervo and Adelman (1970)
Chick atrial cell	0.9–2 × 10^{-8}	Pappano (1972b)

[a] ID_{50} is concentration of TTX that reduced g_{Na} of nerve membranes and $+\dot{V}_{max}$ of chick atrial cells (6th–18th incubation day) by 50%.

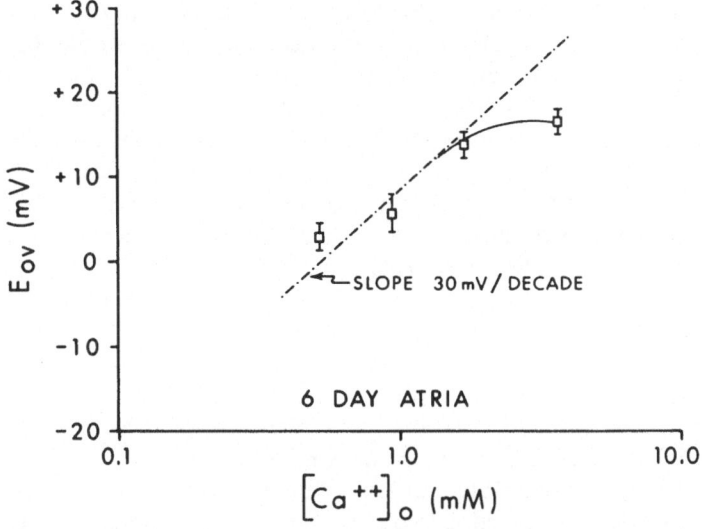

Figure 11. Dependence of action potential overshoot (E_{ov}) **on** $[Ca^{2+}]_0$ **in atrial cells from the 6th incubation day.** Ordinate: E_{ov} (mV); abscissa: $[Ca^{2+}]_0$. Each symbol is the mean ± SEM from 15–20 impalements. The preparations were bathed in Tyrode solution containing 3.1×10^{-6} M TTX. Ideal Ca-electrode properties are marked by the discontinuous line with a slope of 30 mV/10-fold change in $[Ca^{2+}]_0$. (Modified from Pappano, 1972b.)

phase of the action potential and reduced the amplitude by a few millivolts; however, action potentials persisted for at least 35 min. In the presence of 2 mM Mn^{2+}, action potential amplitude diminished very little while the duration was considerably reduced. Complete blockade of action potential generation (within 5 min) required simultaneous addition of TTX and Mn^{2+} at 50–60-hr incubation age. These findings were consistent with the proposal that an early conductance (Na dependent, TTX sensitive) and a late conductance (Na and Ca dependent, Mn sensitive) mechanism were present (see Bernard and Gargouïl, 1970). The conductance mechanisms are similar to those described in chick atria at the 6th incubation day with the exception of the Na dependence of the slow conductance (see above). At the 38–45 somite stage (3–3½-day incubation age) either TTX or Mn^{2+} was sufficient to abolish ventricular action potentials. It was proposed that the early, Na-dependent conductance had become essential for action potential generation at this time during development (Renaud and LeDouarin, 1972).

It is noteworthy that Mn^{2+}, an inhibitor of the slow conductance system, completely eliminated the action potential at a time when the early conductance was essential for initiation of regenerative membrane activity (Renaud and LeDouarin, 1972). The specificity of Mn^{2+} in its ability to inhibit only the slow conductance mechanism is questionable. For example, Mn^{2+} depressed the early inward current (Na dependent, TTX sensitive) in frog atrial fibers (Tarr, 1971). Studies in the chick heart also urged caution in interpreting the effects of Mn^{2+} on action potential components. The Ca-dependent action potentials produced by the catecholamines (see Section IV–B) were blocked by 1 mM Mn^{2+} or La^{3+} (Shigenobu and Sperelakis, 1972). At a concentration of 1 mM, these substances had little or no effect on $+ \dot{V}_{max}$, an index of the early g_{Na}. However, elevation of the concentration to 2 mM was associated with a marked reduction in amplitude, and it was concluded that the effects of this concentration were the result of a greater nonspecific depressant action. The fact that the apparent selectivity of Mn^{2+} and La^{3+} for the "slow channel" system disappears when the concentration is raised from 1 mM to 2 mM certainly warrants caution in use of these compounds as blocking agents of a specific membrane conductance.

Atrial preparations obtained from human embryos in the 7th to 9th week of gestation displayed a two-component action potential (spike and slow wave) when subjected to lower than normal temperature (Tuganowski and Tendera, 1973). The early (spike) component appeared to be Na^+ sensitive whereas the late (slow wave) was sensitive to both Na^+ and Ca^{2+}. No data are available regarding the effects of TTX on the early component; Mn^{2+} blocked both the spike and slow wave. Although the latter observation has been considered a reflection of a Ca^{2+} contribution to both components, it is also possible that blockade by Mn^{2+} is not specifically related either to divalent ion currents or to late currents.

The presence of a two-current mechanism for action potential generation in the embryo heart has also been considered in a study of desensitization to TTX (McDonald et al., 1973). Spontaneous contractions of cellular aggregates prepared from chick hearts isolated on the 4th to the 7th incubation days were depressed by TTX (10^{-5} g/ml). Continued exposure (3 hr) to the drug was associated with a marked recovery of spontaneous contractions in 50–80% of such aggregates from the 4th and 5th day but in less than 20% of those from the 6th and 7th day. Because the drug solutions were still pharmacologically active, the possibility was considered that desensitization arose from a change in cellular electrical activity. The only significant difference between spontaneously contracting control and TTX-treated aggregates was a lower $+ \dot{V}_{max}$ (< 20 V/sec) in the latter group. Moreover, the E_{ov} of the action potential increased 20–25 mV/10-fold change in $[Ca^{2+}]_0$ in cells of TTX-treated aggregates that were contracting spontaneously. This relationship is equivalent to that previously described in TTX-treated atrial cells from the 6th incubation day (Pappano, 1972b). Additional evidence that the resumption of spontaneous contractions in the presence of TTX was referable to the activity of a "slow channel" mechanism was obtained with Mn^{2+} (0.5 mM) and D-600 (1×10^{-6} g/ml), a derivative of verapamil that is alleged to block the late inward current in cardiac muscle (Kohlhardt et al., 1972). Both substances abolished spontaneous contractions that had recovered in TTX; no measurements were made of cellular electrical activity. These measurements would be of assistance in determining the specificity of these compounds in the developing heart; presently available evidence is not very convincing (see above). Desensitization to TTX was prevented if the aggregates were exposed to cycloheximide (5×10^{-6} g/ml) for 4 hr prior to addition of TTX. Accordingly, desensitization was viewed as a process that depended upon protein synthesis. It is not clear how inhibition of protein synthesis by cycloheximide prevented desensitization by TTX. For example, amino acid incorporation into the acid-insoluble fraction of 4-day aggregates was inhibited by 86% at 15 min after addition of cycloheximide. However, prevention of TTX-induced desensitization was observed only after 4 hr exposure to cycloheximide. The possibility that a pool of protein must be exhausted before the effects of cycloheximide became manifest was not verified by study of protein turnover rate. Furthermore, it is not known if cycloheximide has a direct blocking effect on the slow current that has no relationship to inhibition of protein synthesis. The interesting effect of cycloheximide requires additional experimentation to resolve the mechanism involved in the inhibition of TTX-induced desensitization.

The relationship between drug sensitivity and protein synthesis has also been examined in skeletal muscle. The effects of denervation (spread of ACh receptor loci and appearance of TTX-resistant action potentials) have been related to the elimination of a neurotrophic influence on muscle metabolism (Grampp et al., 1972). Since inhibitors of protein synthesis (cycloheximide, chloramphenicol, actinomycin D) prevented the appearance of the effects of denervation, it was suggested that a neurotrophic influence regulated muscle cell metabolism and the reactivity to ACh and TTX. Removal of the neurotrophic influence ultimately caused a change in the pattern of protein synthesis that was sensitive to the inhibitors. As mentioned previously, the sensitivity of the embryo heart to ACh and TTX bore a relationship to functional cholinergic innervation (see Section IV–A). Whether this relationship is causal or coincidental could be determined with experiments done on hearts deprived of functional innervation. In this connection, consideration ought to be given to the possibility that innervation may provide a trophic influence that is effected through protein synthesis. The aforementioned comments regarding careful scrutiny of results obtained with inhibitors of protein synthesis would obviously apply to these experiments.

Cultured heart cells obtained from chick embryo ventricles were found to be insensitive to TTX: the drug had no effect on E_m, E_{ov}, $+\dot{V}_{max}$, and rate of spontaneous contractions, even when the cells were bathed in high concentrations for days (Sperelakis and Lehmkuhl, 1965). The inability of TTX to block excitation does not mean that generation of the action potential is unrelated to g_{Na}, for the E_{ov} of the action potential in cultured heart cells varied about 60 mV/10-fold change in $[Na^+]_0$ over the $[Na^+]_0$ range of 30–100 mM (Pappano and Sperelakis, 1969b). These data suggested that the electrically excitable membrane of chick ventricular cells in culture lacked TTX-sensitive receptors capable of blocking a regenerative increase in g_{Na}. Although the electrically excitable membrane lacked TTX receptors, the toxin exerted a specific pharmacological effect on the chemosensitive membrane. Tetrodotoxin prevented the Na-dependent depolarization of cultured ventricular cells caused by veratrine and veratridine (Sperelakis and Pappano, 1969b). The inward conductance system for action potential generation in cultured heart cells had the characteristics of the "slow channel" described previously. For example, the divalent cations Ba^{2+}, Sr^{2+}, and Ca^{2+} initiated action potentials in cell cultures bathed in a Na-free medium (isotonic replacement of Na^+ by sucrose, choline, and Li^+). Furthermore, Li^+ did not replace Na^+ in allowing action potentials, in contrast to the results obtained in peripheral nerve and skeletal muscle. Uterine smooth muscle cells also are unable to utilize Li^+ as a current carrier to replace Na^+ during spike electrogenesis and have action potentials dependent upon $[Na^+]_0$ over a range of $[Na^+]_0$ similar to that observed in cultured heart cells (Marshall, 1963). It has recently been suggested that the lack of a rapid or early g_{Na} system in cultured heart cells, obtained from chick hearts that display such a system when not cultured, represents a reversion to conditions of an earlier embryonic age (Sperelakis and Shigenobu, 1972). That is, the rapid g_{Na} system may be replaced by a slow g_{Na} system when heart cells are dispersed in cultures. Whether this phenomenon is the result of altered metabolic activity known to occur in cultured cells or a result of treatment with trypsin is unresolved. Others who have used trypsin as a cellular dispersing agent have confirmed that TTX had no effect on the rate of spontaneous contractions even when the cells were obtained directly from tissues that reacted to TTX before being placed in culture (McDonald et al. 1972).

E.   Digitalis Glycosides

Early interest in the actions of the digitalis glycosides on the embryo heart had often centered on toxic effects, particularly the capacity to produce disturbances of cardiac rhythm. Pickering (1893) reported that strophanthin and digitalin usually reduced the rate and increased the vigor of spontaneous contractions in the chick embryo heart (70–85-hr incubation age). The reduction in heart rate was usually associated with a bradyarrhythmia that terminated in cardiac standstill. The similarity between the effects of digitalis glycosides in the chick embryo heart and in the frog heart prompted Pickering to conclude that these drugs were acting directly on cardiac muscle. These observations were amplified in the work of Paff, who reported that isolated chick hearts (48-hr incubation age) responded to ouabain with an initial acceleration followed by varying degrees of atrioventricular (AV) dissociation and terminating in arrest (Paff and Johnson, 1938). Atrial contractions ceased after ventricular contractions; moreover, it was noted that the ability of ouabain to cause AV dissociation occurred in hearts that had not yet developed specialized conduction pathways between atria and ventricles (see Lieberman, 1970). Lower concentrations of ouabain produced cardiac slowing and arrest without AV block. The toxic effects of digitalis could be overcome by removing the drug; reversal of cardiac standstill was especially rapid when calcium chelating agents (hexametaphosphate, citrate, oxalate) were present in the saline solution (Paff, 1940). The effects of digitoxin on atrial and ventricular membrane potentials were first studied by Fingl et al. (1952). Digitoxin produced changes in the electrical properties of atrial and ventricular cells that were essentially the same on the 3rd and 7th incubation day. At low concentrations the drug increased action potential duration by slowing the terminal stages of repolarization. At high concentrations it decreased action potential duration and also reduced the amplitude of the action potential; no change in the resting potential occurred.

1.   Ion Transport and $Na^+ + K^+$-Dependent ATPase

More recently, attention has been given to the ability of the digitalis glycosides to alter transmembrane fluxes of Na^+ and K^+ and to inhibit the $Na^+ + K^+$-dependent, Mg^{2+}-activated ATPase associated with cation transport. Klein and Evans (1961) found that 10^{-4} M ouabain reduced the transfer coefficient for Na^+ efflux by 42% in isolated ventricular preparations taken from animals on the 12th–13th incubation day and at 3 days after hatching. The rate coefficients for K^+ influx were similarly reduced by 27%, 26%, and 37% on the 7th and 12th incubation days and 3 days after hatching, respectively. Further study suggested that the $Na^+ + K^+$-dependent, Mg^{2+}-activated ATPase, associated with the microsomal fraction of cardiac muscle cells, may be induced between the 4th and 7th incubation days (Klein, 1963b). It is noteworthy that significant inhibition of this ATPase by ouabain $(10^{-4}$ M) occurred in preparations from the 7th and 12th, but not from the

4th incubation day. Although no quantitative results were given, it was reported that ouabain had a positive inotropic effect at $10^{-7}-10^{-6}$ M; these concentrations of the glycoside were without inhibitory effects on the Na^+ + K^+-dependent, Mg^{2+}-activated ATPase (Klein and Evans, 1961). The fact that ouabain had a positive inotropic effect in the chick heart (4th incubation day) was noted by McCarty *et al.* (1960). It is noteworthy that the positive effect of the glycoside on cardiac contractions occurred in the presence of DCI which blocks adrenergic receptors.

Additional support for the finding that ATPase inhibition was related to a reduction in active transport of Na^+ and K^+ came from the experiments of McDonald and DeHaan (1973). Ventricular muscle, taken from animals on the 8th incubation day, gained 37.1 mM Na^+ and lost 30.9 mM K^+ when bathed for 1 hr in salt solution containing 10^{-4} M ouabain. At 10^{-5} M, ouabain had no significant effect on the $[Na^+]_i$ and $[K^+]_i$ of ventricular muscle cells. The report of McDonald and DeHaan also corroborates the need for using high concentrations of ouabain to inhibit ion movements. The properties of the enzyme have been described by Sperelakis in a systematic study of the ontogenetic development of the Na^+ + K^+-dependent, Mg^{2+}-activated ATPase. Optimal activation of the Mg-dependent enzyme required 50 mM Na^+ and 8 mM K^+ with 3 mM Mg^{2+} present (Sperelakis and Lee, 1971). Furthermore, half-maximal inhibition of Na^+, K-ATPase activity occurred at 2.7×10^{-6} M ouabain and maximal inhibition required 5×10^{-4} M ouabain. The concentration required for half-maximal inhibition in the chick embryo heart is within the range of concentrations ($10^{-7}-10^{-6}$ M) generally observed to cause half-maximal inhibition in adult vertebrate hearts (Lee and Klaus, 1971). The transport ATPase was not appreciably activated by Li^+, in accordance with the inability of Li^+ to be extruded by the Na pump. However, inhibition of the Na^+ + K^+-dependent, Mg^{2+}-activated ATPase in chick embryo heart cells was not appreciably opposed by elevation of $[K^+]_0$ to 24 mM (Sperelakis and Lee, 1971), in contrast to the findings made in adult hearts (Lee and Klaus, 1971). Using the enzyme prepared with the NaI method, Sperelakis (1972b) reported that the specific activity of the ouabain-sensitive, Na^+, K-ATPase increased during ontogenesis. With the specific activity set at 100% on the 16th incubation day, 43% was observed on the 6th day, 73% on the 13th day, 140% on the 20th day, and 96% in the adult. These observations extend those of Klein (1963b) and demonstrate a large fraction of Na^+, K-ATPase inhibition by ouabain, perhaps owing to a more satisfactory preparation of the enzyme with NaI. Although the increased specific activity of the Na^+, K-ATPase can be attributed to an increased density of enzyme molecules (or active sites per molecule), it is also possible that the ontogenetic increase in specific activity was caused by changes in the ionic requirements for optimal activity of the enzyme.

2. Heart Cells in Culture

Trypsin-dispersed cells from chick embryos displayed marked sensitivity to the digitalis glycosides. Concentrations as low as 10^{-9} M increased the rate of pulsation of spontaneously contracting cells and appeared to increase the force of contractions (Wollenberger, 1964). In addition, digitalis allowed quiescent cells to develop spontaneous contractions. Similar observations have been made on rat heart cells in culture (Harary and Slater, 1965). Arrhythmic contractions, associated with an abrupt increase in pulsation frequency, developed when concentrations greater than 10^{-7} M were used (Wollenberger, 1964). The arrhythmogenic action of digitalis glycosides on heart cells in culture (15–48 hr) was also described by Mercer and Dower (1966) who reported that the percentage of cells contracting arrhythmically increased in the presence of digoxin. Atrial cells appeared to be slightly more sensitive than ventricular cells; a marked increase in the percentage of arrhythmically contracting atrial cells required 1×10^{-6} g/ml digoxin as compared to 2×10^{-6} g/ml in ventricular cells.

Ouabain (1×10^{-6}–1.5×10^{-3} M) depolarized and eventually abolished automaticity (15–30 min) and excitability (60 min) in cultured chick heart cells (Sperelakis and Lehmkuhl, 1968). The reduction in the membrane potential produced by ouabain is consistent with its ability to inhibit Na^+ + K^+-dependent, Mg^{2+}-activated ATPase in such cells (Sperelakis and Lee, 1971). The effects of ouabain on cation content, ATP, and cellular membrane potentials have been compared in neonatal rat heart cells in culture (Cheneval et al., 1972). Typical effects of the glycoside (10 μM/ml) included a reduction in cellular K^+ content by 20% and an increase in Na^+ content of 50% within 15 min. The resting membrane potential (E_m) declined by 20 mV from the control value of -80 mV in accordance with the reduction in E_K. No data are given regarding the effects of ouabain on action potential overshoot which would be expected to decrease as the resting E_m declined and as the driving force for Na ($E_{Na} - E_m$) diminished. Metabolic inhibitors (oligomycin, 2-deoxy-D-glucose) increased cellular Na^+ content and reduced the overshoot (E_{ov}) but did not change K^+ content or the resting E_m. The fact that E_{ov} decreased by more than 20 mV in the presence of oligomycin or 2-deoxy-D-glucose is consistent with a reduction in inward Na^+ current caused by a reduction in the driving force ($E_{Na} - E_m$) for Na^+ (Hyde et al., 1972). It was also noted that cellular ATP content was unchanged by ouabain at a time when marked shifts had occurred in ion contents (Cheneval et al., 1972); this observation is in keeping with the view that the action of ouabain on ion transport was referable to inhibition of transport ATPase. Ouabain (10^{-4} M) increased $[Na^+]_i$ by 36 mM and reduced $[K^+]_i$ by 39 mM in cultured chick heart cells (McDonald and DeHaan, 1973); this concentration of ouabain inhibited transport ATPase by more than 90% (Sperelakis and Lee, 1971).

There are two features that emerge from these studies that bear consideration. First, the effects of ouabain on ion content were not detected at 10^{-5} M, even though half-maximal inhibition of the transport ATPase occurred at 2.7×10^{-6} M (Sperelakis and Lee, 1971). Perhaps nearly complete inhibition of the enzyme is required to produce a significant disturbance of Na^+ and K^+ transport. Alternatively, the contribution of active ion pumping to cellular homeostasis may not be very significant at the time studied (cells isolated from hearts on 8th incubation day; McDonald and DeHaan, 1973); the specific activity of the enzyme reached 100% of adult values at the 16th incubation day (Sperelakis, 1972b). Second, the effects of trypsin on the ion concentration of dispersed heart cells suggest that membrane transport is affected by enzyme treatment since the cells gained Na^+ and lost K^+ (McDonald and DeHaan, 1973). Although there was some recovery, $[Na^+]_i$ continued to remain higher in cultured cells than in intact ventricular tissue, whereas $[K^+]_i$ was about equal in cultured cells and intact tissue. [Estimates of $[K^+]_i$ from electrophysiological measurements in cultured cells gave an average of about 95 mM (Pappano and Sperelakis, 1969a) as compared to the total $[K^+]_i$ of about 142 mM obtained by McDonald and DeHaan (1973). Since the estimated $[K^+]_i$ from these electrophysiological measurements is an index of the concentration of free K^+ within the cell water (activity), an activity coefficient of 0.67 can be calculated from these data. The activity coefficient of 0.1 molal KCl is 0.77 at 25°C (Robinson and Stokes, 1959). Thus, the fraction of K^+ in the myoplasm that is able to participate in physicochemical reactions is about the same as that observed in water.]

Digitalis glycoside-induced changes in developed tension have been measured in cultured heart cells obtained from neonatal rats (Okarma et al., 1972). Digoxin ($ED_{50} = 3 \times 10^{-9}$ M) and dihydrodigoxin ($ED_{50} = 5 \times 10^{-8}$ M) increased the mechanical displacement of single cells (monitored by photoelectric recording of cell images) in a concentration-dependent manner. The glycosides also increased the rate of spontaneous contractions. The role of the positive chronotropic effect in increasing the displacement of muscle cells was discounted because the glycosides were able to increase cell displacement without changing rate when bathed in a salt solution containing 8 mM $[K^+]_o$. Binding of digoxin and dihydrodigoxin to albumin did not interfere with the time to produce maximal effects on displacement (30–60 sec) but did prevent cellular uptake of the glycosides. These findings suggested that the positive inotropic action of the digitalis glycosides was caused by activation of a receptor at the cell surface. It was also concluded that the inotropic action of these compounds may be related to inhibition of $Na^+ + K^+$-dependent, Mg^{2+}-activated ATPase, although the concentrations of the glycosides required to inhibit enzyme activity were 200–700 times greater than those needed to produce 50% of maximum "inotropic" effect (Okarma *et al.*, 1972). This comparison is somewhat limited because the "inotropic" effects were measured in cultured heart cells and the enzyme inhibition was assayed in subcellular fractions of cells derived from intact hearts. In addition, the findings are not easily related to the results of others because the rat heart is relatively insensitive to the inotropic action and ATPase inhibition caused by the glycosides (Repke *et al.*, 1965). Wildenthal (1971b) found that ouabain (10^{-8}–10^{-6} M) had no effect on the rate of spontaneous contractions of fetal mouse hearts in organ culture. Arrhythmias appeared when a high concentration (10^{-4} M) of the glycoside was present for at least several hours. In addition, the survival time was reduced by at least two days when 10^{-4} M ouabain was added to the culture medium. It seems reasonable to conclude that the toxic effects of the digitalis glycosides in cultured heart cells are related to inhibition of transport ATPase, a mechanism consistent with conclusions reached in studies of adult hearts (Lee and Klaus, 1971). However, the possible relationship between transport ATPase inhibition and the positive inotropic effect of digitalis has not been resolved either in the embryonic heart or in the adult heart (Lee and Klaus, 1971).

V. SUMMARY

Cellular reactivity to drugs is ultimately determined by a chemical reaction between the drug and a receptor that is linked to an effector mechanism. This basic scheme is subjected to considerable variation in the embryo heart in which pharmacologic effects are dependent upon the development of both the receptor and effector mechanism. Cardiac innervation, changes in membrane ionic conductance, hormone levels, and concentration and distribution of ions represent some of the naturally imposed factors that can modulate the drug–receptor–effector interaction. The reactivity of the developing heart to a few selected drugs has been viewed in terms of this background.

1. Functional innervation of the sinoatrial pacemaker in the chick embryo heart occurred in two distinct stages: cholinergic neuroeffector transmission appeared on the 12th incubation day and adrenergic neuroeffector transmission appeared on the 21st incubation day. The gap between morphologic ingrowth of autonomic nerves and the onset of transmission was related to a prejunctional factor (amount of transmitter available for release) and a postjunctional factor (transmitter sensitivity).

2. The chick heart displayed an increased sensitivity to ACh around the time of functional cholinergic innervation. Desensitization by ACh and other atropine-sensitive cholinomimetics diminished at the onset of cholinergic neuroeffector transmission. Ontogenetic changes in the membrane effects of

ACh were determined, at least in part, by an increase in specificity of the ionic conductance (g_K) activated by ACh and an increase in K-electrode properties. The existence of a causal relationship between functional innervation and ACh sensitivity remains speculative.

3. The sensitivity of the chick heart to EPI and ISO increased at the onset of adrenergic neuroeffector transmission. The role of cardiac innervation, per se, in this phenomenon is open to question. The subsensitivity of the adrenergic receptor seen just before hatching could be the result of a persistent change in the adrenergic receptor caused by the marked hypoxia of terminal ontogenesis or an increased enzymatic degradation of exogenously applied catecholamines.

4. The ontogenetic appearance of cardioinhibition by nicotine (11th–12th incubation day) and of marked cardioacceleration by tyramine (21st–22nd incubation day) corresponded rather well with the onset of cholinergic and adrenergic neuroeffector transmission, respectively. These findings are consistent with the view that the gap between morphological and functional innervation depends, to a large extent, upon the amount of transmitter available for release. The failure of nicotine to accelerate the pacemaker, at a time when adrenergic neuroeffector transmission appears, cannot be reconciled with existing information.

5. Sensitivity of atrial cells to the depressant action of TTX on g_{Na} did not change during ontogenesis. The increased susceptibility of action potentials to blockade by TTX was owing to an increased contribution of g_{Na} to the regenerative change in membrane potential associated with excitation. As with ACh, the actions of TTX were modified by a change in membrane ionic conductance, specifically related to an increase of the density of g_{Na} sites during maturation. Calcium-dependent action potentials maintained excitation in young hearts when TTX had eliminated the Na-dependent early conductance. Catecholamines can activate g_{Ca} and restore action potentials to older hearts when g_{Na} has been eliminated by TTX or elevated $[K^+]_0$.

6. The digitalis glycosides increased developed tension and produced several types of arrhythmias before and at the time that autonomic nerves appeared in the chick heart. Available evidence strongly supports a causal relationship between transport ATPase activity and ionic balance in embryo heart cells. Inhibition of $Na^+ + K^+$-dependent ATPase by ouabain was associated with an increase in cell Na^+ and a decrease in cell K^+. The resting potential predictably decreased. The possibility that the positive inotropic effect of the glycosides is related to inhibition of transport ATPase has been considered, but there is no strong evidence to support this hypothesis.

7. Cell and organ culture methods have been used to maintain heart cells for extended periods of time *in vitro*. Such procedures have been especially useful in providing cardiac preparations devoid of functional nerves. It

should be noted that the pharmacology of the digitalis glycosides, as determined in trypsin-dispersed heart cell cultures, corresponded very well with the observations in intact heart tissues. The lack of complicating cellular elements, such as nerves, certainly commends the use of cell culture as a system for studying the mechanism of drug action. There has not been uniform success in preparing cell cultures sensitive to some of the other drugs mentioned in this report. It has been suggested that trypsin may be partially responsible for the insensitivity of heart cells to some drugs and that the use of collagenase can obviate this problem. This possibility deserves serious consideration. Pharmacological studies of cardiac cells can benefit considerably from the availability of nerve-free heart cell cultures sensitive to drugs, since these preparations lend themselves readily to environmental manipulations that can be strictly regulated.

ACKNOWLEDGMENTS

The studies conducted in the author's laboratory were supported by Grant HL-13339 from the U.S. Public Health Service and by a grant from the American Medical Association Education and Research Foundation. Dr. Konrad Löffelholz collaborated in a portion of the work, and Carol Skowronek provided skillful assistance.

REFERENCES

Abel, W., 1912, Further observations on the development of the sympathetic nervous system in the chick, *J. Anat. Physiol.* **47**:35.

Barry, A., 1950, The effect of epinephrine on the myocardium of the embryonic chick, *Circulation* **1**:1362.

Bernard, C., and Gargouïl, Y.-M., 1967, Etude électrophysiologique de la sensibilité aux catécholamines du cœur de Rat lors de la croissance embryonnaire, *C.R. Soc. Biol.* **161**:2600.

Bernard, C., and Gargouïl, Y.-M., 1968, Les perméabilités de la membrane myocardique embryonnaire de Rat; étude de leurs évolutions au cours de l'embryogénèse a l'aide d'inhibiteurs: tétrodotoxine, manganèse, tétraéthylammonium, *C.R. Acad. Sci. (Paris)* **267**:1626.

Bernard, C., and Gargouïl, Y.-M., 1970, Acquisitions successives, chez l'embryon de Rat, des perméabilités spécifiques de la membrane myocardique, *C.R. Acad. Sci. (Paris)* **270**:1495.

Blinks, J., 1966, Field stimulation as a means of effecting the graded release of autonomic transmitters in isolated heart muscle, *J. Pharmacol. Exp. Ther.* **151**:221.

Boder, G. B., and Johnson, I. S., 1972, Comparative effects of some cardioactive agents on automaticity of cultured heart cells, *J. Mol. Cell. Cardiol.* **4**:453.

Boder, G. B., Harley, R. J., and Johnson, I. S., 1971, A recording system for monitoring automaticity of heart cells in culture, *Nature* **231**:531.

Bogue, J. Y., 1932, The heart rate of the developing chick, *J. Exp. Biol.* **9**:351.

Bolton, T. B., 1967, Intramural nerves in the ventricular myocardium of the domestic fowl and other animals, *Br. J. Pharmacol.* **31**:253.

Burnstock, G., 1969, Evolution of the autonomic innervation of visceral and cardiovascular systems in vertebrates, *Pharmacol. Rev.* **21**:247.

Callingham, B. A., and Cass, R., 1966, Catecholamines in the chick, in *Physiology of the Domestic Fowl* (C. Horton-Smith and E. C. Amoroso, eds.), pp. 279–285, Oliver and Boyd, London.

Carmeliet, E., and Vereecke, J., 1969, Adrenaline and the plateau phase of the cardiac action potential, *Pfluegers Arch. Gesamte Physiol. Menschen Tiere* **313**:300.

Cheneval, J.-P., Hyde, A., Blondel, B., and Girardier, L., 1972, Heart cells in culture: Metabolism, action potential and transmembrane ionic movements, *J. Physiol. (Paris)* **64**:413.

Coltart, D. J., Davies, G. M., Gillibrand, I. M., and Hamer, J., 1972, Adenyl cyclase activity in the developing human foetal heart, *J. Physiol. (London)* **225**:38P.

Coraboeuf, E., Obrecht-Coutris, G., and LeDouarin, G., 1970a, Acetylcholine and the embryonic heart, *Am. J. Cardiol.* **25**:285.

Coraboeuf, E., LeDouarin, G., and Obrecht-Coutris, G., 1970b, Release of acetylcholine by chick embryo heart before innervation, *J. Physiol. (London)* **206**:383.

Couch, J. R., West, T. C., and Hoff, H. E., 1969, Development of the action potential of the prenatal rat heart, *Circ. Res.* **24**:19.

Cuatrecasas, P., Tell, G. P. E., Sica, V., Parikh, I., and Chang, K.-J., 1974, Noradrenaline binding and the search for catecholamine receptors, *Nature* **247**:92.

Cuervo, L. A., and Adelman, W. J., Jr., 1970, Equilibrium and kinetic properties of the interaction between tetrodotoxin and the excitable membrane of the squid giant axon, *J. Gen. Physiol.* **55**:309.

Cullis, W. C., and Lucas, C. L. T., 1936, Action of acetylcholine on the aneural chick heart, *J. Physiol. (London)* **86**:53P.

Dail, W. G., Jr., and Palmer, G. C., 1973, Localization and correlation of catecholamine-containing cells with adenyl cyclase and phosphodiesterase activities in the human fetal heart, *Anat. Rec.* **177**:265.

Deguchi, T., and Axelrod, J., 1973, Supersensitivity and subsensitivity of the β-adrenergic receptor in pineal gland regulated by catecholamine transmitter, *Proc. Natl. Acad. Sci.* **70**:2411.

DeHaan, R. L., 1967, Introduction: Spontaneous activity of cultured heart cells, in *Factors Influencing Myocardial Contractility* (R. D. Tanz, F. Kavaler, and J. Roberts, eds.), pp. 217–243, Academic Press, New York.

DeHaan, R. L., 1970, The potassium-sensitivity of isolated embryonic heart cells increases with development, *Dev. Biol.* **23**:226.

Dufour, J. J., and Posternak, J. M., 1960, Effects chronotropes de l'acétylcholine sur le cœur de l'embryon du poulet, *Helv. Physiol. Acta* **18**:563.

Enemar, A., Falck, B., and Håkanson, R., 1965, Observations on the appearance of norepinephrine in the sympathetic nervous system of the chick embryo, *Dev. Biol.* **11**:268.

Ertel, R. J., Clarke, D. E., Chao, J. C., and Franke, F. R., 1971, Autonomic receptor mechanisms in embryonic chick myocardial cell cultures, *J. Pharmacol. Exp. Ther.* **178**:73.

Faber, J. J., 1968, Mechanical function of the septating embryonic heart, *Am. J. Physiol.* **214**:475.

Fänge, R., Persson, H., and Thesleff, S., 1956, Electrophysiologic and pharmacological observations on trypsin-disintegrated embryonic chick hearts cultured *in vitro*, *Acta Physiol. Scand.* **38**:173.

Feltz, A., and Mallart, A., 1971a, An analysis of acetylcholine responses of junctional and extrajunctional receptors of frog muscle fibres, *J. Physiol. (London)* **218**:85.

Feltz, A., and Mallart, A., 1971b, Ionic permeability changes induced by some cholinergic agonists on normal and denervated frog muscles, *J. Physiol. (London)* **218**:101.

Fingl, E., Woodbury, L. A., and Hecht, H. H., 1952, Effects of innervation and drugs upon direct membrane potentials of embryonic chick myocardium, *J. Pharmacol. Exp. Ther.* **104**:103.

Fleming, W. W., McPhillips, J. J., and Westfall, D. P., 1973, Postjunctional supersensitivity and subsensitivity of excitable tissues to drugs, *Ergeb. Physiol.* **68**:55.

Friedman, W. F., 1972, The intrinsic physiologic properties of the developing heart, *Prog. Cardiovasc. Dis.* **15**:87.

Furness, J. B., McLean, J. R., and Burnstock, G., 1970, Distribution of adrenergic nerves and changes in neuromuscular transmission in the mouse vas deferens during postnatal development, *Dev. Biol.* **21**:491.

Gennser, G., and Nilsson, E., 1970, Response to adrenaline, acetylcholine and change of contraction frequency in early human foetal hearts, *Experientia* **26**:1105

Gifford, P., Ouyang, G., Franke, F. R., Clarke, D. E., and Ertel, R. J., 1973, Choline acetyltransferase (CAT) in hearts of developing embryos, *Pharmacologist* **15**:198.

Girard, H., 1973, Adrenergic sensitivity of circulation in the chick embryo, *Am. J. Physiol.* **224**:461.

Girard, H., and Muffat-Joly, M., 1971, Evolution de la pression partielle d'oxygene et du pH sanguins chez l'embryon de Poulet au cours de la croissance, *Pfluegers Arch.* **328**:21.

Grampp, W., Harris, J. B., and Thesleff, S., 1972, Inhibition of denervation changes in skeletal muscle by blockers of protein synthesis, *J. Physiol.* **221**:743.

Gyevai, A., 1969, Comparative histochemical investigations concerning prenatal and postnatal cholinesterase activity in the heart of chickens and rats, *Acta Biol. Acad. Sci. Hung.* **20**:253.

Harary, I., and Farley, B., 1960, *In vitro* studies of single isolated beating heart cells, *Science* **131**:1674.

Harary, I., and Slater, E. C., 1965, Studies *in vitro* on single beating heart cells: VIII. The effect of oligomycin, dinitriphenol, and ouabain on the beating rate, *Biochim. Biophys. Acta* **99**:227.

Harris, J. B., and Marshall, M. W., 1973, Tetrodotoxin-resistant action potentials in newborn rat muscle, *Nature (London), New Biol.* **243**:191.

Harsch, M., and Green, J. W., 1963, Electrolyte analysis of chick embryonic fluids and heart tissues, *J. Cell. Comp. Physiol.* **62**:319.

Hauswirth, O., Noble, D., and Tsien, R. W., 1968, Adrenaline: Mechanism of action on the pacemaker potential in cardiac Purkinje fibers, *Science* **162**:916.

Hertting, G., 1964, The fate of ^{3}H-iso-proterenol in the rat, *Biochem. Pharmacol.* **13**:1119.

Hille, B., 1970, Ionic channels in nerve membranes, *Prog. Biophys. Mol. Biol.* **21**:1.

Hollman, M., and Green, R. D., 1973, The development of sensitivity of the embryonic chick heart to the inotropic and cAMP-elevating effects of isoproterenol, *Fed. Proc.* **32**:711 (abstract).

Hsu, F.-Y., 1933, The effect of adrenaline and acetylcholine on the heart rate of the chick embryo, *Chin. J. Physiol.* **7**:243.

Hyde, A., Cheneval, J.-P., Blondel, B., and Girardier, L., 1972, Electrophysiological correlates of energy metabolism in cultured rat heart cells, *J. Physioi. (Paris)* **64**:269.

Ignarro, L. J., and Shideman, F. E., 1968a, Appearance and concentrations of catecholamines and their biosynthesis in the embryonic and developing chick, *J. Pharmacol. Exp. Ther.* **159**:38.

Ignarro, L. J., and Shideman, F. E., 1968b, The requirement of sympathetic innervation for the active transport of norepinephrine by the heart, *J. Pharmacol. Exp. Ther.* **159**:59.

Ignarro, L. J., and Shideman, F. E., 1968c, Catechol-o-methyl transferase and monoamine oxidase activities in the heart and liver of the embryonic and developing chick, *J. Pharmacol. Exp. Ther.* **159**:29.

Ishima, Y., 1968, The effect of tetrodotoxin and sodium substitution on the action potential in the course of development of the embryonic chick heart, *Proc. Jpn. Acad.* **44**:170.

Iversen, L. L., de Champlain, J., Glowinski, J., and Axelrod, J., 1967, Uptake, storage and metabolism of norepinephrine in tissues of the developing rat, *J. Pharmacol. Exp. Ther.* **157**:509.

Jaffee, O. C., 1972, Effects of propranolol on the chick embryo heart, *Teratology* **5**:153.

Johnson, E. A., and Lieberman, M., 1971, Heart: Excitation and contraction, *Ann. Rev. Physiol.* **33**:479.

Kao, C. Y., 1966, Tetrodotoxin, saxitoxin and their significance in the study of excitation phenomena, *Pharmacol. Rev.* **18**:997.

Karczmar, A. G., Srinivasan R., and Bernsohn, J., 1973, Cholinergic function in the developing fetus, in *Fetal Pharmacology* (L. Boreus, ed.), pp. 127–176, Raven Press, New York.

Kaufmann, R., Tritthart, H., Rodenroth, S., and Rost, B., 1969, Das mechanische und elektrische Verhalten isolierter embryonaler Herzmuskelzellen in Zellkulturen, *Pfluegers Arch.* **311**:25.

Kent, K. M., Goodfriend, T. L., McCallum, Z. T., Dempsey, P. J., and Cooper, T., 1972, Inotropic agents in hypoxic cat myocardium: Depression and potentiation, *Circ. Res.* **30**:196.

Klein, R. L., 1960, Ontogenesis of K and Na fluxes in embryonic chick heart, *Am. J. Physiol.* **199**:613.

Klein, R. L., 1963a, High Na content of early embryonic chick heart, *Am. J. Physiol.* **205**:370.

Klein, R. L., 1963b, The induction of a transfer adenosine triphosphate phosphohydrolase in embryonic chick heart, *Biochim. Biophys. Acta* **73**:488.

Klein, R. L., and Evans, M. L., 1961, Effects of ouabain, hypothermia and anoxia on cation fluxes in embryonic chick heart, *Am. J. Physiol.* **200**:735.

Kohlhardt, M., Bauer, B., Krause, H., and Fleckenstein, A., 1972, Differentiation of the transmembrane Na and Ca channels in mammalian cardiac fibres by the use of specific inhibitors, *Pfluegers Arch.* **335**:309.

Krause, E.-G., Halle, W., Kallabis, E., and Wollenberger, A., 1970, Positive chronotropic response of cultured isolated rat heart cells to $N^6,2'-O$-dibutyryl-$3',5'$-adenosine monophosphate, *J. Mol. Cell. Cardiol.* **1**:1.

Kuntz, A., 1910, The development of the sympathetic nervous system in birds, *J. Comp. Neurol.* **20**:283.

Langer, G. A., and Frank, J. S., 1972, Lanthanum in heart cell culture: Effect on calcium exchange correlated with its localization, *J. Cell. Biol.* **54**:441.

Langer, G. A., Sato, E., and Seraydarian, M., 1969, Calcium exchange in a single layer of rat cardiac cells studied by direct counting of cellular activity of labeled calcium, *Circ. Res.* **24**:589.

Lee, K. S., and Klaus, W., 1971, The subcellular basis for the mechanism of inotropic action of cardiac glycosides, *Pharmacol. Rev.* **23**:193.

Lee, W. C., McCarty, L. P., Zodrow, W. W., and Shideman, F. E., 1960, The cardiostimulant action of certain ganglionic stimulants on the embryonic chick heart, *J. Pharmacol. Exp. Ther.* **130**:30

Lefkowitz, R. J., O'Hara, D. S., and Warshaw, J., 1973, Binding of catecholamines to receptors in cultured myocardial cells, *Nature (London), New Biol.* **244**:79.

Lieberman, M., 1970, Physiologic development of impulse conduction in embryonic cardiac tissue, *Am. J. Cardiol.* **25**:279.

Lieberman, M., and Paes de Carvalho, A., 1965, The spread of excitation in the embryonic chick heart, *J. Gen. Physiol.* **49**:365.

Lieberman, M., Roggeveen, A. E., Purdy, J. E., and Johnson, E. A., 1972, Synthetic strands of cardiac muscle: Growth and physiological implication, *Science* 175:909

Lissák, K., Törö, I., and Pásztor, J., 1942, Untersuchungen über den Zusammenhang des Acetylcholingehaltes und der Innervation des Herzmuskels in Gewebskulturen, *Pfluegers Arch.* 245:794.

Löffelholz, K., and Pappano, A. J., 1974a, Ontogenetic changes in pacemaker activity in chick heart, *Life Sci.* 14:1755.

Löffelholz, K., and Pappano, A. J., 1974b, Increased sensitivity of sinoatrial pacemaker to acetylcholine and to catecholamines at the onset of autonomic neuroeffector transmission in chick embryo heart, *J. Pharmacol. Exp. Ther.* 191:479.

Magazanik, L. G., and Vyskočil, F., 1970, Dependence of acetylcholine desensitization on the membrane potential of frog muscle fibre and on the ionic changes in the medium, *J. Physiol. (London)* 210:507.

Manasek, F. J., 1968, Embryonic development of the heart. I. A light and electron microscopic study of myocardial development in the early chick embryo, *J. Morphol.* 125:329.

Manukhin, B. N., Pustovoitova, Z. E., and Vyaz'mina, N. M., 1969, The content of catecholamines and DOPA in tissues of chick embryo and chicken, *Zh. Evol. Biokhim. Fiziol.* 5:42.

Markowitz, C., 1931, Response of explanted embryonic cardiac tissue to epinephrine and acetylcholine, *Am. J. Physiol.* 97:271.

Marshall, J. M., 1963, Behavior of uterine muscle in Na-deficient solutions; effects of oxytocin, *Am. J. Physiol.* 204:732.

McCarty, L. P., Lee, W. C., and Shideman, F. E., 1960, Measurement of the inotropic effects of drugs on the innervated and noninnervated embryonic chick heart, *J. Pharmacol. Exp. Ther.* 129:315.

McDonald, T. F., and DeHaan, R. L., 1973, Ion levels and membrane potential in chick heart tissue and cultured cells, *J. Gen. Physiol.* 61:89.

McDonald, T. F., Sachs, H. G., and DeHaan, R. L., 1972, Development of sensitivity to tetrodotoxin in beating chick embryo hearts, single cells, and aggregates, *Science* 176:1248.

McDonald, T. F., Sachs, H. G., and DeHaan, R. L., 1973, Tetrodotoxin desensitization in aggregates of embryonic chick heart cells, *J. Gen. Physiol.* 62:286.

Mercer, E. N., and Dower, G. E., 1966, Normal and arrhythmic beating in isolated cultured heart cells and the effects of digoxin, quinidine and procaine amide, *J. Pharmacol. Exp. Ther.* 153:203.

Michal, F., Emmett, F., and Thorp, R. H., 1967, A study of drug action on the developing avian cardiac muscle, *Comp. Biochem. Physiol.* 22:563.

Moore, J. W., and Narahashi, T., 1967, Tetrodotoxin's highly selective blockage of an ionic channel, *Fed. Proc.* 26:1655.

Nakanishi, H., and Takeda, H., 1969, Effect of acetylcholine on the electrical activity of cultured chick embryonic heart, *Jpn. J. Pharmacol.* 19:543.

Nastuk, W. L., Manthey, A. A., and Gissen, A. J., 1966, Activation and inactivation of postjunctional membrane receptors, *Ann. N.Y. Acad. Sci.* 137:999.

Noble, D., and Tsien, R. W., 1968, The kinetics and rectifier properties of the slow potassium current in cardiac Purkinje fibres, *J. Physiol. (London)* 195:185.

Obrecht-Coutris, G., and Coraboeuf, E., 1967, Sensibilité à la noradrénaline et à l'acétylcholine du myocarde embryonnaire de Poulet. *J. Physiol. (Paris)* 59:275.

Okarma, T. B., Tramell, P., and Kalman, S. M., 1972, The surface interaction between digoxin and cultured heart cells, *J. Pharmacol. Exp. Ther.* 183:559.

Paff, G. H., 1940, Detoxification of digitalis in the embryonic chick heart, *J. Pharmacol. Exp. Ther.* 70:235.

Paff, G. H., and Glander, T. P., 1968, The time of appearance of sympathomimetic receptors in the embryonic chick heart, *Anat. Rec.* 160:405.

Paff, G. H., and Johnson, J. R., 1938, The behavior of the embryonic heart in solutions of ouabain, *Am. J. Physiol.* **122**:753.

Pager, J., Bernard, C., and Gargouïl, Y., 1965, Evolution, au cours de la croissance foetale, des effets de l'acétylcholine au niveau de l'oreillette du rat, *C. R. Soc. Biol. (Poitiers)* **159**:2470.

Pappano, A. J., 1970, Calcium-dependent action potentials produced by catecholamines in guinea pig atrial muscle fibers depolarized by potassium, *Circ. Res.* **27**:379.

Pappano, A. J., 1972a, Sodium-dependent depolarization of non-innervated embryonic chick heart by acetylcholine, *J. Pharmacol. Exp. Ther.* **180**:340.

Pappano, A. J., 1972b, Action potentials in chick atria: Increased susceptibility to blockade by tetrodotoxin during embryonic development, *Circ. Res.* **31**:379.

Pappano, A. J., and Löffelholz, K., 1974, Ontogenesis of adrenergic and cholinergic neuro-effector transmission in chick embryo heart, *J. Pharmacol. Exp. Ther.* **191**:468.

Pappano, A. J., and Skowronek, C., 1974, Reactivity of chick embryo heart to cholinergic agonists during ontogenesis: Decline in desensitization at the onset of cholinergic transmission, *J. Pharmacol. Exp. Ther.* **191**:109.

Pappano, A. J., and Sperelakis, N., 1969a, Spontaneous contractions of cultured heart cells in high K$^+$ media, *Exp. Cell. Res.* **54**:58.

Pappano, A. J., and Sperelakis, N., 1969b, Spike electrogenesis in cultured heart cells, *Am. J. Physiol.* **217**:615.

Patten, B. M., and Kramer, T. C., 1933, The initiation of contraction in the embryonic chick heart, *Am. J. Anat.* **53**:349.

Pickering, J. W., 1893, Observations on the physiology of the embryonic heart, *J. Physiol. (London)* **14**:383.

Pickering, J. W., 1896, Experiments on the hearts of mammalian and chick embryos, with special reference to action of electric currents, *J. Physiol. (London)* **20**:165.

Plattner, F., and Hou, Ch. L., 1931, Zur Frage des angriffspunktes vegetativer Gifte. Versuche am Embryonalherzen und am Flimmerepithel, *Pfluegers Arch. Gesamte Physiol. Menschen Tiére* **228**:281.

Rang, H. P., and Ritter, J. M., 1970, On the mechanism of desensitization at cholinergic receptors, *Mol. Pharmacol.* **6**:357.

Renaud, D., and LeDouarin, G., 1972, Mise én evidence par l'emploi d'inhibiteurs, d'une évolution des perméabilités membranaires cardiaques aux jeunes stades du développement chez l'embryon de poulet, *C.R. Acad. Sci. (Paris)* **274**:418

Repke, K., Est., M., and Portius, H. J., 1965, Über die Ursache der Speciesunterschiede in der Digitalisempfindlichkeit, *Biochem. Pharmacol.* **14**:1785.

Reuter, H., 1966, Strom-Spannungsbeziehungen von Purkinje-Fasern bei verschiedenen extracellulären Calcium-Konzentration und unter Adrenalineinwirkung, *Pfluegers Arch. Gesamte Physiol. Menschen Tiére* **287**:357.

Robinson, R. A., and Stokes, R. H., 1959, *Electrolyte solutions*, 2nd edition (revised), Butterworths, London.

Romanoff, A. L., 1960, *The Avian Embryo: Structural and Functional Development*, The Macmillan Company, New York.

Schümann, H. J., Wagner, J., and Reinhardt, D., 1972, Sensitivity changes of adrenergic β-receptors induced by alterations of the metabolic state of isolated organs, *Naunyn Schmiedeberg's Arch. Pharmacol.* **275**:105.

Shigenobu, K., and Sperelakis, N., 1971, Development of sensitivity to tetrodotoxin of chick embryonic hearts with age, *J. Mol. Cell. Cardiol.* **3**:271.

Shigenobu, K., and Sperelakis, N., 1972, Calcium current channels induced by catecholamines in chick embryonic hearts whose fast sodium channels are blocked by tetrodotoxin or elevated potassium, *Circ. Res.* **31**:932.

Shimizu, Y., and Tasaki, K., 1966, Electrical excitability of developing cardiac muscle in chick embryos, *Tohoku J. Exp. Med.* **88**:49.

Sissman, N. J., 1970, Developmental landmarks in cardiac morphogenesis: Comparative chronology, *Am. J. Cardiol.* **25**:141.

Sperelakis, N., 1972*a*, Electrical properties of embryonic heart cells, in *Electrical Phenomena in the Heart* (W. C. DeMello, ed.), pp. 1–61, Academic Press, New York.

Sperelakis, N., 1972*b*, (Na$^+$, K$^+$)-ATPase activity of embryonic chick heart and skeletal muscles as a function of age, *Biochim. Biophys. Acta* **266**:230.

Sperelakis, N., and Lee, E. C., 1971, Characterization of (Na$^+$, K$^+$)-ATPase isolated from embryonic chick hearts and cultured chick heart cells, *Biochim. Biophys. Acta* **233**:562.

Sperelakis, N., and Lehmkuhl, D., 1965, Insensitivity of cultured chick heart cells to autonomic agents and tetrodotoxin, *Am. J. Physiol.* **209**:693.

Sperelakis, N., and Lehmkuhl, D., 1968, Ba^{2+} and Sr^{2+} reversal of the inhibition produced by ouabain and local anesthetics on membrane potentials of cultured heart cells, *Exp. Cell. Res.* **49**:396.

Sperelakis, N., and Pappano, A. J., 1969*a*, Depolarization of cultured heart cells by a lipid-soluble acetylcholine analogue, *Am. J. Physiol.* **217**:625.

Sperelakis, N., and Pappano, A. J., 1969*b*, Increase in P_{Na} and P_K of cultured heart cells produced by veratridine, *J. Gen. Physiol.* **53**:97.

Sperelakis, N., and Shigenobu, K., 1972, Changes in membrane properties of chick embryonic hearts during development, *J. Gen. Physiol.* **60**:430.

Sturkie, P. D., and Poorvin, D. W., 1973, The avian neurotransmitter, *Proc. Soc. Exp. Biol. Med.* **143**:644.

Sun, T. P., 1932, Histo-physiogenesis of the glands of internal secretion—thyroid, adrenal, ·parathyroid, and thymus—of the chicken embryo, *Physiol. Zool.* **5**:384.

Szantroch, Z., 1929, L'histogénèse des ganglions nerveux du cœur, *Bull. Int. Acad. Pol. Sci. Lett. Ser. B* **2**:417.

Szepsenwol, J., and Bron, A., 1936, L'origine et la nature de l'innervation primitive du cœur chez les embryons d'Oiseaux, (Canard et Poulet), *Rev. Suisse Zool.* **43**:1.

Tarr, M., 1971, Two inward currents in frog atrial muscle, *J. Gen. Physiol.* **58**:523.

Toda, N., and West, T. C., 1967, Interactions of K, Na, and vagal stimulation in the S-A node of the rabbit, *Am. J. Physiol.* **212**:416.

Trautwein, W., 1963, Generation and conduction of impulses in the heart as affected by drugs, *Pharmacol. Rev.* **15**:277.

Trautwein, W., 1973, Membrane currents in cardiac muscle fibers, *Physiol. Rev.* **53**:793.

Tuganowski, W., and Tendera, M., 1973, Components of the action potential of human embryonic auricle, *Am. J. Physiol.* **224**:803.

Tummons, J., and Sturkie, P. O., 1968, Cardio-accelerator nerve stimulation in chickens, *Life Sci.* **7**:377.

Tummons, J. L., and Sturkie, P. O., 1970, Beta adrenergic and cholinergic stimulants from the cardioaccelerator nerve of the domestic fowl, *Z. Vgl. Physiol.* **68**:268.

Van Mierop, L. H. S., 1967, Location of pacemaker in chick embryo heart at the time of initiation of heartbeat, *Am. J. Physiol.* **212**:407.

Vassalle, M., 1966, Analysis of cardiac pacemaker potential using a "voltage clamp" technique, *Am. J. Physiol.* **210**:1335.

Vassalle, M., 1970, Electrogenic suppression of automaticity in sheep and dog Purkinje fibers, *Circ. Res.* **27**:361.

Vassort, G., Rougier, O., Garnier, D., Sauviat, M. P., Coraboeuf, E., and Gargouïl, Y.-M., 1969, Effects of adrenaline on membrane inward currents during the cardiac action potential, *Pfluegers Arch. Gesamte Physiol. Menschen Tiére* **309**:70.

Vincenzi, F. F., and West, T. C., 1963, Release of autonomic mediators in cardiac tissue by direct subthreshold electrical stimulation, *J. Pharmacol. Exp. Ther.* **141**:185.

Waud, D. R., 1968, Pharmacological receptors, *Pharmacol. Rev.* **20**:49.

Waymouth, C., 1965, Construction and use of synthetic media, in *Cells and Tissues in Culture* (E. N. Willmer, ed.), Vol. 1, pp. 99–142, Academic Press, New York.

Wekstein, D. R., and Zolman, J. F., 1968, Sympathetic control of homeothermy in the young chick, *Am. J. Physiol.* **214**:908.

Wenzel, D. G., Wheatley, J. W., and Byrd, G. D., 1970, Effects of nicotine on cultured rat heart cells, *Toxicol. Appl. Pharmacol.* **17**:774.

Wildenthal, K., 1971a, Long-term maintenance of spontaneously beating mouse hearts in organ culture, *J. Appl. Physiol.* **30**:153.

Wildenthal, K., 1971b, Responses to cardioactive drugs of fetal mouse hearts maintained in organ culture, *Am. J. Physiol.* **221**:238.

Wildenthal, K., 1973, Maturation of responsiveness to cardioactive drugs: Differential effects of acetylcholine, norepinephrine, theophylline, tyramine, glucagon, and dibutyryl cyclic AMP on atrial rate in hearts of fetal mice, *J. Clin. Invest.* **52**:2250.

Wollenberger, A., 1964, Rhythmic and arrhythmic contractile activity of single myocardial cells cultured in vitro, *Circ. Res.* **14** (Suppl. 2); **15**:184.

Yeh, B. K., and Hoffman, B. F., 1968, The ionic basis of electrical activity in embryonic cardiac muscle, *J. Gen. Physiol.* **52**:666.

Zachs, S. I., 1954, Esterases in the early chick embryo, *Anat. Rec.* **118**:509.

4

Analysis of Dose–Response Relationships

DOUGLAS R. WAUD

I. SOME COMMENTS ON GENERAL PHARMACOLOGY

The discipline of pharmacology is currently going through an important stage in its development. It is at that point where it is appropriate to begin to shift emphasis from what has been essentially a descriptive approach to one tied to a more general framework. The "aspirin through zinc paste" approach has reached the point where, if for no other reason, limitations of memory make it necessary to begin to codify the overall area. In other words, one must begin to focus on the similarities among drugs rather than their differences. This is what general pharmacology is all about.

Now I am sure that many pharmacologists would say they have been doing this for years. But this has generally been true only to a limited extent. For example, the physiological pharamacologist will consider similarities between acetylcholine and epinephrine (mechanisms for synthesis, storage, release, removal, etc.) but how often will these "general principles" extend to, say, penicillin or estradiol? While "short-range" generalizations are, of course, still better than none, one must not stop at this level. It is clearly important to build a framework that is as general as possible. To this end, it is

DOUGLAS R. WAUD · Department of Pharmacology, University of Massachusetts Medical Center, Worcester, Massachusetts 01605.
Supported by U.S. Public Health Service Research Grant NS 04618 from NINDS.

useful periodically to ask oneself "How broad is this idea?" A simple test is to consider another drug and see if the idea is useful there. The more drugs you can consider, the more likely you are getting at a part of the basic structure of pharmacology, i.e., at the framework from which you approach drug action. Consider a few examples. A chance observation that tubocurarine produces a marked pressor response in the ferret (Evans and Waud, 1973) illustrates one extreme end of the spectrum; change the drug, the variable measured, or the species, and you will probably see something different. The well-known similarities in behavior of acetylcholine and epinephrine represent a more general level of approach. For example, the interaction of atropine with acetylcholine provided a very useful model when propranolol came along [see, for example, Blinks's (1967) use of Arunlakshana and Schild's (1959) approach]. Finally, since all drugs exhibit a relationship between the magnitude of response to the dose administered, an approach to analysis of such a relationship is an important component of general pharmacology. While many of the ideas relevant to looking at the dose–response relationship are simple once you have seen them, they are not trivial. For example, as will be discussed below, ignorance of the pitfalls of reading too much into the shape of a dose–response curve can lead to incorrect or ambiguous conclusions. And, although the general approach has been with us for quite some time [the classic papers by Stephenson (1956) and Arunlakshana and Schild (1959) can be considered the fountainhead], even the elementary aspects are often not very widely appreciated. For example, the closest approach to a decent text on general pharmacology, Goldstein, Aronow, and Kalman's *Principles of Drug Action* (1974), still contains a reciprocal plot type of analysis of a histamine dose–response curve (their Figure 1–69).

We shall now turn, therefore, to a consideration of how to look at dose–response curves. The general aspects will be considered to give the overall framework, but some more specific topics of somewhat less general applicability, of particular interest in some particular areas of cellular pharmacology, will also be considered.

II. EMPIRICAL EXAMINATION OF DOSE–RESPONSE CURVES

A. Classification of Dose–Response Curves

Dose–response curves are two-dimensional relationships and therefore can be classified with respect to the abscissae or the ordinates. Before turning to the more important ordinates, a few comments on conventions for abscissae are in order because the phrase "dose" in dose–response curve is often used loosely to mean other than dose in the strict sense. Originally, when dealing with a whole organism pharmacologists gave various *amounts* of drug, i.e., *doses*, and observed the corresponding responses. However, except in rare or contrived situations, it is not the amount of drug given but its *concentration* at the site of action that is the meaningful independent variable. The pharmacologist recognizes this and either explicitly (cf. the units "mg/kg" for example) or implicitly recognizes that the dose is distributed through a volume to produce an effective concentration at the site of action but, either because that concentration may not be known precisely or because dose is easier to say than concentration, continues to use the word dose. This has even carried over to dose–response relationships determined *in vitro* where the concentration applied is usually known.

The reader should be warned about another convention. If you ask a pharmacologist to draw a typical dose–response curve he will in all probability unconsciously draw a sigmoid curve like that in the right-hand panel of Figure 1. This is the form taken by most dose– (or concentration–) response relationships when a logarithmic scale of abscissae is used. However, if concentration, not its logarithm, is plotted, most curves will be the shape shown in the left panel of Figure 1 (a few may still be sigmoid, but this is not too common). This latter form of plotting is rarely used because the dependence of response on concentration is such that most of the curve is crowded over against the scale of ordinates; generally the logarithmic plot is used to spread the observations out.

Thus, one ends up with the rather odd convention that the term dose in dose–response curve more often than not will really mean log concentration. The reader may prefer to use the more precise terminology; however, he should still be warned that there is a large number of publications where terminology is loose, *caveat lector*. (Incidentally, there is still a small fraction

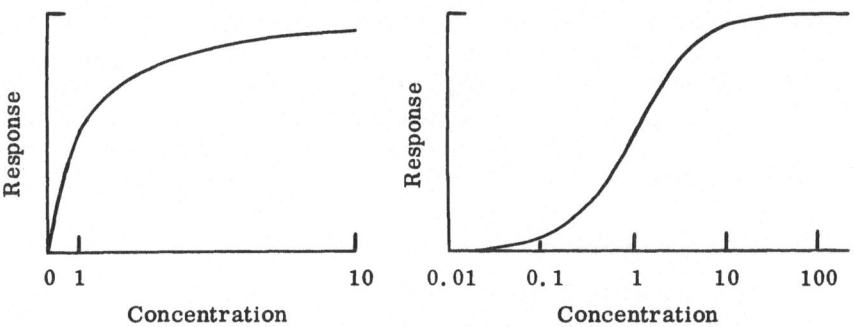

Figure 1. The concentration– (or dose–) response relationship (left), compared to the log concentration–response relationship (right).

of biologists who measure concentrations in units such as mg/ml or, even more irritatingly, mg %. If you happen to be one, come out of the Middle Ages; don't be an isolationist; use molar units.)

The preceding dose/concentration/log concentration distinctions are more semantic than anything. When we turn to the scale of ordinates of a dose–response relationship, we encounter more meaningful distinctions. There are two general types of dose–response curves—graded and quantal— depending on the nature of the response. Since the two types of response are fundamentally different, it is important to recognize which type you are dealing with whenever you encounter a dose–response curve. A third type of curve, which may be called ordered, can also be pictured. Although strictly not a distinct entity (see below), the ordered dose–response relationship can occasionally form a convenient frame of reference.

1. Graded Dose–Response Curves

These are the most common types of relationship. The scale of ordinates is any variable that can be measured on a continuously graded scale, for example, tension exerted by a muscle, membrane potential change produced by a drug, rate of beating of heart tissue, etc.

2. Quantal Dose–Response Curves

Here we are dealing with an all-or-none response. The prototype example is death. The organism or cell is either dead or not dead; responses like three-eighths dead or 90% dead are not possible. Thus, the dose–response relationship takes the form shown in the left-hand panel of Figure 2; only responses of 0 or 1 are allowed. Now such a diagram as this causes considerable anxiety among editors and pharmacologists ("look at all that empty space in the middle," "it's not sigmoid") and, until recently, was hard to analyze quantitatively. Therefore, one generally finds that groups of individuals are tested at each dose level so that one can obtain a fraction responding which can then be plotted against concentration to give something resembling the more familiar sigmoid shape of the graded dose–response curve as in the right-hand panel of Figure 2. Thus, at first glance, the quantal curve may look like a graded curve. However, the underlying model is quite different and is analyzed differently.

3. Ordered Dose–Response Curves

Guedel's stages of ether anesthesia provide the prototype example. As the concentration of ether in the brain is raised, one sees a reproducible

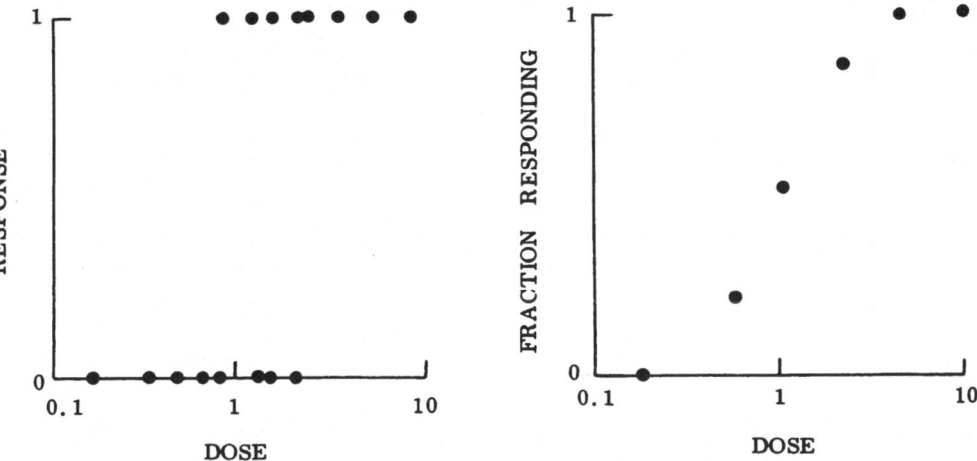

Figure 2. **The form of quantal dose–response curves.** Left panel: the fundamental form of a quantal dose–response curve. Right panel: the form taken when subjects are grouped.

progression of signs—unconsciousness, settling down of respiration, eye movements, relaxation of various groups of muscles in a particular order, respiratory arrest, and finally death. These various indicators define a series of "stages" and "planes" (I, II, III_1–III_4, IV) so one can picture a relationship as in Figure 3a; as the ether concentration rises one passes progressively through the sequence of end points. Such a diagram appears to have the general form of a dose–response relationship, but this is somewhat misleading. In fact, there is no significance to distance along the scale of ordinates. In other words, a patient in stage II is not twice as deep as in stage I. Thus, the dose–response curve is better pictured as in Figure 3b where the scale of ordinates is removed. All one can say is that stage I is reached before stage II, i.e., the order of response end points is regular.

The notion of an ordered curve can be useful heuristically in situations where a regular progression of events occurs. However, note that the ordered dose–response curve is not a distinct entity; it is really just a collection of quantal dose–response curves associated with a sequential series of end points. Thus, the ordered dose–response curve of Figure 3a or b can be viewed as in Figure 3c or, more fundamentally, Figure 3d.

This section on empirical classification of dose–response curves may be summarized by saying there is more than one type of dose–response curve and interpretation or quantitative analysis depends on the type.

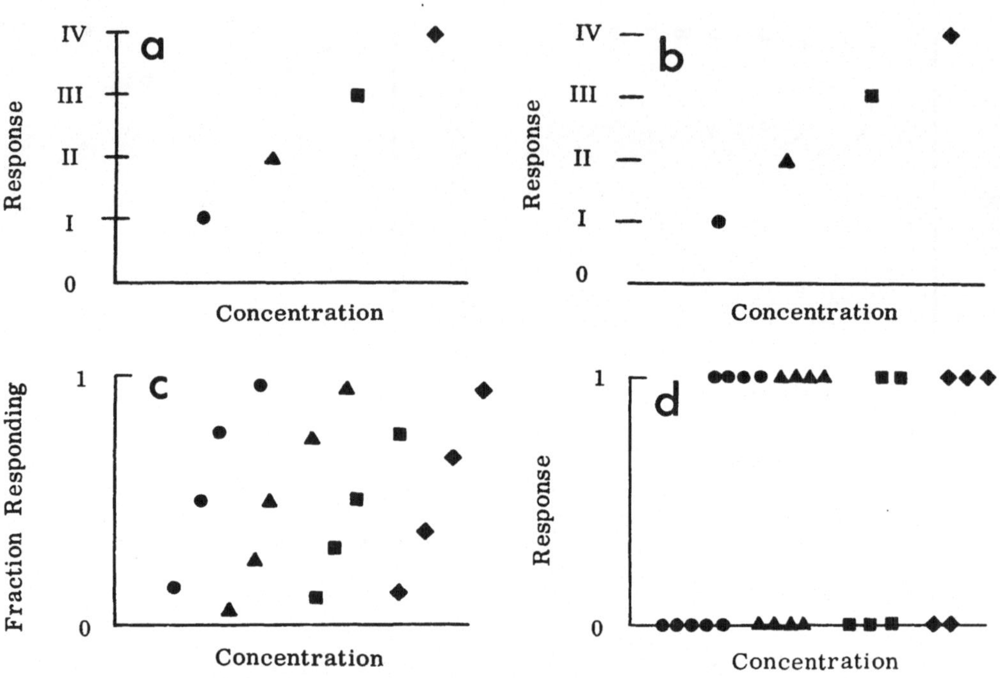

Figure 3. Diagrams to illustrate the nature of the ordered dose–response curve. a: the usual form of plotting; b: plotted to emphasize the ordered aspect; c: equivalent set of quantal dose–response curves (grouped data); d: equivalent set of quantal dose–response curves (more fundamental form).

B. Classification of Antagonists

The availability of a specific antagonist greatly facilitates analysis of mechanism of action of a drug. Therefore, sensible use of antagonists is an important part of pharmacological investigation. However, as is so often the case, it is easy to get in trouble at a very elementary level if a systematic approach is not used. Therefore, a few comments on antagonism are in order.

1. Descriptive Classification

First, recognize that there are three principal classes of antagonist—chemical, physiological (or functional), and pharmacological. A chemical antagonist is one that acts by reacting directly with the drug in question; a chelating agent is a good example. Physiological antagonists are agents that oppose each other because they act on systems that are opposed physiologically; for example, epinephrine, by activating radial muscle fibers in the pupil of the eye, antagonizes the action of acetylcholine to constrict the pupil by activating circularly arranged fibers. The third group, pharmacological antagonists, includes those drugs that interact by a more intimate mechanism—for example, competitive antagonists.

Now the pharmacological antagonists are generally the most interesting. However, it is inappropriate, when you first encounter an antagonism, to assume automatically and without good evidence that the interaction is pharmacological. A common error, for example, is to observe a "parallel shift" of the dose–response curve to the right and to conclude the interaction is competitive, i.e., to leap immediately to one of the subtypes of pharmacological antagonism. This conclusion may or may not be right. To be in such an ambiguous situation is a poor beginning. Many years ago, Gaddum recognized this pitfall and proposed a terminology that is very useful. He suggested that one talk of *surmountable* and *unsurmountable* antagonism, depending on whether it was still possible in the presence of the antagonist to regain a maximal response by increasing the dose of agonist (Gaddum *et al.*, 1955). Thus, in Figure 4, the antagonist in the top panel would be

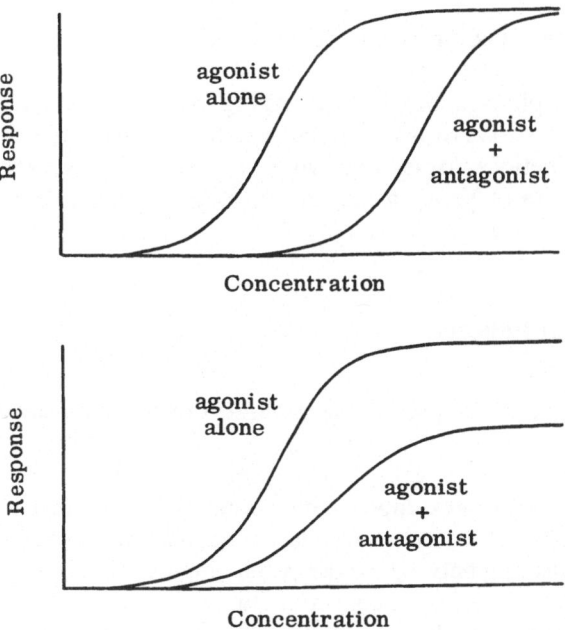

Figure 4. The dose–response relationships in a surmountable antagonism (top) and an unsurmountable antagonism (bottom).

termed surmountable, that in the bottom, unsurmountable. We may now return to the situation mentioned at the beginning of this paragraph; when that parallel shift of the dose–response curve was observed, a surmountable antagonism could have been reported and thus nothing more than appropriate would have been read into the observations and nobody would have been misled. Admittedly the term surmountable antagonist sounds less elegant than competitive antagonist, but accuracy should take precedence over the possibility of a false claim.

2. Kinetic Classification of Antagonism

Suppose now that we have ruled out a chemical or physiological antagonism and wish further to subdivide what seems to be a pharmacological antagonism. At this point kinetic studies become of interest, and one begins to think in terms of competitive or uncompetitive interactions. These are already defined in chemistry, so the classification need not be repeated here. However, we shall soon discuss in detail the approach to kinetic analyses in complicated systems such as an intact cell.

3. Mechanistic Classification of Antagonism

Again, the pharmacologist has nothing to add to conventional chemical terminology here. There is one point worth emphasizing, however: do not forget that kinetic analyses may rule out some mechanisms, but kinetic experiments cannot prove a mechanism is operative. Mechanistic experiments are necessary.

C. Empirical Indices

As indicated in the previous section, it is important not to overstep the limitations of your experimental design and try to read more than is appropriate into your results. This caveat extends to numbers you may put on your observations. For example, many people (unfortunately, including those responsible for writing many standard pharmacological texts) are sloppy about distinguishing between a dose producing a half-maximal response and a drug-receptor dissociation constant. But, just as it is useful to emphasize the distinction between the empirical and the kinetic or mechanistic by appropriate terminology, it is helpful to do the same for indices. Therefore, we may now briefly indicate the empirical indices relevant to dose–response curves.

1. Agonists*

The great majority of dose–response relationships are symmetrical sigmoid curves when response is plotted against logarithm of the dose or concentration administered, i.e., the form is similar to that in the right-hand diagram of Figure 1 (Figure 5, gives a specific example). Consequently, although the overall relationship is two dimensional, it is possible to summarize the shape of the curve reasonably closely by specifying just three numbers—a scale factor for the ordinates and a location and scale factor for the abscissae. The vertical scale is usually given in terms of the height of the maximal response, and a drug which produces a greater maximal response is said to be more effective or more powerful. The location parameter for the abscissae is usually taken to be the ED_{50}—the dose or concentration that produces a half-maximal response. The reciprocal of the ED_{50} is then used as a measure of potency (as opposed to effectiveness or power). There is no general agreement as to scale factor for the abscissae; various measures of "slope" have been used. One might work in terms of the concentration difference between, say, 20% and 80% response levels (for example, Langer and Trendelenburg, 1969); one can make the relationship linear by appropriate plotting to get a Hill coefficient (Brown and Hill, 1923), or one can fit an explicit function to the observations and use the parameter appropriate to that model as a measure of slope, for example, work in terms of the standard deviation of a normal distribution (Gaddum, 1933) or the scale factor of the logistic distribution (Berkson, 1944; Parker and Waud, 1971).

2. Antagonists

Just as it avoids ambiguity to have the terms surmountable and unsurmountable to describe curves without reading more than is appropriate into experimental results, it is also useful to be able to put a number on the extent of the antagonism. For example, consider a surmountable antagonism. What measure of antagonistic potency corresponds to an ED_{50}? Well, the effect of a surmountable antagonist is to shift the log dose–response curve to the right. Thus, this shift can be used as a measure of effect. Specifically, one can work in terms of the so-called "dose ratio" (Gaddum et al., 1955), since a shift to the right on a logarithmic axis amounts to an increase in dose by a constant factor to match any given control response. However, the maximal response is potentially infinite, so one cannot define a half-maximal response but has to work instead in terms of somewhat arbitrarily chosen response

* The term agonist, derived from antagonist, is used simply to refer to a drug that produces a response as opposed to a drug, the antagonist, that blocks that response.

levels, say a dose ratio of 2 or 10. Thus, Schild (1947) has introduced an index pA_x defined in this frame of reference. Specifically, the pA_x is the negative logarithm (to base 10) of the (molar) concentration of antagonist that produces a dose ratio of x. If the mechanism is competitive, the pA_2 will give the logarithm of the association constant of the antagonist–receptor complex. However, such a specific interpretation need not be read into the measure. Like the terms surmountable and unsurmountable the pA_x index allows you to state precisely what you observed without implying more.

A corresponding index, the pD_2 has been proposed for the unsurmountable case (cf. Ariens and van Rossum, 1957), i.e., the pD_2 is the negative logarithm (to base 10) of the (molar) concentration of antagonist that scales the curve down twofold. One should be particularly careful about reading anything mechanistic into a pD_2 since this would involve attaching mechanistic significance to the shape of the dose–response curve—a dangerous route to travel (see below).

This concludes the introductory discussion of terminology and empirical presentation of results. We may turn now to the central part of this paper, kinetic analysis of dose–response curves.

III. KINETIC ANALYSIS OF DOSE–RESPONSE CURVES

A.   Models

If one considers any system where action of a drug is examined, the input is application of a drug and the output is some observed response. It is convenient to split the overall sequence of events into three stages—*access* of the drug to the receptor, *reaction* with the receptor, and *actuation* of the sequence of events leading to the observed response. We may consider these in turn.

1.   Access

Generally, problems of uptake and distribution of drugs are greatest in the whole organism; however, it is important not to ignore access in a simple *in vitro* cellular system. Although flow limitations occasionally come up, for example in perfused or superfused tissues, most of the time one has to deal only with diffusional limitations and/or the problems associated with unstirred layers. Analysis of the kinetics of drug access is a major topic in itself and so will not be considered explicitly here. [The reader can get a good introduction to diffusional kinetics in Crank's monograph (1957); the paper by Dainty (1963) will indicate some of the problems of unstirred layers.] Thus, in what follows, it will be assumed that appropriate consideration of access limitations has been built into the experimental design so that the kinetics observed are not just those of factors like diffusion. This is not to say that access problems cannot slip in where not expected nor be interesting—cf. Katz and Miledi's (1973) "pipette artifact" and their final picture of factors controlling the duration of a miniature end-plate potential in the presence of an anticholinesterase.

2. Reaction with the Receptor

Various models have been proposed for this stage of the process. The classical model (Clark, 1926; Stephenson, 1956) corresponds to the Michaelis–Menton analysis of enzyme kinetics. Many other models have been put forth, for example, allosteric/cooperative variants (Changeux and Podleski, 1968; Karlin, 1967; Thron, 1973; or Colquhoun, 1973) or an ion-exchange formalism (Taylor *et al.*, 1970, see also Waud, 1974a). For simplicity, the present discussion will be restricted to one particular model as an illustration of how to approach a kinetic analysis. The extension to whatever alternative or variant takes the reader's fancy should be reasonably straightforward.

There is general agreement that a larger number of drugs react chemically with some specific site or "receptor" as the first stage in their interaction with the cell. It is hard to escape such a conclusion. For example, how else can one explain the common observation of drug action at micromolar concentrations, sensitivity of potency of subtle changes in structure, and selective antagonism by drugs again active at low concentrations and again with potency very sensitive to structure?

Thus one can picture the model

$$A + R \rightleftharpoons AR \tag{1}$$

as a reasonable starting point. A represents an agonist, R the receptor. Note that this model is not necessarily applicable to all drugs. For example, it most likely is *not* relevant to the action of anesthetics like ether.

Given the model (1) as a starting point, then one can characterize this stage of the process in the usual way with a macroscopic dissociation constant

$$K_A = \frac{[A][R]}{[AR]} \tag{2}$$

This, in combination with the relation

$$[AR] + [R] = [R_t] \tag{3}$$

(i.e., the receptor is either occupied by drug or not) allows one readily to write an explicit relation between the dependent variable receptors occupied and the independent variable drug concentration $[A]$. The usual situation in living tissues is that the total concentration of receptors $[R_t]$ is not known so it is convenient to work in terms of fractional receptor occupancy $y_A = [AR]/[R_t]$. Thus, one can use equation (2) to eliminate $[R]$ from equation (3), divide by $[R_t]$ and rearrange to get the familiar expression

$$y_A = \frac{[AR]}{[R_t]} = \frac{[A]}{[A] + K_A} \tag{4}$$

In general, modeling the drug–receptor reaction stage is quite straightforward; the relation of receptors occupied to drug concentration can be derived with little trouble from whatever model is chosen to represent the reaction.

3. Actuation

We can now consider subsequent events leading to the observed response; these events can be conveniently lumped under the label "actuation." Here we encounter the converse of the situation in the preceding step. In general an explicit model is not available. Thus, one must start with the position emphasized by Stephenson (1956). The existence of a reproducible dose–response relationship allows us to write

$$E = f(y_A) \tag{5}$$

but, in general no more, i.e., the effect E is some function f of the fraction of receptors occupied by the agonist A, but the shape of this function is not available *a priori*. This is a very important point. It means that the shape of the dose–response curve can reflect unknown factors, and therefore it is inappropriate to attach kinetic (or mechanistic) significance to the shape of the dose–response curve. In particular, it is dangerous (if not silly) to interpret blindly an ED_{50} as the K_A.

Now there are specific situations in which the nature of f can reasonably be predicted. For example, if you consider a competitive antagonist and choose to define occlusion of receptors as the response, then $E = y_A$. Or, if you are measuring transmembrane electrical changes produced by a drug, membrane electrical models make it reasonable to expect that change in conductance will be directly proportional to the number of receptors occupied (Werman, 1969, gives an example of use of such a model). However, the safest approach is to assume the general case (5), in the absence of a reason to be more specific, rather than arbitrarily to choose an explicit model which may not be justified.

To illustrate how one uses models such as (4) and (5) in kinetic analysis, in particular to show how one can live with (5), we may turn now to a particular problem.

B. Estimation of Dissociation Constants

As mentioned already, there are many models which can be used to describe various systems, so it is not practical to discuss each in detail. Instead, I shall focus in on a couple of examples to illustrate the general approach in the hope that the reader will then be able to make the appropriate modifications or construct the appropriate new model and analysis relevant to his or her particular system. Specifically, I shall consider estimation of the dissociation constant of a competitive antagonist. This is probably the best example of a useful kinetic analysis in intact cells. I shall also mention briefly the corresponding analysis for an agonist, in particular to illustrate the problems involved with this more difficult problem.

1. Competitive Antagonists

We may begin with a statement of the problem. Given that one has reason to believe that an antagonist B interacts competitively with an agonist A, how does one measure the dissociation constant K_B between B and the receptor in question? And how does one do this in intact cells?

The solution to be described is that of Arunlakshana and Schild (1959). To illustrate, consider the results summarized in Figure 5. In this experiment, an isolated guinea pig lumbrical muscle was used as a sample of mammalian skeletal muscle. The lumbrical was mounted vertically in Krebs' solution at 37°C. The surface of the muscle was scanned electrically by Fatt's moving fluid electrode technique (Fatt, 1950). Normally, the muscle surface is equipotential but, in the presence of carbachol, an area of negativity is recorded over the end-plate region. Graded doses of carbachol produce graded responses (see the control curve at the left in Figure 5), and the responses are reproducible (the open circle is the response to a repeat dose at the end of the day). Thus, the preparation fulfills the two primary criteria for a bioassay. The experimental design amounts simply to determining a control

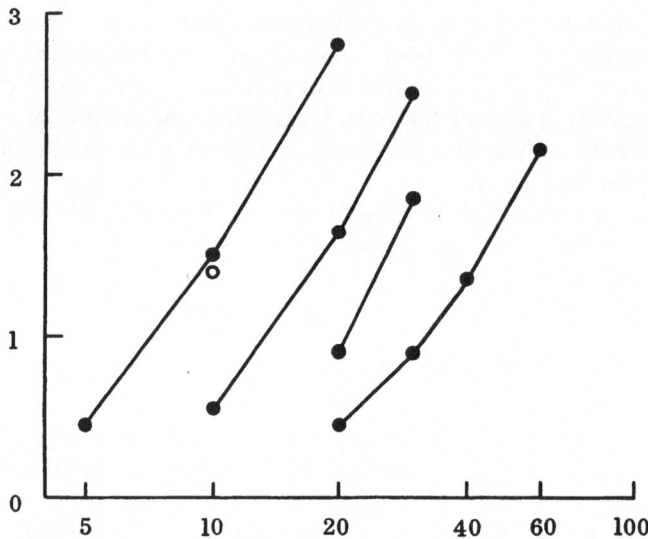

Figure 5. Example of experimental results that might be used to estimate the dissociation constant of the reaction between a competitive antagonist and the receptor *in situ*. The preparation was an isolated guinea pig lumbrical muscle. Depolarization (ordinates, mV) was recorded extracellularly (moving fluid electrode technique) during application of various concentrations (abscissae) of carbachol. The left-hand dose–response curve represents the control response (the open circle was obtained at the end of the day to demonstrate reproducibility of response). The other three curves were obtained in the presence of 10^{-7}, 2×10^{-7}, and 4×10^{-7} M tubocurarine.

dose–response curve and then one or more curves in the presence of one or more concentrations of the antagonist, tubocurarine in this experiment.

How does one analyze such results? The first step is to get an explicit model. The control curve can be represented by (4) and (5) above, i.e.,

$$E = f(y_A) \quad (5) \qquad \text{and} \qquad y_A = \frac{A}{A + K_A} \quad (4)$$

(The square brackets representing concentration of drug A—carbachol—have been dropped for simplicity.) In the presence of tubocurarine (B), an analogous model obtains. One can start with the equations (6) and (7) corresponding to (2) and (3) above:

$$K_B = \frac{B \cdot R}{BR} \tag{6}$$

$$AR + BR + R = R_t \tag{7}$$

use (2) and (6) to eliminate BR and R in (7), and rearrange to get

$$y'_A = \frac{A'}{A' + K_A(1 + B/K_B)} \tag{8}$$

where the primes indicate values for A in the presence of B. [Note in passing the form of (8). It is identical to (4) except for a larger K_A. This larger effective K_A means the frame of reference for concentration of A has been increased. In other words, to get back to any given effect, E, the dose of A has to be increased by a constant amount. Thus, simple inspection of (8) shows why a competitive antagonist produces the characteristic "parallel shift of the curve to the right."]

In turn, corresponding to (5) we have

$$E' = f(y'_A) \tag{9}$$

Note that the f will be unchanged by B. If B is on a receptor, the receptor does not react with A so f is irrelevant, while if B is not on the receptor the receptor is normal so the normal f obtains.

We may now illustrate the beauty of appropriate experimental design. Specifically, we can now get around our problem of not knowing the nature of the actuation function f, for if we match effects (i.e., compare concentrations producing matching effects) we have

$$E = E' \tag{10}$$

in other words,

$$f(y_A) = f(y'_A) \tag{11}$$

or

$$y_A = y'_A \tag{12}$$

and the f's cancel out. From here on the analysis is straightforward. Equation (12) implies

$$\frac{A}{A + K_A} = \frac{A'}{A' + K_A(1 + B/K_B)} \tag{13}$$

With a little rearranging this can be put in the form

$$\frac{A'}{A} - 1 = \text{dose ratio} - 1 = \frac{B}{K_B} \tag{14}$$

If only the control curve and one curve in the presence of antagonist are available, one can read off the dose ratio—for example, about 1.8 with the left-hand two curves in Figure 5—and obtain K_B from (14) as

$$K_B = \frac{B}{\text{Dose ratio} - 1}$$

$$= \frac{10^{-7} \text{ M}}{1.8 - 1} = 1.25 \times 10^{-7} \text{ M} \tag{15}$$

Arunlakshana and Schild (1959) proceeded more elegantly. They took the logarithmic form of (14):

$$\log(\text{dose ratio} - 1) = -\log K_B + \log B \tag{16}$$

and obtained $\log K_B$ from the intercept of a plot of $\log(\text{dose ratio} - 1)$ against $\log B$. Such a "Schild plot" from the results of Figure 5 is given in Figure 6. The intercept gives an estimate of about 1.2×10^{-7} M for K_B. The Schild plot gives a form of weighted average of the estimates of K_B that would have been obtained if one had separately compared each of the three tubocurarine curves with the control curve. However, the Schild plot also provides a check of how consistent the results are with the model. Equation (16) indicates that the slope of the plot should be unity.

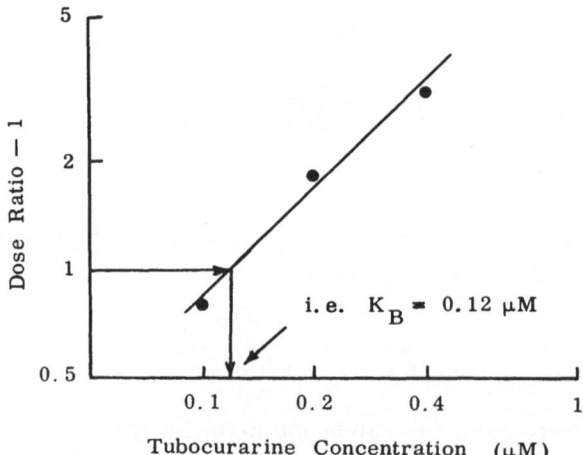

Figure 6. Schild plot of the results of Figure 5. Ordinates: log (carbachol dose–ratio − 1). Abscissae: log (concentration of tubocurarine).

2. Agonists

Estimation of K_B was considered before that of K_A because the analysis is somewhat easier. However, it is of considerable interest not to look at antagonists only. Several methods have been used to measure K_A (they are listed in Waud, 1969), but a discussion of the approach of Furchgott and Bursztyn (1967) will illustrate the problem and the sort of solution that is possible. These authors used an irreversible antagonist to occlude permanently enough receptors to reduce the maximal response to the agonist and then compared the control curve and this depressed curve. The model for the control curve was the usual one, i.e., (4) and (5) above;

$$E = f(y_A) \quad (5) \qquad y_A = \frac{A}{A + K_A} \quad (4)$$

In the presence of the irreversible receptor blocking agent, (4) becomes

$$y'_A = \frac{A}{A + K_A}(1 - y_I) \tag{17}$$

where y_I is the function of receptors occluded by the irreversible antagonist. Thus, equation (5) is just a scaled down version of (4). Corresponding to (5), we have

$$E' = f(y'_A) \tag{18}$$

where again the function f is unchanged.

Furchgott and Bursztyn (1967) then matched responses before and in the presence of the antagonist, i.e., they matched effects

$$E = E' \tag{19}$$

which amounted to

$$f(y_A) = f(y'_A) \tag{20}$$

or

$$y_A = y'_A \tag{21}$$

or

$$\frac{A}{A + K_A} = \frac{A'}{A' + K_A}(1 - y_I) \tag{22}$$

This can be rearranged to the linear form

$$\frac{1}{A} = \frac{y_I}{1 - y_I} \cdot \frac{1}{K_A} + \frac{1}{1 - y_I} \cdot \frac{1}{A'} \tag{23}$$

which is convenient for graphical analysis. Thus, if one plots $1/A$ against $1/A'$, one can get an estimate of K_A as

$$K_A = \frac{\text{Slope} - 1}{\text{Intercept on } (1/A) \text{ axis}} \tag{24}$$

As with the Schild plot, the reciprocal plot here gives a test of how consistent the results are with the model; the plot should be linear.

The preceding discussion illustrates the approach, but before leaving the topic it is interesting to mention one result obtained by Furchgott and Bursztyn. Consider carbachol. The ED_{50} was about 10^{-8} M while the estimate of K_A was about 2×10^{-6} M. Thus, in this system anyone who chose to use the ED_{50} as a measure of K_A would have been off by a factor of about 200. This just confirms explicitly the folly of trying to read too much into the shape of a dose–response curve!

C.   Statistical Aspects

In both the method for estimation of K_B and that for estimation of K_A, the final results took the form of a graph from which the estimate of the parameter was obtained. Furthermore, the values used for these final graphs generally have been obtained as visual estimates from the observed dose–response relationship. For example, to get the dose ratios plotted in Figure 6, one would traditionally sketch a set of parallel curves through the observations of Figure 5 and read off visual estimates of the dose ratios. It is generally recognized that fitting even a straight line by eye to a set of points can be treacherous. To do the corresponding maneuver with a curvilinear relationship can be expected to increase even more the subjectivity of the estimates of parameters. Thus, it is very desirable to have an objective statistical procedure for doing the job. In addition, a statistical analysis can provide error estimates as well as tests of appropriateness of the model. [For example, it is convenient to be able to test the curves in Figure 5 to see if they deviate from parallelism. As discussed earlier, comparison of equations (4) and (13) indicates parallel curves should result if the competitive model is correct.]

I have discussed the analysis of quantal dose–response curves fully elsewhere (Waud, 1973), and quantal responses are more often encountered in whole organisms than in cellular pharmacology so the interested reader is referred to the earlier paper. Parker and I (Parker and Waud, 1971; Waud and Parker, 1971) have presented analyses corresponding to the Arunlakshana and Schild approach to K_B and the Furchgott and Bursztyn approach to K_A. Since that work with Parker, I have begun to realize that there is an even better way to handle the analysis objectively. The point is to start from the original model rather than try to operate within the frame of reference provided by the traditional graphical analysis. The technique is important if one is to have an objective analysis and one that will provide values for the error of the estimates of the parameters. The approach may now be described.

On one hand, we have a set of observations such as those in Figure 5. On the other hand, we have a model. What we want is to find the values of the model's parameters, in particular those most consistent with the observations (so-called maximum-likelihood estimates, see Kendall and Stuart, 1961; in fact, these values are equivalent to those obtained by fitting the observations to the model by least squares). First we need to put the model in a suitable form. In particular we must choose some function empirically to use for the f of equation (5). It is not essential that the function be mechanistically correct but simply that its shape is consistent with the sigmoid shape of a dose–response curve. Various functions have been used this way (see Winsor, 1932, for example), and all seem to give as good a fit as the next one. The logistic function (Berkson, 1944) has a computational advantage, however, and will be used here to illustrate the method. Specifically, we can represent the control dose–response curve by the function

$$E = M \frac{A^P}{A^P + K^P} \tag{25}$$

This representation says nothing more than that we are going to fit the observations to a sigmoid-shaped function with a maximum of M, an ED_{50} of K, and a slope determined by P (which corresponds to a Hill coefficient).

Now what do we use for a curve in the presence of tubocurarine? As indicated already in connection with equation (8), the effect of tubocurarine is simply to change the frame of reference for A [compare equations (4) and (8)]. Thus, the K of equation (25) will become $K(1 + B/K_B)$ in the presence of the competitive antagonist. Or, we could write

$$E = M \frac{A^P}{A^P + [K(1 + B/K_B)]^P} \tag{26}$$

as a general expression for a dose–response curve with equation (25) representing the special case when $B = 0$.

It is convenient finally to generalize equation (26) by replacing B by B^Q:

$$E = M \frac{A^P}{A^P + [K(1 + B^Q/K_B)]^P} \tag{27}$$

This will allow us later to test whether the kinetics of the reaction of B with the receptor are consistent with a one-to-one reaction.

As long as the logistic function provides a reasonable fit to observed dose–response curves (which it does), we need not be concerned about the specific form of the function other than the term $(1 + B^Q/K_B)$, and that term was derived on solid kinetic grounds.

Our next step is to fit equation (27) to the observations. Unfortunately, this is a rather cumbersome process since equation (27) is not linear in the parameters (i.e., P comes in as a power and K and K_B appear in the denominator). The significance of this feature is that if you set up normal equations for a least-squares fit, the equations cannot be solved explicitly for M, P, Q, K, and K_B. An iterative approach is necessary. Fortunately, a computer can be used to handle the menial aspect.

The expression (27) is expanded in a Taylor series in each parameter (the linear one M can be included as well so that it will not have to be handled differently). Thus, one can make initial estimates of M, K_B, K, Q, and P (call these values M_1, K_{B_1}, K_1, Q_1, and P_1) and can then write:

$$E \approx M_1 \frac{A^{P_1}}{A^{P_1} + [K_1(1 + B^{Q_1}/K_{B_1})]^{P_1}} + (M - M_1) \left.\frac{\partial E}{\partial M}\right|_{M_1, K_{B_1}, K_1, Q_1, P_1}$$

$$+ (K_B - K_{B_1}) \left.\frac{\partial E}{\partial K_B}\right|_{M_1, K_{B_1}, K_1, Q_1, P_1}$$

$$+ \text{ corresponding terms in } K, Q, \text{ and } P \tag{28}$$

This is of the form

$$E = E_1 + (M - M_1)\left(\frac{\partial E}{\partial M}\right)_1 + (K_B - K_{B_1})\left(\frac{\partial E}{\partial K_B}\right)_1 + \cdots \tag{29}$$

This can be written

$$E - E_1 = E_{\text{res}} = B_1 X_1 + B_2 X_2 + \cdots \tag{30}$$

which is of the form of a multiple linear regression (with five independent variables X_i in this case), and can be fitted by least squares to yield estimates of the five slopes B_i. These estimates can be used to improve the first round of estimates of M, K_B, K, Q, and P. For example, the second round estimate of M becomes

$$M_2 = M_1 + B_1 \tag{31}$$

Similarly,

$$K_{B_2} = K_{B_1} + B_2 \tag{32}$$

and so on.

Armed with this new set of estimates, we can try another cycle starting at equation (28) but with subscripts 2 instead of 1. The B_i we calculate can be used to get a third set of estimates of M, K_B, K, P, and Q. Thus, we can continue improving our estimates until no further change occurs. At this point, we will have the maximum likelihood (or least-squares) estimates we seek. Furthermore, the statistical fitting process yields errors of estimate as a by-product (cf. Kendall and Stuart, 1961, equation 19.16, or Snedecor and Cochran, 1968, Section 13.5).

Although simple to use once the relevant computer program has been written, the process is not easy to follow the first time through. Therefore, a numerical illustration may be helpful. I have already provided one for the full model of equation (28) (Waud, 1975), so this time let us work with a variant of (28), in fact, one that is useful for responses such as those in Figure 5. In those experiments, large depolarizations were avoided so as to minimize the extent of development of desensitization (the complete recovery indicated by the open circle testifies to the success of this strategy). However, this means that the curves have not been followed high enough that they would begin to flatten out. In turn, this means that the curves cannot be used to estimate M. Thus, we must modify the analysis to the extent that we will simply fix M at some reasonable value and just estimate K_B, K, P, and Q. The reader may object that the choice of M will affect the result. However, Waud and Parker (1971) found that the estimate of K_B can be amazingly insensitive to the choice of M (in fact, this observation is one reason I am not particularly concerned what function is chosen empirically to model the dose–response curve). In any case, later we can try several values of M and see what happens.

We start with the values in Table 1. First we need initial estimates of K_B, K, P, and Q and the permanent estimate of M. Inspection of Figure 5 (the source of the values in Table 1) suggests an M of 5 would not be outrageous, so let us start there. The ED_{50} of the control curve would then be about 15 μM so that will be our K_1. To get an initial estimate of K_B, we can compare the first two curves. Their ED_{50}'s (with an assumed maximum M of 5) would be about 15 and 25 so, from equation (14), we can start K_B at $B/(\text{dose ratio} - 1) = 0.1/(25/15 - 1) = 0.15 \, \mu M$. We expect Q to be 1. Finally, we need a starting

TABLE 1. Numerical Values of Concentrations and Responses
of Figure 5

	Concentration of carbachol (μM)	Depolarization response (mV)
Control curve	5	0.45
	10	1.5
	10	1.4
	20	2.8
10^{-7} M tubocurarine	10	0.55
	20	1.65
	30	2.5
2×10^{-7} M tubocurarine	20	0.9
	30	1.85
4×10^{-7} M tubocurarine	20	0.45
	30	0.9
	40	1.35
	60	2.15

value for P. One could guess, try a Hill plot, or work from past experience with the system. The last route leads me to try 2.5 as an initial value for P.

We now have to set up our normal equations for the linear approximation. This approximation will be of the form of equation (30), i.e.,

$$X_5 = B_1 X_1 + B_2 X_2 + B_3 X_3 + B_4 X_4$$

where

$$X_5 = E_{\text{obs}} - 5 \frac{A^{2.5}}{A^{2.5} + [15(1 + B^1/0.15]^{2.5}} \tag{33}$$

and

$$\begin{array}{ll} B_1 = K_B - K_{B_1}; & B_2 = K - K_1; \\ B_3 = Q - Q_1; & B_4 = P - P_1 \end{array} \tag{34}$$

If we write $K' = K(1 + B^Q/K_B)$, then

$$X_1 = \frac{\partial E}{\partial K_B} = \frac{\partial E}{\partial K'} \cdot \frac{\partial K'}{\partial K_B} = \frac{\partial E}{\partial K'} \cdot \frac{-KB^Q}{K_B^2} \tag{35}$$

$$X_2 = \frac{\partial E}{\partial K} = \frac{\partial E}{\partial K'} \cdot \frac{\partial K'}{\partial K_B} = \frac{\partial E}{\partial K'} \cdot (1 + B^Q/K_B) \tag{36}$$

$$X_3 = \frac{\partial E}{\partial Q} = \frac{\partial E}{\partial K'} \cdot \frac{\partial K'}{\partial Q} = \frac{\partial E}{\partial K'} \cdot \frac{K}{K_B} \cdot B^Q \cdot \ln_e (B) \tag{37}$$

$$X_4 = \frac{\partial E}{\partial P} = M \frac{A^P K'^P \ln_e (A/K')}{(A^P + K'^P)^2} \tag{38}$$

with

$$\frac{\partial E}{\partial K'} = M \frac{-A^P P K'^{(P-1)}}{(A^P + K'^P)^2} \tag{39}$$

These expressions appear very complicated but one line in the computer program disposes of each of them (see Appendix).

The normal equations for finding the least-squares estimate of $B_1 - B_4$ then take the form (cf. Snedecor and Cochran, 1968, Chapter 13)

$$\begin{bmatrix} \Sigma X_1^2 & \Sigma X_1 X_2 & \Sigma X_1 X_3 & \Sigma X_1 X_4 \\ \Sigma X_1 X_2 & \Sigma X_2^2 & & \\ \vdots & & \ddots & \\ \Sigma X_1 X_4 & & & \Sigma X_4^2 \end{bmatrix} \cdot \begin{bmatrix} B_1 \\ B_2 \\ B_3 \\ B_4 \end{bmatrix} = \begin{bmatrix} \Sigma X_1 X_5 \\ \Sigma X_2 X_5 \\ \Sigma X_3 X_5 \\ \Sigma X_4 X_5 \end{bmatrix} \tag{40}$$

which are equations of the form

$$\mathbf{MB} = \mathbf{Y} \tag{41}$$

the solution of which is

$$\mathbf{B} = \mathbf{M}^{-1}\mathbf{Y} \tag{42}$$

In other words, to get $B_1 - B_4$ we calculate $X_1^2, X_1 X_2, \ldots, X_4 X_5$ in equation (40) and then solve the equation by inverting the matrix $\mathbf{M}$. The elements of $\mathbf{M}$ are formed in a straightforward fashion. For example, to get the term $\Sigma X_1 X_2$ we start with the first point on the control curve (5, 0.45) and put $A = 5$ in (33) and (34) [and (37)] along with our initial estimates of K_B, K, P, and Q to calculate the values of X_1 and X_2 at the point $K_{B_1}, K_1, P_1,$ and Q_1. These values of X_1 and X_2 are multiplied together and saved. Now we move to the next point on the control curve (10, 1.5), repeat the process, and add the product obtained to the product just saved. We continue doing this until the contributions from all the points have been added. While calculating X_1 and X_2, we do X_3, X_4, and $X_5 (= E_{\text{obs}} - E_1)$, as well, and accumulate all the relevant sums of products as we go from point to point. When we are done, we have the equations

$$
\begin{bmatrix}
808.831 & -13.2913 & 157.82 & -15.0831 \\
-13.2913 & 0.320624 & -2.84585 & 0.328731 \\
157.82 & -2.84585 & 35.763 & -2.92462 \\
-15.0931 & 0.328731 & -2.92462 & 1.45051
\end{bmatrix}
\cdot
\begin{bmatrix}
B_1 \\ B_2 \\ B_3 \\ B_4
\end{bmatrix}
=
\begin{bmatrix}
-19.7926 \\ 0.401535 \\ -4.14138 \\ -0.382651
\end{bmatrix}
\quad (43)
$$

which, when solved give

$$
\begin{aligned}
B_1 &= -0.0189331 \\
B_2 &= 1.36974 \\
B_3 &= 0.0163773 \\
B_4 &= -0.738213
\end{aligned}
\quad (44)
$$

The values can now be used to get better estimates of K_B, K, P, and Q, i.e.,

$$
\begin{aligned}
\text{new } K_B &= \text{old } K_B + B_1 = 0.15 - 0.0189331 = 0.131067 \\
\text{new } K &= \text{old } K + B_2 = 15 + 1.36974 = 16.3697 \\
\text{new } Q &= \text{old } Q + B_3 = 1 + 0.0163773 = 1.01638 \\
\text{new } P &= \text{old } P + B_4 = 2.5 - 0.738213 = 1.76179
\end{aligned}
\quad (44)
$$

We can calculate a new set of equations, solve for a new set of B_i's, and readjust the estimates of the parameters. Thus, one gets the sequence of estimates

Cycle	K_B	K	Q	P
0	0.15	15	1	1
1	0.131067	16.3697	1.01638	1.76179
2	0.126677	16.9191	1.01702	1.80973
3	0.126594	16.9285	1.01869	1.81037
4	0.126593	16.9287	1.01871	1.81037
5	0.126594	16.9287	1.01871	1.81037
6	0.126594	16.9287	1.01871	1.81037
7	0.126594	16.9287	1.01871	1.81037

Obviously, the final value is reached about the fourth or fifth cycle. The remaining iterations were just included to illustrate the convergence. Thus, we conclude that our estimate of K_B is 1.27×10^{-7} M, a value consistent with the graphical estimate obtained earlier. Now all we need is a standard error. This comes from the $\mathbf{M}^{-1}$ of equation (42). Thus, when we stop at the end of the fourth cycle, we estimate $\mathbf{B}$ as $\mathbf{M}^{-1}\mathbf{Y}$ but save $\mathbf{M}^{-1}$. It is

$$
\mathbf{M}^{-1} = \begin{bmatrix} 0.0122326 & 0.0659336 & -0.0534215 & 0.0200054 \\ 0.0659332 & 28.382 & 1.09886 & -1.8815 \\ -0.0534215 & 1.09885 & 0.379781 & -0.057592 \\ 0.0200054 & -1.8815 & -0.0575921 & 0.722669 \end{bmatrix} \quad (45)
$$

Next, we estimate the sum of squares of deviations about the fitted curves, i.e., we calculate the sum

$$
\Sigma = \sum_i \left\{ E_{obs_i} - M \frac{A_i^P}{A_i^P + [K(1 + B^Q/K_B)]^P} \right\}^2 \quad (46)
$$

over all points i to get an error sum of squares of 0.0527814. Then the standard errors of the parameters are given by

$$
\begin{aligned}
SE\,(K_B) &= [M^{-1}(1,1)/(N - 4)]^{1/2} \\
SE\,(K) &= [M^{-1}(2,2)/(N - 4)]^{1/2} \\
SE\,(Q) &= [M^{-1}(3,3)/(N - 4)]^{1/2} \\
SE\,(P) &= [M^{-1}(4,4)/(N - 4)]^{1/2}
\end{aligned} \quad (47)
$$

where $M^{-1}(1,1)$ through $M^{-1}(4,4)$ are the diagonal elements of $\mathbf{M}^{-1}$, and $(N - 4)$ is the degrees of freedom associated with the error sum of squares and is equal to the total number of points $N (= 13$ here) minus the number of parameters estimated, 4.

Thus, in the present example

$$
\begin{aligned}
SE\,(K_B) &= [0.0527814 \times 0.0122326/9]^{1/2} = 0.0085 \\
SE\,(K) &= [0.0527814 \times 28.382/9]^{1/2} = 0.41 \\
SE\,(Q) &= [0.0527814 \times 0.379781/9]^{1/2} = 0.047 \\
SE\,(P) &= [0.0527814 \times 0.722669/9]^{1/2} = 0.065
\end{aligned} \quad (48)
$$

Besides K_B, only Q is of particular interest. Its value, 1.02 ± 0.05, includes unity and so the drug–receptor reaction is first-order with regard to tubocurarine. This test of Q corresponds to comparing the slope of a Schild plot (like that in Figure 6) with unity. Finally, we can repeat the calculations with various values of M. When this is done, the result is

M	K_B	SE (K_B)	$K_B - $ SE (K_B)	$K_B + $ SE (K_B)
3	0.125	0.011	0.114	0.136
4	0.125	0.006	0.119	0.131
5	0.127	0.008	0.119	0.135
6	0.128	0.010	0.118	0.138
7	0.128	0.011	0.117	0.139
8	0.129	0.012	0.117	0.141
9	0.129	0.013	0.116	0.142
10	0.129	0.013	0.116	0.142
15	0.130	0.014	0.116	0.144
20	0.131	0.015	0.116	0.146
30	0.131	0.016	0.115	0.147
40	0.131	0.016	0.115	0.147
60	0.132	0.016	0.116	0.148
80	0.132	0.016	0.116	0.148
100	0.132	0.016	0.116	0.148

Clearly, even over a ridiculously large range of choices of M, the estimate of K_B does not change much. The M of 5 used in the calculations does not appear quite so good as one of 4 would have been, i.e., the latter value yields a slightly smaller standard error of K_B. However, the difference is negligible compared to the standard error of estimate. It is interesting to note that even if we had been so silly as to choose an M of, say, 60, the only price we would have paid would have been a slightly larger error band; however, the range 0.116–0.148 still would have included the 0.119–0.131 obtained with an M of 4. Thus, the only price we would have had to pay for being clumsy would have been a slightly reduced efficiency of the experiment; our error limits would still be expected to include the right answer.

These calculations illustrate the general approach but should not be taken to mean this is the only way to handle these data. For example, one might wish to fit the curves first with separate slopes and then with a common slope as above so that the two error sums of squares may be tested to see if the curves are parallel (cf. Waud and Parker, 1971). Such an extension is straightforward. An example is given in the reference mentioned earlier (Waud, 1975).

By this point, the reader may be asking whether the result is worth all the effort. It is for several reasons. First, the objectivity avoids reading biases into the results. Second, the availability of error limits is very useful. Third, once the program is written, the calculations just take a few seconds, i.e., the method is faster than the graphical method. Finally, the time taken to write the program is less than the extra time that would be needed for extra experiments required to get the same degree of precision of estimate if one were restricted to the inefficient method of using graphical estimates and making up for their greater imprecision by doing more experiments. I prefer to give the dull repetitive tasks to the computer.

Incidentally, once you get the hang of it, writing the program is not a lengthy procedure. The one in the appendix was written in about 40 minutes while I was supposed to be listening to a lecture. It took about 10 or 15 minutes more for debugging [a $K(1)$ inadvertently had become a $K(2)$]. Thus, the total expenditure of effort getting "tooled up" is not much of an argument against doing the job properly.

IV. MECHANISTIC ANALYSIS OF THE DOSE–RESPONSE RELATIONSHIP

We come now to the final level at which one can approach the analysis of the dose–response relationship. Generally, mechanistic studies will be done on simple systems which may not even include an intact cell. In other words, one will typically be working with a system that will be similar to those used in chemistry or biochemistry, and thus the techniques will not be peculiar to pharmacology but rather will be those relevant to a general mechanistic analysis of a reasonably pure system. Thus, a specific discussion of all the tools at one's disposal would be extremely lengthy and redundant. It will be sufficient to give a few examples and then leave the reader to his own devices.

A. Access

As indicated earlier, this aspect of pharmacology is somewhat peripheral to the analysis of mechanism of action. However, a simple example may be given. When faced with the question of determining whether acetylcholine acted on the inside or outside of the cell, del Castillo and Katz (1957) attacked the problem directly by injecting the drug intracellularly by a microiontophoretic method. Similarly, Narahashi et al. (1970) bypassed a long series of kinetic studies designed to determine whether local anesthetics acted inside or outside the nerve axon by applying the drug directly to the inside and outside of a perfused giant axon.

B. Reaction with the Receptor

Here one mechanistic approach involves preparing a reasonably pure preparation of isolated receptor material and then doing binding studies on this purified system (cf. Changeux *et al.*, 1971). For example, one can use such a system to answer specific questions unambiguously (like, is the cholinergic receptor the same as the cholinesterase molecule?—the answer is no, Changeux *et al.*, 1971). It is also beginning to be possible to work with reconstituted model systems (Kasai and Changeux, 1971).

One can also study mechanism *in situ*. For example, Rang and Ritter (1969), by looking at uptake of a labeled irreversibly binding antagonist, were able to provide direct evidence of an alteration in the receptor *in situ*.

C. Actuation

Katz and Miledi (1972) have recently introduced a method for probing the mechanisms underlying the permeability change produced by acetylcholine. By examining the frequency spectrum of the increase in membrane noise associated with the action of various drugs, they were able to detect evidence that the duration of the elementary conductance change produced by depolarizing agents can vary from drug to drug.

V. SUMMARY

Ways to analyze dose–response relations have been discussed. Approaches have been grouped as descriptive, kinetic and mechanistic. Kinetic approaches, in particular, have been discussed and appropriate experimental design and statistical evaluation have been emphasized.

REFERENCES

Ariens, E. J., and van Rossum, J. M., 1957, pD_x, pA_x and pD'_x values in the analysis of pharmacodynamics, *Arch. Int. Pharmacodyn.* **110**:275.
Arunlakshana, O., and Schild, H. O., 1959, Some quantitative uses of drug antagonists, *Br. J. Pharmacol.* **14**:48.
Berkson, J., 1944, Application of the logistic function to bio-assay, *J. Am. Stat. Assoc.* **39**:357.
Blinks, J. R., 1967, Evaluation of the cardiac effects of several beta adrenergic blocking agents, *Ann. N.Y. Acad. Sci.* **144**:882.

Brown, W. E. L., and Hill, A. V., 1923, The oxygen-dissociation curve of blood and its thermodynamical basis, *Proc. R. Soc. London, Ser. B.* **94**:297.

Changeux, J.-P., and Podleski, T. R., 1968, On the excitability and cooperativity of the electroplax membrane, *Proc. Natl. Acad. Sci. USA* **59**:944.

Changeux, J.-P., Meunier, J. C., and Huchet, M., 1971, Studies on the cholinergic receptor protein of *Electrophorus electricus*, *Mol. Pharmacol.* **7**:538.

Clark, A. J., 1926, The reaction between acetyl choline and muscle cells, *J. Physiol. (London)* **61**:530.

Cleland, W. W., 1967, The statistical analysis of enzyme kinetic data, *Adv. Enzymol.* **29**:1.

Colquhoun, D., 1973, The relation between classical and cooperative models for drug action, in *Drug Receptors* (H. P. Rang, ed.), University Park Press, London.

Crank, J., 1957, *The Mathematics of Diffusion*, Clarendon Press, Oxford.

Dainty, J., 1963, Water relations of plant cells, *Adv. Bot. Res.* **1**:279.

Evans, C. A., and Waud, D. R., 1973, A pressor effect of high doses of tubocurarine in the ferret, *Pharmacology* **10**:32.

del Castillo, J., and Katz, B., 1957, A study of curare with an electrical micromethod, *Proc. R. Soc. London, Ser. B.* **146**:339.

Fatt, P., 1950, The electromotive action of acetylcholine at the motor end-plate. *J. Physiol. (London)* **111**:408.

Furchgott, R. F., and Bursztyn, P., 1967, Comparison of dissociation constants and of relative efficacies of selected agonists acting on parasympathetic receptors, *Ann, N.Y. Acad. Sci.* **144**:882.

Gaddum, J. H., 1933, Methods of biological assay depending on a quantal response, *Med. Res. Counc. (G.B.) Spec. Rep. No.* 183.

Gaddum, J. H., Hameed, K. A., Hathway, D. E., and Stephens, F. F., 1955, Quantitative studies of antagonists for 5-hydroxytryptamine, *Quart. J. Exp. Physiol.* **40**:49.

Goldstein, A., Aronow, L., and Kalman, S. M., 1974, *Principles of Drug Action*, 2nd edition, Wiley, New York.

Karlin, A., 1967, On the application of "a plausible model" of allosteric proteins to the receptor for acetylcholine, *J. Theoret. Biol.* **16**:306.

Kasai, M., and Changeux, J.-P., 1971, *In vitro* excitation of purified membrane fragments by cholinergic agonists, *J. Membr. Biol.* **6**:1.

Katz, B., and Miledi, R., 1972, The statistical nature of the acetylcholine potential and its molecular components, *J. Physiol.* **224**:665.

Katz, B., and Miledi, R., 1973, The binding of acetylcholine to receptors and its removal from the synaptic cleft, *J. Physiol.* **231**:549.

Kendall, M. G., and Stuart, A., 1961, *The Advanced Theory of Statistics*, Griffin, London.

Langer, S. Z., and Trendelenburg, U., 1969, The effect of a saturable uptake mechanism on the slopes of dose–response curves produced by a competitive antagonist, *J. Pharmacol. Exp. Ther.* **167**:117.

Narahashi, T., Frazier, D. T., and Yamada, M., 1970, The site of action and active form of local anesthetics. I. Theory and pH experiments with tertiary compounds, *J. Pharmacol. Exp. Ther.* **171**:32.

Parker, R. B., and Waud, D. R., 1971, Pharmacological estimation of drug-receptor dissociation constants. Statistical Evaluation. I. Agonists, *J. Pharmacol. Exp. Ther.* **177**:1.

Rang, H. P., and Ritter, J. M., 1969, A new kind of drug antagonism: Evidence that agonists cause a molecular change in acetylcholine receptors, *Mol. Pharmacol.* **5**:394.

Schild, H. O., 1947, pA, a new scale for the measurement of drug antagonism, *Br. J. Pharmacol.* **2**:189.

Snedecor, G. W., and Cochran, W. G., 1968, *Statistical Methods*, 6th edition, Iowa State University Press, Ames, Iowa.

Stephenson, R. P., 1956, A modification of receptor theory, *Br. J. Pharmacol.* **175**:213.

Taylor, D. B., Steinborn, J., and Lu, T., 1970, Ion exchange processes at the neuromuscular junction of voluntary muscle, *J. Pharmacol. Exp. Ther.* **175**:213.

Thron, C. D., 1973, On the analysis of pharmacological experiments in terms of an allosteric receptor model, *Mol. Pharmacol.* **9**:1.

Waud, D. R., 1969, On the measurement of the affinity of partial agonists for receptors, *J. Pharmacol. Exp. Ther.* **170**:117.

Waud, D. R., 1973, On biological assays involving quantal responses, *J. Pharmacol. Exp. Ther.* **183**:577.

Waud, D. R., 1974a, Adsorption isotherm vs. ion-exchange models for the drug-receptor reaction. *J. Pharmacol. Exp. Ther.* **188**:520.

Waud, D. R., 1975, Analysis of dose–response curves, in *Methods in Pharmacology* (E. E. Daniel and D. M. Paton, eds.), Plenum Press, New York.

Waud, D. R., and Parker, R. B., 1971, Pharmacological estimation of drug-receptor dissociation constants. Statistical evaluation. II. Competitive antagonists, *J. Pharmacol. Exp. Ther.* **177**:13.

Werman, R., 1969, An electrophysiological approach to drug-receptor mechanisms, *Comp. Biochem. Physiol.* **30**:997.

Winsor, C. P., 1932, A comparison of certain symmetrical growth curves, *J. Wash. Acad. Sci.* **22**:73.

APPENDIX

Example of a computer program to estimate the dissociation constant of a competitive antagonist.

The program below is written in the language BASIC and was run on a Digital Equipment Corporation PDP-8e. The version of BASIC available did not have matrix commands so a subroutine (pirated from Cleland, 1967) is inserted (lines 3500–3900) to perform the matrix inversion involved in solving the normal equations.

The computer listing of the program is given below, along with a few comments to illustrate the roles of the various statements.

```
10  DIM M(5,8),C(5,10),E(5,10)
20  LET N=0
30  READ C
40  FOR I=1 TO C
50  READ N(I),B(I),K(I)
60  LET N=N+N(I)
70  FOR J=1 TO N(I)
80  READ C(I,J),E(I,J)
90  NEXT J
100 NEXT I
110 READ M,K(3),K(4)
120 LET I=K(1)
```

```
130 LET K(1)=B(2)/(K(2)/K(1)-1)
140 LET K(2)=I
150 LET B(1)=1E-15
160 LET R=4
170 GOSUB 1000
180 PRINT
190 GOSUB 2000
200 PRINT"PARAMETER          VALUE              S.E."
210 PRINT
220 PRINT"        KB        ",K(1),SQR(S*M(1,2)/(N-4))
230 PRINT"        K         ",K(2),SQR(S*M(2,3)/(N-4))
240 PRINT"        Q         ",K(3),SQR(S*M(3,4)/(N-4))
250 PRINT"        P         ",K(4),SQR(S*M(4,5)/(N-4))
260 PRINT
270 PRINT"(M WAS   ";M;"   )"
280 PRINT
290 STOP
1000 FOR I=1 TO 5
1010 FOR J=1 TO 8
1020 LET M(I,J)=0
1030 NEXT J
1040 NEXT I
1050 PRINT K(1),K(2),K(3),K(4)
1060 FOR I=1 TO C
1070 FOR J=1 TO N(I)
1080 LET U=C(I,J)↑K(4)
1090 LET K=K(2)*(1+B(I)↑K(3)/K(1))
1100 LET D=U+K↑K(4)
1110 LET E=-M*U*K(4)*K↑(K(4)-1)/D↑2
1120 LET X(1)=-E*K(2)*B(I)↑K(3)/K(1)↑2
1130 LET X(2)=E*K/K(2)
1140 LET X(3)=E*K(2)*B(I)↑K(3)*LOG(B(I))/K(1)
1150 LET X(4)=M*U*K↑K(4)*LOG(C(I,J)/K)/D↑2
1160 LET X(5)=E(I,J)-M*U/D
1170 FOR K=1 TO 4
1180 FOR L=1 TO 5
1190 LET M(K,L)=M(K,L)+X(K)*X(L)
1200 NEXT L
1210 NEXT K
1220 NEXT J
1230 NEXT I
1240 GOSUB 3500
1250 LET K=0
1260 FOR I=1 TO 4
1270 LET K(I)=K(I)+M(I,1)
1280 LET K=K+ABS(M(I,1)/K(I))
```

```
1290 NEXT I
1300 IF K>0.001 THEN 1000
1310 PRINT K(1),K(2),K(3),K(4)
1320 PRINT
1330 RETURN
2000 LET S=0
2010 FOR I=1 TO C
2020 FOR J=1 TO N(I)
2030 LET E=C(I,J)↑K(4)
2040 LET E=M*E/(E+(K(2)*(1+B(I)↑K(3)/K(1)))↑K(4))
2050 LET S=S+(E(I,J)-E)↑2
2060 NEXT J
2070 NEXT I
2080 RETURN
3000 DATA 4
3010 DATA 4,0,15
3020 DATA 5,.45,10,1.5,10,1.4,20,2.8
3030 DATA 3,0.1,25
3040 DATA 10,.55,20,1.65,30,2.5
3050 DATA 2,0.2,35
3060 DATA 20,.9,30,1.85
3070 DATA 4,0.4,60
3080 DATA 20,.45,30,.9,40,1.35,60,2.15
3090 DATA 5,1,2.5
3500 FOR I=1 TO R
3510 LET M(I,R+4)=1/SQR(M(I,I))
3520 NEXT I
3530 LET M(R+1,R+4)=1
3540 FOR I=1 TO R
3550 FOR J=1 TO R+1
3560 LET M(I,J)=M(I,J)*M(I,R+4)*M(J,R+4)
3570 NEXT J
3580 NEXT I
3600 LET M(R+1,R+3)=-1
3610 LET M(1,R+2)=1
3620 FOR K=1 TO R
3630 FOR I=1 TO R
3640 LET M(I,R+3)=M(I,1)
3650 NEXT I
3660 FOR J=1 TO R+1
3670 FOR I=1 TO R
3680 LET M(I,J)=M(I+1,J+1)-M(I+1,R+3)*M(1,J+1)/M(1,R+3
3690 NEXT I
3700 NEXT J
3710 NEXT K
3800 FOR J=2 TO R+1
```

```
3810 FOR I=1 TO R
3820 LET M(I,J)=M(I,J)*M(I,R+4)*M(J-1,R+4)
3840 NEXT I
3850 LET M(J-1,1)=M(J-1,1)*M(J-1,R+4)
3860 NEXT J
3900 RETURN
4000 END
```

Comments on Program

Line	
10	Sets aside space for arrays (M will be used for the normal equations, C for concentration, and E for effect).
20, 60	Compute N, the total number of points.
30	Gets the number of curves, C, from the top of the DATA list in lines 3000–3090.
40–110	Read the rest of the data. $N(I)$ is the number of points, $B(I)$ is the tubocurarine concentration, and $K(I)$ is the ED_{50} estimate, of the Ith curve. $C(I,J)$ and $E(I,J)$ are the concentration and effect for the Jth point in the Ith curve. $K(3)$ and $K(4)$ will be Q and P.
120	Saves ED_{50} of first curve temporarily.
130	Sets $K(1)$ to initial estimate of K_B.
140	Sets $K(2)$ to initial estimate of K.
150	Avoids taking LOG (0) at line 1140 (i.e., makes $B(1)$ nearly, but not quite equal to 0).
160	Sets R to the number of parameters being estimated.
170	Calls the 1000 subroutine that carries out the iterative fitting process.
190	Calls the 2000 subroutine that calculates the error sum of squares [equation (46)].
200–280	Print out the estimates and their standard errors [the latter are calculated as indicated in equations (47) and (48) of the main text].
1000–1330	Subroutine that carries out the fitting process.
1000–1040	Set all elements of M to zero initially.
1050	Prints out current estimates of the parameters as you go along (for entertainment value).
1060–1230	Fill in **M** (first four columns of M in the program) and **Y** (next column of M) of equation (41).

1080–1160	Calculate X_1–X_5 of equations (33) and (35)–(39).
1170–1210	Calculate and accumulate the appropriate sums of squares and products that are the elements of M.
1240	Calls the 3500 subroutine that inverts M. Upon return, $\mathbf{M}^{-1}$ is in the second through fifth columns of M and $\mathbf{B}$ is in the first column.
1250–1290	Calculate the new estimates of the parameters and accumulate K, a measure of how much change there has been in the last cycle.
1300	Unless K has become negligible, we go back for another iteration.
1310	Prints out our final values.
2000–2080	Calculate S, the error sum of squares [cf. equation (46)].
3000–3090	The data arranged in the order in which they are sought by the READ statements in lines 30–110.
3500–3900	The subroutine that inverts M (cf. Cleland, 1967).

5

Cellular Pharmacology of Ganglionic Transmission

SYOGORO NISHI

I. GENERAL CHARACTERISTICS OF AUTONOMIC GANGLIA

A. Morphological Aspects

Sympathetic and parasympathetic ganglia are made up of neurons which lie outside the central nervous system. They appear either as a macroscopic fusiform lump with clearly recognizable pre- and postganglionic branches or as a microscopic meshwork with indistinct input–output relationships. In contrast to central neurons which are protected in important biochemical respects and maintained in a complete homeostasis by the blood–brain barrier, the neurons in autonomic ganglia are exposed to the common interstitial fluid through a loose layer of satellite cells (gliocytes). Thus the ganglion neurons will be affected much more readily by the drugs applied either systemically or locally.

Sympathetic ganglion cells are adrenergic and liberate norepinephrine at their axon terminals. There are some exceptions; sympathetic ganglion cells that innervate sweat glands, and some of those that innervate the blood

SYOGORO NISHI · Department of Physiology, Kurume University School of Medicine, Kurume, 830, Japan.

vessels of skeletal muscle, are cholinergic. Parasympathetic ganglion cells are cholinergic and release acetylcholine (ACh) at their axon terminals. These ganglion neurons are either multipolar, protruding several processes (mammalian and reptilian ganglia), or unipolar, sending off a single axon (reptilian and amphibian ganglia) (Huber, 1899; Pick, 1970). The size of ganglion cells varies. Nevertheless, three subdivisions have been described for the mammalian ganglion cells; large cells with a diameter of 33–35 μm, medium-sized cells with a diameter of 25–32 μm, and small cells with a diameter of 15–22 μm (De Castro, 1932). From 50–70% of all ganglion cells are of medium size. Their axons, which constitute the postganglionic fibers, are as a rule nonmyelinated and measure not more than 1.5 μm in diameter.

The preganglionic nerve fibers of both sympathetic and parasympathetic systems liberate ACh. The majority of them are myelinated (2–3 μm in diameter) and are classified physiologically as the B-type nerve. The rest are nonmyelinated (< 1.3 μm in diameter) and belong to the C-type nerve. In many ganglia, the preganglionic fibers are outnumbered by the ganglion cells. In the cat superior cervical ganglion, Billingsley and Ranson (1918) found that the ratio of myelinated preganglionic fibers to ganglion cells was 1:32. When, however, the nonmyelinated fibers in the preganglionic nerve are also counted, the ratio of preganglionic fibers to postganglionic neurons falls to between 1:11 and 1:17 (Wolf, 1941). This corresponding ratio in the cat ciliary (parasympathetic) ganglion is, however, only 1:2 (Wolf, 1941).

The preganglionic end fibers usually have a diameter of about 0.1–0.3 μm. Along their path, they exhibit widened portions at which they establish synaptic contacts with the ganglion cells. In the cat superior cervical ganglion the great majority of the synapses are axodendritic; a few axosomatic synapses have also been observed (Elfvin, 1963). The preganglionic end fibers usually run parallel to or wind around the dendrites and establish synaptic contacts with the dendrites at several points. The most common organelles of the preganglionic nerve terminals (synaptic knobs; 1–6 μm in diameter) are small nongranulated vesicles, about 300–500 Å in diameter, vesicles with a dense core about 700–1000 Å in size, and mitochondria. The specialized zones of the pre- and postsynaptic membranes have a triple-layered asymmetric structure, and the interspace (synaptic cleft) between the synaptic membrane is about 60–80 Å (Elfvin, 1963).

Since the original work of de Robertis and Bennett (1954) the submicroscopic features of amphibian sympathetic synapses have been reported by several investigators (Taxi, 1961; Pick, 1963; Yamamoto, 1963; de Robertis, 1964; Uchizono, 1964; Hunt and Nelson, 1965; Nishi et al., 1967). As illustrated in Figure 1, synaptic knobs are seen on the cell body, axon hillock, and proximal part of the axon (Uchizono, 1964; Nishi et al., 1967). Synaptic knobs are mostly of the invaginated type with varying circumferences of up to 4.5 μm.

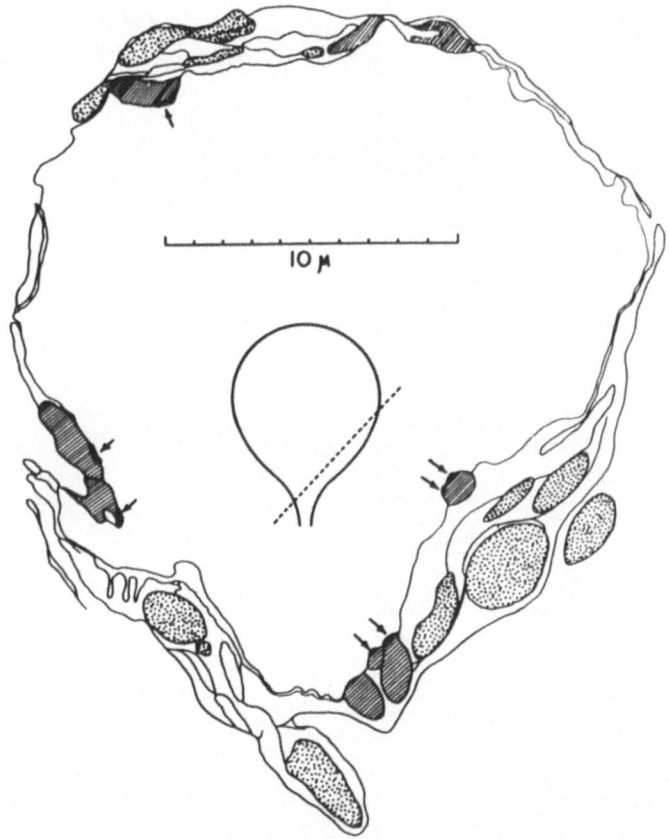

Figure 1. Outline of a section of toad sympathetic ganglion cell and its presynaptic endings. Hatched parts represent presynaptic knobs attached to the ganglion cell. Arrows indicate area of dense synaptic membranes. Stippled parts represent presynaptic fibers and knobs. The latter's attachment to the ganglion cell was intervened by Schwann cytoplasm. The inset illustrates the most probable direction of section (dotted line) made to the ganglion cell. Scale: 10 μm shown with 1-μm interval marks. (From Nishi *et al.*, 1967.)

In synapses which have a relatively large circumference in the section plane, approximately 1/5–1/3 of the pre- and postsynaptic membranes, show increased density (Figure 2A). The width of the cleft, which is approximately 200 Å, seems to be almost uniform in all synapses in an amphibian ganglion. Almost all vesicles in the knobs are nongranulated, having a mean diameter of 500 Å, and tend to be concentrated behind the region of increased density of the pre- and postsynaptic approximation (Figure 2A, B). Small numbers of vesicles are granulated and confined mainly to the proximal part of the

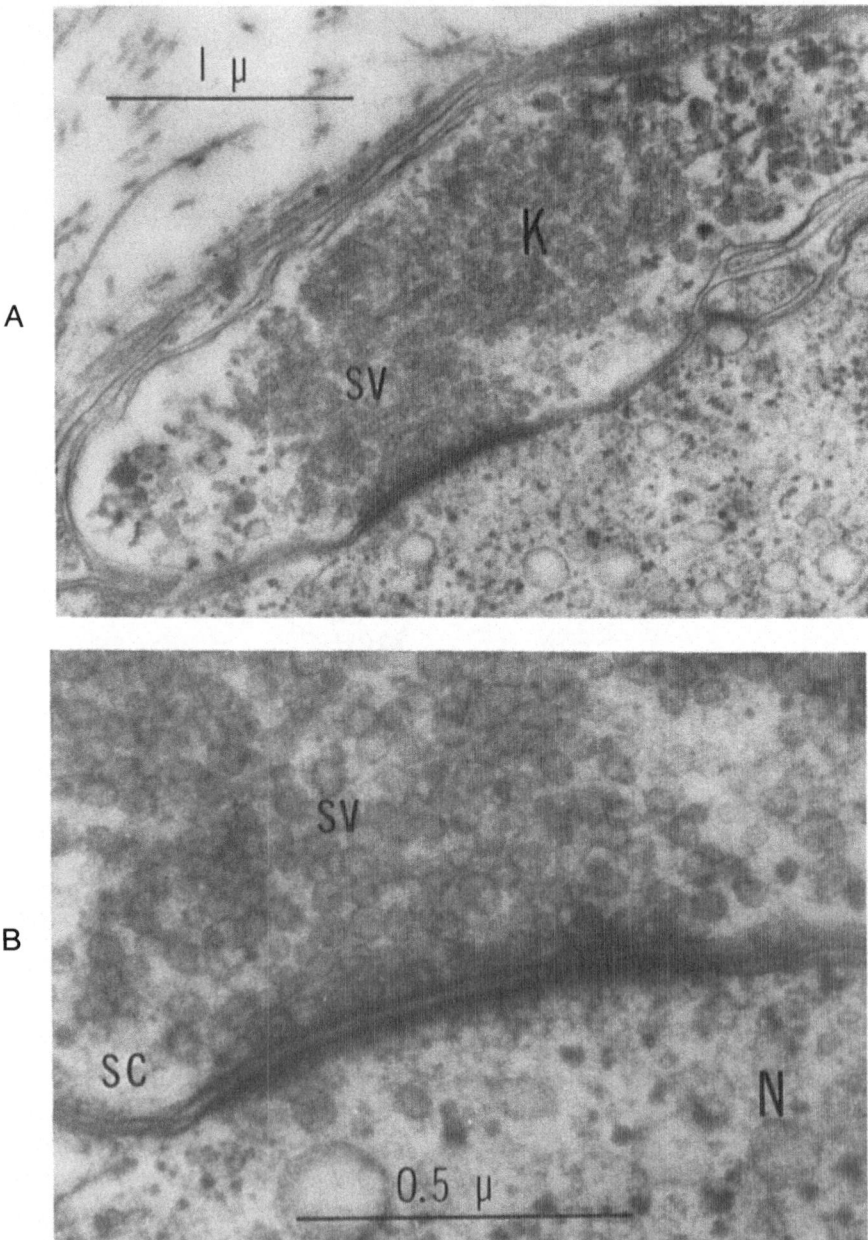

Figure 2. A: Electron micrograph showing a presynaptic knob (K) terminating on a toad sympathetic ganglion cell (N). SV, synaptic vesicles. B: A higher magnification of the junctional area in A. N, postsynaptic neuron; SV, synaptic vesicles; SC, synaptic cleft. (From Nishi *et al.*, 1967.)

knobs and do not appear close to the increased density area of the presynaptic membrane (Figure 2A).

In addition to the typical large ganglion cells, small (6–12 μm in diameter), granule-containing cells are found in the sympathetic ganglion (Siegrist *et al.*, 1966; Grillo, 1966; Fujimoto, 1967; Williams, 1967*a, b;* Elfvin, 1968; Matthews and Raisman, 1968, 1969; Jacobowitz, 1970). The granule-containing cells occur in small clusters (Figure 3A) which lie singly or in groups (Fujimoto, 1967; Matthews and Raisman, 1969). These cells appear, by general structure and location, to be identical (Siegrist *et al.*, 1966; Matthews and Raisman, 1969; Williams, 1967*b*) with the small, intensely fluorescent chromaffin-like cells that were reported by Norberg and Hamberger (1964). The important feature of these chromaffin-like cells is the possession of both afferent and efferent synaptic contacts (Figure 3B). Processes containing many nongranulated (probably cholinergic) vesicles establish specialized contacts with the chromaffin-like cells, which are regarded as afferent synapses. In addition the chromaffin-like cells or their processes show areas of specialized contact with other profiles, which are interpreted as being efferent synapses. Based on these findings Matthews and Raisman (1969) proposed that the small granule-containing cells are capable of acting as interneurons within the ganglion.

B. Functional Aspects

It is generally accepted that the transmission of impulses at ganglionic synapses is chemical and that the principal transmitter is ACh. Some avian ganglia are, however, capable of performing chemical as well as electrical transmission (Martin and Pilar, 1963*a, b*). Recent electrophysiological and pharmacological investigations revealed that many sympathetic ganglion cells possess nicotinic, muscarinic (Eccles and Libet, 1961; Volle and Koelle, 1961; Volle, 1962*a*), and noncholinergic (Nishi and Koketsu, 1968*a*; Chen, 1969, 1971, 1972; Alkadhi and McIsaac, 1971) excitatory postsynaptic sites, as well as adrenergic inhibitory postsynaptic site (Eccles and Libet, 1961). Thus, the prevailing concept that the pre- and postsynaptic elements in autonomic ganglia form a simple excitatory synapse of nicotinic nature is no longer valid.

In response to the ACh liberated from the presynaptic nerve terminals, the subsynaptic nicotinic site generates an excitatory postsynaptic potential (EPSP), which resembles in many respects the end-plate potential of skeletal muscle, and is blocked by common ganglionic blocking agents. Normally, this EPSP plays an essential role in impulse transmission at the ganglion and

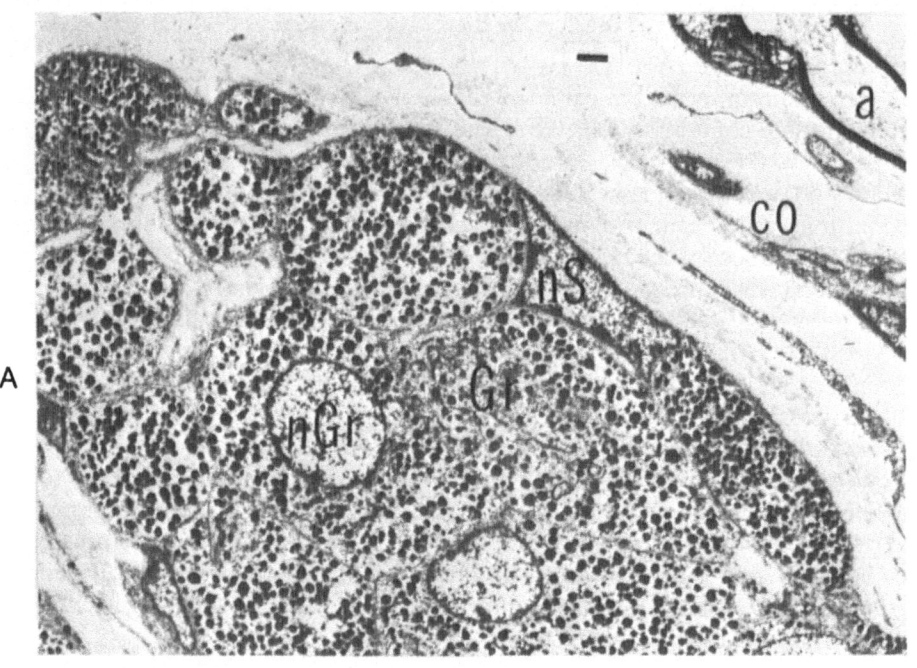

A

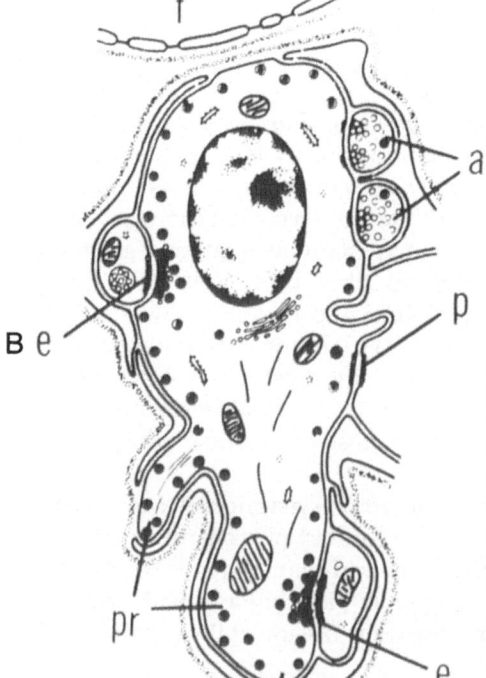

B

Figure 3. A: A cluster of the granular cells (Gr) in the sympathetic ganglion of the toad. The cytoplasm of the granular cells is filled with large numbers of electron dense granules. nS, nucleus of the satellite cell; nGr, nucleus of the granular cell; a, axon; Co, collagen matrix. (× 4400.) (From Fujimoto, 1967.) B: A small granule-containing chromaffin-like cell in the superior cervical ganglion of the rat: a, afferent synapses; e, efferent synapses; f, fenestrated capillaries; p, attachment plaques; pr, cytoplasmic prolongations. (From Matthews and Raisman, 1969.)

is now referred to as the "fast" EPSP in order to differentiate it from the slow
EPSP (see below) of ganglion cells. The extracellularly recorded counterpart
of the fast EPSP has been called the N wave (Eccles and Libet, 1961). The
liberated ACh also activates the muscarinic site on ganglion cells and elicits a
slow postsynaptic depolarization, the slow EPSP, which is selectively blocked
by atropine. Its extracellular counterpart is named the late negative (LN)
wave (Eccles and Libet, 1961). A noncholinergic substance, which has not yet
been chemically identified, is also liberated by presynaptic volleys and generates an extremely long-lasting postsynaptic depolarization. This response
was first found in bullfrog paravertebral sympathetic ganglia by Nishi and
Koketsu (1968a) and termed as the late slow EPSP, or the late late negative
(LLN) wave for its extracellular counterpart. Its existence has also been recognized in the mammalian ganglia by Chen (1969, 1971, 1972) and Alkadhi
and McIsaac (1971). The slow and late slow EPSPs, when induced by repetitive stimuli, trigger the afterdischarges of ganglion cells (Nishi and Koketsu,
1968a).

The inhibitory system in the sympathetic ganglion has been postulated
to be disynaptic and mediated by the intraganglionic chromaffin-like cells
which liberate an adrenergic substance (Eccles and Libet, 1961). The adrenergic substance activates the inhibitory postsynaptic site on ganglion cells
which is alpha-adrenoceptive in nature and induces a slow inhibitory postsynaptic potential (slow IPSP; Eccles and Libet, 1961). Its extracellular
counterpart is called the positive (P) wave. The slow IPSP is in general too
small to counteract the fast EPSP, but it can effectively suppress both the slow
and late slow EPSPs and thereby decreases the afterdischarges of ganglion
cells (Koketsu and Nishi, 1967; Nishi and Koketsu, 1968a).

Recent investigations demonstrated that the preganglionic nerve terminals are endowed with cholinoceptive (Koketsu and Nishi, 1968; Ginsborg,
1971), as well as adrenoceptive, sites (Nishi, 1970; Christ and Nishi, 1971a, b;
Dun and Nishi, 1974), which directly and indirectly influence the liberation
of transmitter. For example, the activation of the presynaptic adrenoceptive
site by a catecholamine induces a depression of ganglionic transmission
which is much greater than that elicited by its postsynaptic hyperpolarizing
action (Nishi, 1970; Christ and Nishi, 1971a; Dun and Nishi, 1974).

The sympathetic ganglion thus seems now to be more complex than considered hitherto, and these newly discovered properties reflect the intricacy
and flexibility of its functional role as a center of the peripheral autonomic
function.

In contrast to the recent advance in the study of sympathetic ganglia,
the neurons in parasympathetic ganglia have been scarcely investigated, and
most of their synaptic functions are very poorly understood. This is because
parasympathetic ganglia are not readily accessible for electrical recording.
There are, in fact, only a few anatomically recognizable parasympathetic

ganglia which are deeply located in the head, and all other parasympathetic ganglia are scattered diffusely throughout the effector organs. In addition, synaptic transmission at both the parasympathetic ganglia and neuroeffector junctions is cholinergic. Drugs possessing a cholinomimetic or cholinolytic property may influence the two junctional sites, thereby complicating the analysis of ganglionic function with pharmacological agents.

II. POSTSYNAPTIC RECEPTOR SITES

A. Excitatory Cholinoceptive Sites

1. Nicotinic Site

a. Synaptic Response and Its Functional Role. Upon arrival of an impulse, the small nonmyelinated terminal boutons of preganglionic nerve fibers liberate packets of ACh from their storage sites. The liberated ACh diffuses across the synaptic cleft and impinges on the subsynaptic membrane which is thought to be the site of receptors susceptible to the nicotinic action of ACh. The resulting interaction between ACh and the receptor sites greatly increases the ionic permeability of the subsynaptic membrane, and gives rise to a local graded depolarization of the ganglion cell membrane. The amplitude of this depolarization, namely the fast EPSP, is dependent upon the amount of liberated ACh and the number of individual synapses activated. As the synapses of mammalian ganglion cells are mainly of axodendritic type (Elfvin, 1963), the EPSP spreads electrotonically along the dendrites to the soma, where an all-or-none propagating impulse is generated as soon as the tonically spreading EPSP is large enough to excite the soma membrane. The impulse so generated at the soma conducts along the axon down to the postganglionic nerve terminals.

b. Pattern of Innervation. The nicotinic sites of a mammalian superior cervical ganglion cell receive a multiterminal and polyneuronal innervation. Indeed as seen in Figure 4, a maximal presynaptic stimulus applied away from the ganglion induces multiple synaptic potentials owing to the difference in conduction time of each innervating fiber, and lowering the stimulus strength reduces the number of synaptic potentials (Erulkar and Woodward, 1968). The conduction velocities of the several components of the cat cervical preganglionic nerve trunk are $18-25$ (S_1), $10-12$ (S_2), $7-10$ (S_3) and $1-5$ (S_4) m/sec (Eccles, 1935); S_1-S_3 groups belong to the B-type nerve and S_4 to the

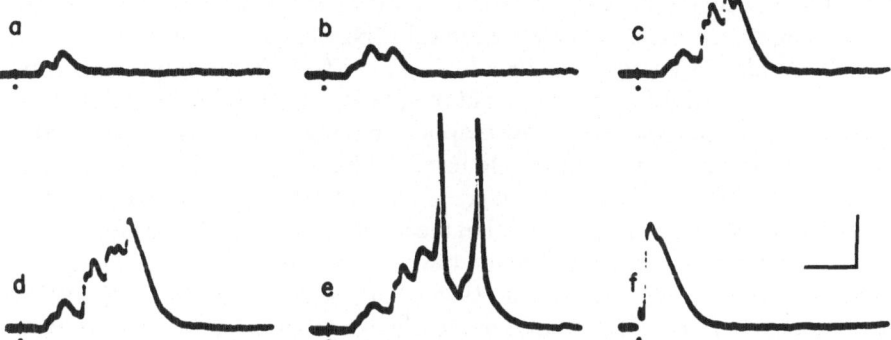

Figure 4. Fast EPSPs of a rabbit superior cervical ganglion cell induced by single preganglionic stimuli (dots) which were applied 4 cm (a–e) and 6 mm (f) away from the cell. Relative stimulus intensities: 1.0 (a), 1.5 (b), 2.8 (c), 3.9 (d), and 5.2 (e and f). Stimulus duration: 0.1 msec. Calibrations: 20 mV and 20 msec.

C-type nerve. Shaw *et al.* (1951) have shown that the relative degrees of blockade of the impulse transmission via S_1 group to the nictitating membrane and via S_2 to the blood vessels in the ear differed in intensity and duration with different blocking compounds. Volle (1962a) has observed that the postganglionic response to stimulation of the preganglionic fibers with the highest conduction velocity and lowest threshold is the most resistant to modification by drugs.

In contrast to the superior cervical ganglion cells, the neurons in the stellate (Bronk, 1939; Larrabee and Posternak, 1952) and the inferior splanchnic ganglia (Lloyd, 1937, 1939) receive only one main fiber type belonging to the B group. The neurons in lumbar sympathetic ganglia are innervated by a variety of B and C fibers (Obrador and Odoritz, 1936). The ciliary (parasympathetic) ganglion consists of a large number of B-type neurons which have myelinated axons and a small number of C-type neurons which have nonmyelinated axons. The B neurons are innervated exclusively by preganglionic B fibers, while the C neurons are innervated by preganglionic C fibers (Nishi and Christ, 1971). Such a characteristic pattern of innervation of the ciliary ganglion is quite similar to that of the amphibian sympathetic ganglia (Nishi *et al.*, 1965). Furthermore, many ciliary neurons receive only one or two presynaptic fibers. The B-type neurons of amphibian sympathetic ganglion cells are very specific in this respect; all the nicotinic sites of a single neuron are innervated by a single presynaptic B fiber. This is a typical multiterminal and unineuronal innervation. The fast EPSP in these neurons never shows multiple peaks and appears in an all-or-none manner, if its small random fluctuation in amplitude is disregarded.

On the other hand the pattern of innervation of C ganglion cells is similar to that of mammalian ciliary ganglion cells (Nishi *et al.*, 1965).

c. Mode of Generation of Impulse by Fast EPSP. In the amphibian sympathetic ganglion cells, the threshold membrane potential for the initiation of the orthodromic spike response is approximately -40 mV which is usually 10–20 mV lower than the threshold level for the soma membrane excitation (Nishi and Koketsu, 1960). This difference suggests that the synaptic potential initially evokes the action potential of the axon hillock and the proximal part of the axon where threshold may be lower, as has been proposed for spinal motoneurons (Araki and Otani, 1955; Fatt, 1957; Fuortes *et al.*, 1957; Coombs *et al.*, 1957*a*, *b*). A similar mode of spike generation was also found in both B and C neurons of the cat ciliary ganglion (Nishi and Christ, 1971). In the rabbit superior cervical ganglion cells, however, the synaptically evoked spike seems to arise anywhere from the soma–dendritic membrane and not specifically from the axon hillock and/or the proximal part of the axon (Eccles, 1963).

Although mammalian ganglion cells are able to fire at a high rate (80–170 Hz) in response to direct intracellular stimulation (Blackman and Purves, 1969; Crowcroft and Szurszewski, 1971; Nishi and North, 1973), they are incapable of responding with such a high rate to repetitive preganglionic stimulation. For example, the superior cervical ganglion cells of the rabbit respond faithfully to preganglionic volleys at 35 Hz or less; these cells show at most only abortive spike responses except for the first spike when stimulus frequencies are greater than 35 Hz (Eccles, 1955). However, even at a frequency of 160 Hz, a small synaptic potential appears following each preganglionic volley, indicating that some preganglionic fibers are capable of responding to this frequency (Eccles, 1955).

d. Synaptic Delay and Time Course of Fast EPSP. Classical experiments showed that the synaptic delay for the fast EPSP in the mammalian sympathetic ganglia is 1–2 msec (Brown, 1934) or 0.5–4 msec (Eccles, 1936). These values were obtained from the estimated arrival time of an impulse at the presynaptic nerve terminals and the onset time of the postsynaptic depolarization. A recent experiment on single superior cervical ganglion cells of the rabbit (Christ and Nishi, 1971*b*) showed that the synaptic delay measured between the time of direct stimulation of presynaptic terminals and the onset of the fast EPSP is 1.5–2.0 msec. The values obtained with a similar method from toad B and C sympathetic ganglion cells are 1.6 msec and 2.6 msec, respectively (Nishi and Soeda, unpublished observations).

The fast EPSP recorded from the surface of curarized mammalian superior cervical ganglion shows a peak time of about 10 msec and a decay half-time of 60–90 msec (Eccles, 1943). This time course is much slower than that of the intracellularly recorded fast EPSP, which shows a peak time of about

4 msec and a decay half-time of about 4 msec (Eccles, 1955). The slowness of the surface records is probably a result of summation and fusion of the fast EPSPs dispersed temporally by the difference in conduction velocity of presynaptic fibers. Perri *et al.* (1970) reported that the average time constant of decay of the fast EPSP is 6.7 msec in rat superior cervical neurons, and the corresponding value is 8.5 msec in guinea pig superior cervical neurons. They found that the time constant of EPSP decay is much larger than that of the electrotonic potential of cell membrane, with the difference of 148% in the rat and 93% in the guinea pig.

Because of the much simpler geometrical feature of amphibian sympathetic neurons, which are spherical and devoid of dendrites, comparison of the EPSP and membrane time constants can be made more accurately in these neurons than in mammalian neurons (Nishi and Koketsu, 1960). In toad sympathetic ganglion cells, the fast EPSP declines with an exponential time course having an average time constant of 10.4 msec for the B neurons and 13.9 msec for the C neurons. These values are 1.3 (B neurons) to 2 times (C neurons) larger than the membrane time constant, suggesting that the decay of the fast EPSP is slowed down by a residual transmitter action which probably results from some diffusional barriers or a lower activity of acetylcholinesterase (AChE) at the strategic sites.

e. Membrane Current During Activation of Nicotinic Sites. When one comes to consider the synaptic events responsible for the fast EPSP, it is evident that the decreased charge on the ganglion cell membrane must be caused by an electric current inwardly directed across the activated nicotinic subsynaptic membrane and outwardly directed across the remainder of the cell membrane, so depolarizing it. Since the amphibian sympathetic neurons are unipolar with the synaptic boutons confined chiefly to the lower hemisphere of the soma, a direct recording of synaptic current of these neurons can be made accurately by a voltage-clamp technique (Kuba and Nishi, 1971). In Figure 5, the nicotinic excitatory postsynaptic current (fast EPSC) as so determined is shown in comparison with the fast EPSP which was recorded in the same cell before clamping the membrane potential. The synaptic current rises rapidly, reaching its summit much earlier than that of EPSP, while it shows a slow decline which is still observable during the early phase of potential decay. This residual flow of synaptic current may explain the slower falling phase of the fast EPSP than expected from the membrane time constant (Nishi and Koketsu, 1960). Thus the activation of nicotinic receptor site by the liberated ACh is impulsive at its beginning and declines relatively slowly with a decay half-time of approximately 4 msec.

f. Ionic Permeability During Active State. Figure 6 shows the typical relationship between the peak amplitude of fast EPSP and the initial membrane potential obtained from two amphibian (*Rana pipiens*) sympathetic

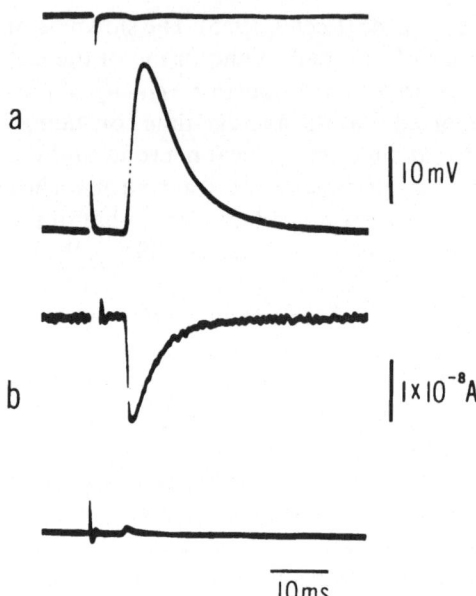

a

b

|10mV

|1×10⁻⁸A

10ms

Figure 5. Fast EPSP (a) and the associated membrane current (EPSC) (b)
recorded from a bullfrog sympathetic
ganglion cell. Both the EPSP and EPSC
were induced at a hyperpolarized level
of the membrane potential at which the
EPSP failed to trigger an action potential. Upper trace: membrane current.
Lower trace: membrane potential.

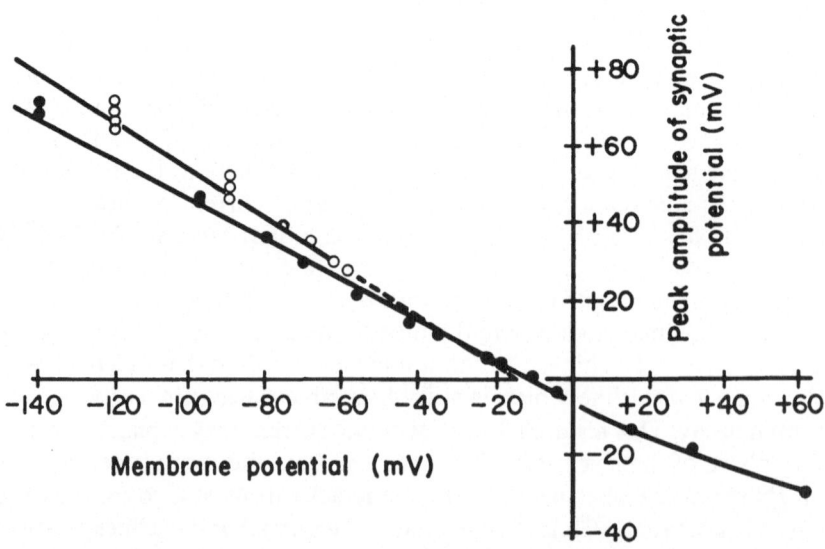

Figure 6. Relationship between peak amplitude of fast EPSP (ordinate) and initial level of membrane potential (abscissa) of two cells in frog sympathetic ganglion. Membrane potential was
altered by delivering long hyperpolarizing or depolarizing currents through the cell membrane.
Open circles plotted from EPSP of one cell, while closed circles obtained from another cell.
(From Nishi and Koketsu, 1960.)

ganglion cells. The amplitude of fast EPSP is increased by increasing the membrane potential. When the membrane is progressively depolarized, the synaptic potential is reduced accordingly and finally reverses when depolarization exceeds a certain level; the deflection of EPSP is always directed toward the level at which it is nullified. The relationship between the amplitude of fast EPSP and the displacement of the membrane potential is almost linear over a wide extent; in the two cases shown in Figure 6, the EPSP is zero at about -10 mV, which is thus the equilibrium potential for the ionic mechanisms that produce it. The mean value of this equilibrium potential for frog sympathetic ganglion cells is -14 mV (range -8 to -20 mV) (Nishi and Koketsu, 1960). Similar experiments on the fast EPSPs of toad sympathetic ganglion cells indicate that the equilibrium potential is about -10 mV for B neurons and -6 mV for C neurons (Nishi et al., 1965). In the B neurons of bullfrog sympathetic ganglia, the fast EPSC equilibrium potential which was determined by a voltage-clamp technique is -9.4 ± 7.0 mV (SD, $n = 27$; Kuba and Nishi, unpublished observations). The fast EPSP of rabbit superior cervical ganglion cells shows the equilibrium potential of -10 to -15 mV (Nishi and Tashiro, unpublished observations). A much lower value (-30 mV) has been reported for cat superior cervical ganglion cells (Skok, 1968).

In amphibian sympathetic ganglion cells, the equilibrium potential of the fast EPSP is not altered when the perfusing Ringer solution is changed to a Cl-free solution (Nishi and Koketsu, 1967; Koketsu, 1969). A decrease in the external Na concentration shifts the equilibrium potential toward the resting potential. An increase or decrease in the K concentration shifts the equilibrium potential toward zero or resting potential level, respectively. These findings imply that the fast EPSP is generated by an increased Na and K conductance of the subsynaptic membrane, as in the case of the end-plate potential (Takeuchi and Takeuchi, 1960). The ratio of the increased Na and K conductance ($\Delta G_{Na}/\Delta G_{K}$) of the activated ganglionic nicotinic membrane appears to be $1.99-1.69$ in rabbit superior cervical neurons whose Na and K equilibrium potentials have been estimated to be $+33.6$ mV and -96.9 mV (Woodward et al., 1969). This ratio is considerably larger than that (1.23) of the activated end-plate membrane (Takeuchi and Takeuchi, 1960).

g. Activation of Nicotinic Receptors by Exogenous ACh. Iontophoretic application of ACh from a micropippette to the surface of an amphibian ganglion cell (Figure 7A) produces a depolarization of the cell membrane (Figure 7B) which is composed of a fast (fast ACh potential) and a slow (slow ACh potential) component resembling, electrophysiologically and pharmacologically, the fast and slow EPSPs (see below), respectively (Koketsu et al., 1968; Nishi et al., 1969b). The fast ACh potential is selectively blocked by d-tubocurarine, hexamethonium, or nicotine, while the slow ACh potential is selectively blocked by atropine. Apparently, the fast and slow ACh potentials are generated respectively at the nicotinic and muscarinic receptor sites.

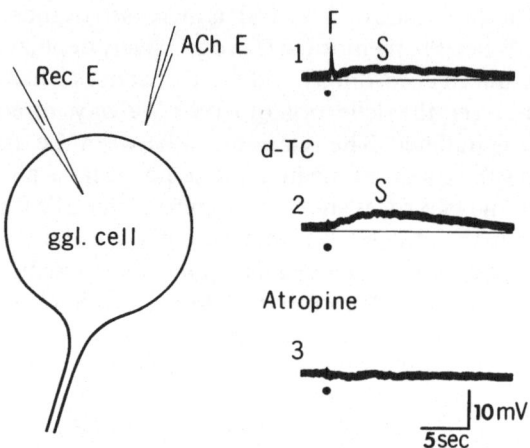

Figure 7. Fast (F) and slow (S) ACh potentials (record 1) evoked by iontophoretic application of ACh to a bullfrog sympathetic ganglion cell. The strength of iontophoretic pulses (marked by dots) was 5×10^{-7} A with a duration of 15 msec. d-Tubocurarine (0.015 mM) was given 3 min before record 2 was taken, and atropine (0.0014 mM) was added 5 min before record 3 was taken. The scheme illustrates a superficially located ganglion cell and the position of recording and ACh-containing microelectrodes. (From Koketsu *et al.*, 1968.)

Figure 8A and B show the fast ACh potential and the fast EPSP obtained from a single cell in which the membrane potential was altered stepwise in a range between -150 and $+60$ mV. When the cell membrane was hyperpolarized, the ACh potential usually showed a greater increment than the fast EPSP (Figure 8C). However, the reversal levels of both the fast ACh potential and EPSP were found to be identical (Nishi *et al.*, 1969b).

The peak time of the fast ACh potentials ranged from 15 to 500 msec. In the cells most sensitive to the applied ACh, a brief (about 1 msec) current pulse of 6×10^{-6} C produced a fast ACh potential of 10 mV which rose to a peak within 15 msec; the quantity of ACh released in these cases was estimated to be approximately 1.8×10^{-5} moles, on the assumption that the transport number of ACh is approximately 0.3. It was also estimated that the distance between the tip of the ACh micropipette and the idealized point ACh receptor was about 10 μm by assuming the diffusion coefficient of ACh to be 8×10^{-6} cm^2/sec (del Castillo and Katz, 1955). Application of ACh from an ACh pipette in close contact with the outer edge (proximal surface) of superficially located cells evoked the fast ACh potentials having peak times between 80–150 msec or no response at all. Such long peak times and the occasional failure of evoking the response indicate that the ordinary cell-body membrane is not responsible for production of the fast ACh potential. The peak times of

80–150 msec of evoked responses yield the distances (r) between the tip of ACh pipette and the nicotinic receptors of approximately 20–27 μm. Based on both the calculated r values and the localization of nicotinic receptors in the lower hemisphere of the ganglion cells, the large peak times must be caused by diffusion of ACh to the distal surface of the cells. This is additional evidence

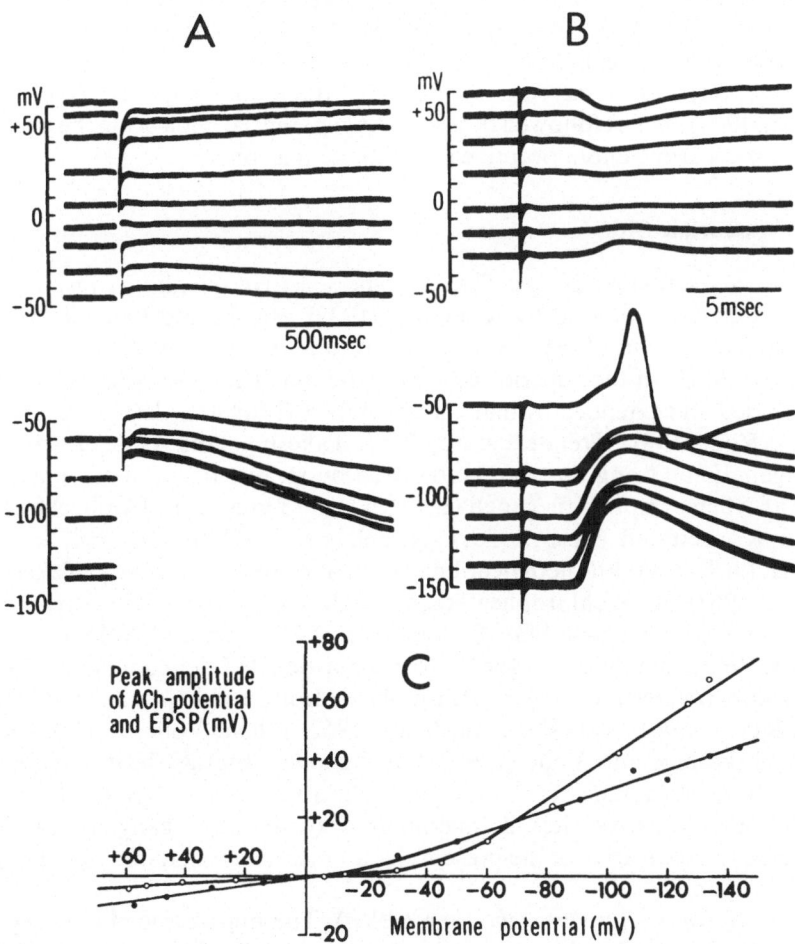

Figure 8. Fast ACh potentials (A) and fast EPSP (B) of a bullfrog sympathetic ganglion cell set up at various levels of membrane potential. The original resting membrane potential was −60 mV; other membrane potential levels were obtained by application of electric currents through one barrel of a double-barreled microelectrode. C: Relationship between peak amplitude of ACh potentials (open circles) and EPSP (closed circles) and displacement of membrane potential. (From Nishi *et al.*, 1969*b*.)

to support the idea that the subsynaptic nicotinic receptors are responsible for generation of both the fast ACh potential and fast EPSP.

The fast ACh potential induced in the rabbit superior cervical ganglion cells is in general similar to that of amphibian sympathetic ganglion cells (Nishi, 1970; Christ and Nishi, 1971a). However, its rates of rise and fall are much smaller than those of amphibian ganglion cells. This is probably owing to the dendritic distribution of nicotinic receptors (subsynaptic membranes, Elfvin, 1963). Unlike the sympathetic ganglion cells, the majority of ciliary (parasympathetic) ganglion cells of the cat (Christ and Nishi, unpublished observation) and the myenteric neurons of the guinea pig ileum (Nishi and North, 1973) are not followed by a slow ACh potential, indicating the absence of the muscarinic cholinoceptive site in these neurons.

2. Muscarinic Site

a. Activation by Drugs. The atropine-sensitive ganglionic response to drugs was first reported by Koppanyi (1932). He showed that pilocarpine caused contraction of the nicitating membrane of the cat when injected into the circulation of the superior cervical ganglion. This observation has been confirmed and extended by many investigators (Marrazzi, 1939b; Ambache, 1949; Root, 1951; Trendelenburg, 1954; Takeshige and Volle, 1964). The postganglionic firing that can be blocked by minute doses of atropine also occurs when sympathetic ganglia are exposed to muscarine (Ambache *et al.,* 1956; Konzett and Waser, 1956; Gyermek *et al.,* 1963; Jones, 1963; Sanghvi *et al.,* 1963), acetyl-β-methylcholine (Pappano and Volle, 1962; Takeshige *et al.,* 1963), 4-(m-chlorophenylcarbamoyloxy)-2-butynyl-trimethylammonium chloride (McN-A-343) (Roszkowski, 1961; Levy and Ahlquist, 1962; Jones, 1963; Sanghvi *et al.,* 1963), oxotremorine (De Groat and Volle, 1963), or an anticholinesterase agent (Hilton, 1961; Long and Eckstein, 1961; Volle and Koelle, 1961; Takeshige and Volle, 1962, 1963a; Volle, 1962b). Moreover, Takeshige and Volle (1962, 1963b) showed that ACh, in contrast to these drugs, is capable of activating both the atropine-sensitive and the hexamethonium-sensitive sites in mammalian sympathetic ganglia. All these findings are indicative of the presence of a muscarinic excitatory site in sympathetic ganglia.

b. Synaptic Response (the slow EPSP). The muscarinic cholinoceptive site can be activated by preganglionic impulses. Eccles and Libet (1961) demonstrated that a long-lasting, surface negative (the late negative, LN) synaptic potential which is sensitive to blockade by atropine can be recorded following suitable orthodromic stimulation of curarized sympathetic ganglia. It was found later (Libet, 1964) that uncurarized ganglia are also capable of producing the LN response, and that the LN response in such ganglia contributes postsynaptically to the well-known, long-lasting posttetanic potentiation of orthodromic responses as described by Larrabee and Bronk (1947).

Using intracellular recording in curarized ganglia of both frog and rabbit, Tosaka and Libet (1965) and Libet and Tosaka (1966) showed that the LN wave is in fact a depolarizing postsynaptic response. It was also demonstrated that an atropine-sensitive facilitation of orthodromic discharges of ganglion cells roughly matched the time course and amplitude of the LN response (Libet, 1964). The LN wave has since been referred to as the slow excitatory postsynaptic potential (slow EPSP) (Libet, 1967).

The slow EPSP can be recorded from the majority of neurons in the rabbit superior cervical ganglion and from the majority of B and C neurons in the bullfrog sympathetic ganglia (Figure 9a). In case of the latter preparation, the preganglionic B nerve alone should be stimulated to record the slow EPSP, since the slow EPSP as well as the late slow EPSP (the intracellular counterpart of LLN wave; see below) would be evoked when both the preganglionic B and C nerves were stimulated (cf. Figure 9e) (Nishi and Koketsu, 1968a).

The slow EPSP has a latency of 100–400 msec and may last more than 20 sec after a tetanic (10–50 Hz) train of stimuli lasting for 1–5 sec (Libet, 1967; Libet et al., 1968; Nishi and Koketsu, 1968a). This large synaptic delay had been explained earlier (Eccles and Libet, 1961; Libet, 1967) by the concept that the liberated ACh might have taken a long time to diffuse to the muscarinic (LN) postsynaptic sites on the ganglion cell. However, with the iontophoretic application of ACh to the very close vicinity of a ganglion cell, Koketsu et al. (1968) have shown that there is a similar time lag for the onset of the atropine-sensitive slow depolarization (slow ACh potential) of the ganglion cell. This implies that the large synaptic delay of the slow EPSP is due mainly to a postsynaptic process underlying the initiation of the slow EPSP. The amplitude of the slow EPSP varies considerably (5–25 mV) from cell to cell in both frog and rabbit ganglia, indicating that the area occupied by the muscarinic postsynaptic receptors also differs between individual cells.

c. *Electrogenesis of slow EPSP.* The slow EPSP does not behave like a postsynaptic depolarization generated by an increased ion permeability. Libet and Kobayashi (1968, 1969; see also Kobayashi and Libet, 1968, 1970) found no decrease in membrane resistance during the slow EPSP in frog or rabbit ganglion cells. Actually there is an increase in membrane resistance in the frog ganglion cells. Similarly, the depolarization elicited by the muscarinic action of ACh is accompanied by no appreciable change in membrane resistance in curarized rabbit cells and by an increase in membrane resistance in nicotinized frog cells. (Libet and Kobayashi, 1969; Kobayashi and Libet, 1970). In frog ganglion cells, the slow EPSP is enhanced by moderate depolarization of 10–20 mV, and it is depressed by moderate hyperpolarization of

10–20 mV (Kobayashi and Libet, 1968; Libet and Kobayashi, 1968), the reverse of the findings for the fast EPSP. In contrast to the slow EPSP in frog cells, the slow EPSP in rabbit cells is depressed by depolarization and enhanced by moderate hyperpolarization of 10–15 mV. However, even in these cells, stronger hyperpolarization of 20–30 mV depresses and abolishes the slow EPSP even though the fast EPSP is appropriately enhanced under these conditions (Kobayashi and Libet, 1968).

Nishi *et al.* (1969a) found in frog ganglia that the effect of changes in membrane potential on the slow EPSP differs considerably between cells. For example, hyperpolarization of the cell membrane (by approximately 30 mV) causes either a decrease, an increase, or even no change in size of the slow EPSP, depending upon the individual cell. However, the membrane current associated with the slow EPSP (slow EPSC), which can be obtained by a manually controlled voltage-clamp method (cf. Nishi *et al.*, 1969a), shows in most cells a decrease during hyperpolarization and an increase during depolarization (10–15 mV). The increase of membrane resistance during the slow EPSP is found only when the cell membrane is depolarized. Nishi *et al.* (1969a) also found that the size of the slow EPSP and EPSC are not appreciably altered when the external K concentration is reduced to $\frac{1}{10}$ or when the external NaCl concentration is lowered to $\frac{1}{2}$.

Kobayashi and Libet (1968) showed that metabolic inhibitors such as dinitrophenol, azide, and anoxia all depress the slow EPSP preferentially over the fast EPSP and slow IPSP (the intracellular counterpart of the P wave, see below). They also demonstrated that the slow EPSP is not specifically depressed by ouabain, K-free Ringer or Cl-free Ringer, or by iontophoretic reduction of the intracellular Cl ions. Kobayashi and Libet then proposed that the slow EPSP is probably generated by a metabolically based electrogenic mechanism, but one other than the electrogenic Na pump or Cl pump.

An alternative hypothesis that the slow EPSP is caused by a synaptic inactivation of K conductance of the postsynaptic membrane was suggested by Weight and Votava (1970). Their conclusion was based on the following results (Weight and Votava, 1970). Firstly, the size of the slow EPSP in frog ganglion cells varies inversely with the membrane potential. Secondly, the slow EPSP reverses from a depolarization to a hyperpolarization at a membrane potential close to K equilibrium potential. Thirdly, a significant decrease in membrane conductance is also found during the slow EPSP.

The results of Weight and Votava are not all in agreement with those of others (Kobayashi and Libet, 1968; Nishi *et al.*, 1969a). One of the crucial points is that the slow EPSP or its membrane current is not always associated with a decrease in membrane resistance (Nishi, *et al.*, 1969a). The other point is that a partial or total removal of the external K does not significantly affect the size of slow EPSP (Kobayashi and Libet, 1968; Nishi, *et al.*,

1969*a*). According to Weight and Votava (1970), the slow EPSP should be enhanced under such conditions. Furthermore, Nishi *et al.* (1969*a*) failed to observe the reversal of the slow EPSP.

Since the electrogenesis of the slow EPSP is still controversial, further investigation is required.

B. Excitatory Noncholinoceptive Site

1. Afterdischarge Mediated by a Noncholinergic Synaptic Mechanism

Nishi and Koketsu (1966, 1968*a*) studied the afterdischarge of the isolated bullfrog sympathetic ganglia with regard to its physiological and pharmacological nature and its relation to the slow postsynaptic potentials. They found that under normal conditions the afterdischarge of postganglionic fibers is elicited only when the preganglionic fibers are stimulated with a train of supramaximal pulses of relatively high frequency (50 Hz). The afterdischarge is enhanced and prolonged after nicotinization or curarization of the ganglion. The appearance of a weak afterdischarge in the physiological condition is ascribed to the presence of a prolonged posttetanic hyperpolarization which suppresses the triggering potentials. The afterdischarge elicited by tetanic stimulation of preganglionic B fibers in the presence of nicotine or *d*-tubocurarine (Figure 9b) is relatively short-lived (less than 1 min) and can be abolished by addition of atropine (Figure 9d). However, the afterdischarge triggered by tetanic B and C nerve stimulation (Figure 9f) is sustained for a much longer period (up to several min) and cannot be completely blocked by atropine in a high concentration. Its initial part is eliminated while its later part remains unaffected when atropine or ACh is added (Figure 9h). Thus it is evident that the afterdischarge has two different components. The component which is sensitive to atropine is termed the early afterdischarge (EAD), and that which is insensitive to atropine and ACh is termed the late afterdischarge (LAD). Recording of the deeply nicotinized or curarized ganglia with the sucrose-gap method of Kosterlitz *et al.* (1968) reveals that tetanic presynaptic B nerve stimulation produces only an atropine-sensitive slow depolarization (LN wave; the extracellular counterpart of the slow EPSP), while the tetanic presynaptic B and C nerve stimulation induces a large LN wave which is followed by an extremely long-lasting slow depolarization which is insensitive to atropine. The atropine-insensitive slow depolarization is termed the late late negative (LLN) wave. It is concluded that the EAD and LAD are respectively triggered by the LN response and the LLN response and the LLN wave is generated at a specific postsynaptic site in response to a noncholinergic transmitter substance which is released when the preganglionic stimulation is strong enough to stimulate the C fibers.

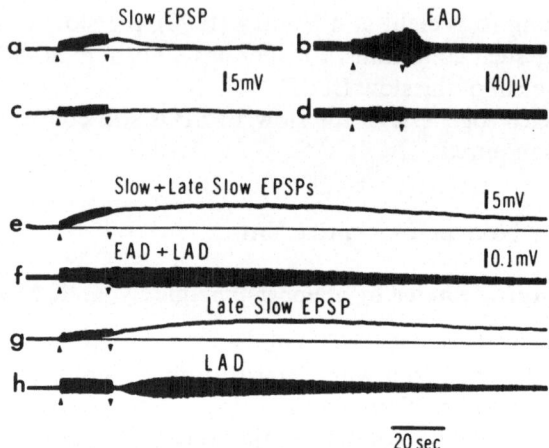

Figure 9. Intracellular slow depolarization and postganglionic afterdischarges obtained from nicotinized bullfrog sympathetic ganglia. Tetanic stimulation of preganglionic B fibers induces the slow EPSP (*a*) and the early afterdischarge (EAD) (*b*). Atropine (0.014 mM) abolishes both the slow EPSP (*c*) and EAD (*d*). Tetanic stimulation of preganglionic B and C fibers induces the slow EPSP plus the late slow EPSP (*e*) and the early and late afterdischarges (EAD + LAD) (*f*). Atropine (0.014 mM) depresses selectively the initial part (slow EPSP) of the postsynaptic depolarization and that (EAD) of the afterdischarge, leaving the late slow EPSP (*g*) and LAD (*h*). Both the slow and late slow EPSP were recorded intracellularly from the same B-type ganglion cell, and the afterdischarges were recorded extracellularly from a postganglionic branch. All recordings were made after ganglion preparations had been superfused with a nicotine-containing (0.12 mM) Ringer solution for over 30 min. Stimulation (marked by arrow) was 10 Hz for 20 sec in all records. (From Nishi and Koketsu, 1968*a*.)

2.   Late Slow EPSP and Its Electrogenesis

Several experimental facts support the synaptic origin of the LLN wave. The response can be recorded intracellularly from both B and C ganglion cells. The response in the presence of nicotine (or *d*-tubocurarine) and atropine is induced without any detectable preceding potential that could act as its generator. The response is reversibly abolished by Ca-free Ringer solution. The response, as will be mentioned below, is accompanied by an increased membrane conductance. For these reasons and because of its delayed onset (1–5 sec) and extremely prolonged time course (5–10 min), the response has been referred to as the late slow EPSP (Nishi and Koketsu, 1968*a*).

Unlike the slow EPSP, the late slow EPSP is always accompanied by a decrease in membrane resistance. This can be seen even when the late slow EPSP is nullified by delivering an anodal countercurrent through the intracellular recording electrode (Figure 10), indicating that the reduction of membrane resistance is not a result of the membrane depolarization (Nishi, 1973). The membrane current associated with the late slow EPSP (late slow EPSC) is enhanced when the membrane potential is increased and depressed when the membrane potential is decreased: The relationship between the amplitude of the late slow EPSC and membrane potential is almost linear, and the equilibrium potential obtained by extrapolation is approximately -35 mV. This level is not significantly altered by total replacement of the external Cl ions with glutamate ions, while it is shifted to the level of approximately -45 mV by reducing the external K concentration to $\frac{1}{10}$ or by reducing the external NaCl concentration to $\frac{1}{2}$. The results suggest that the late slow EPSP is produced by a slow and sustained permeability increase of the noncholinoceptive membrane to Na and K ions (Nishi, 1973).

3. The Noncholinergic Transmission in Mammalian Sympathetic Ganglia

Chen (1969, 1971, 1972) found in the superior cervical and lumbosacral ganglia of the dog a noncholinergic synaptic transmission. Using the contraction of the nicitating membrane and the retractor penis muscle as indicators, he demonstrated that tetanic preganglionic stimulation induces a biphasic response consisting of the early and late response in the ganglia

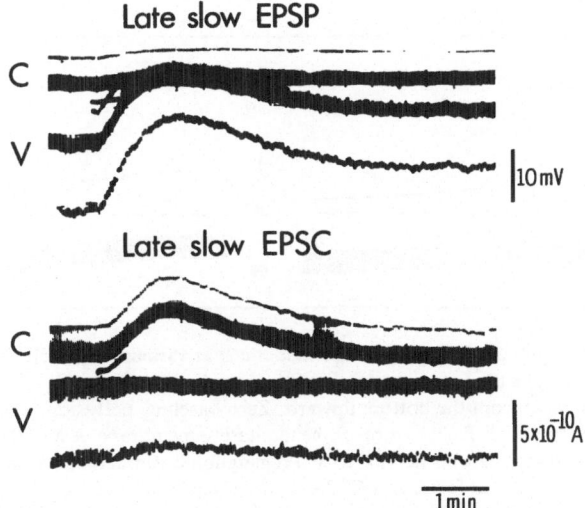

Figure 10. Late slow EPSP and the associated membrane current (late slow EPSP) recorded from a bullfrog sympathetic ganglion cell pretreated with nicotine (0.12 mM) and atropine (0.014 mM). Upper record: late slow EPSP superimposed by repetitive hyperpolarizing electrotonic potentials (trace V), and current pulses (trace C). Lower record: late slow EPSC superimposed by repetitive anodal current pulses (trace C) and electrotonic potentials (trace V). Both EPSP and EPSC were elicited by a train of tetanic stimuli (10 Hz) applied to preganglionic B and C fibers for 20 sec. Electrotonic potentials were induced by anodal current pulses (50 msec) delivered at 0.5 Hz (From Nishi, 1973.)

(Figure 11). Hexamethonium and tetraethylammonium selectively blocked the early response. The remaining late response was not affected by atropine and anticholinesterases. Obviously, this late response is quite different from the atropinesensitive late response of the superior cervical ganglion of the rabbit (Eccles and Libet, 1961; Libet, 1964) and the cat (Emmelin and Mac-Intosh, 1956; Volle, 1962a; Takeshige and Volle, 1962, 1964; Trendelenburg,

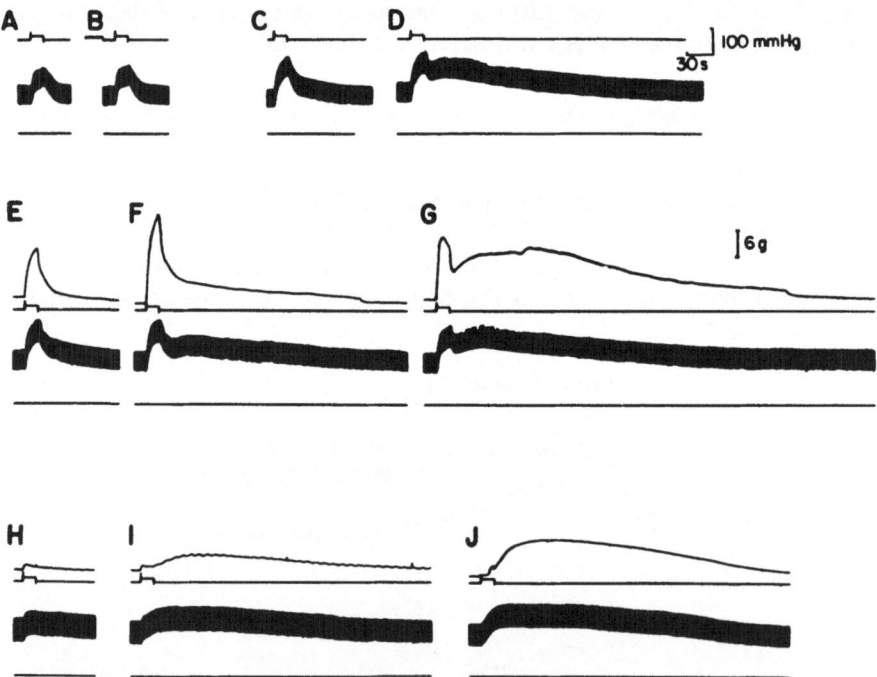

Figure 11. **Effect of pre- and postganglionic stimulations at various frequencies on the perfusion pressure of the ear and on the tension of the nictitating membrane.** All records were obtained from one dog. In each panel from the bottom upward: Zero baseline, perfusion pressure of the ear, event marker, and in panels E–J, tension of the nictitating membrane. A and B: postganglionic stimulation (the external carotid nerve). C–J: Preganglionic stimulation. Stimulus frequency: 3.75 Hz for E and H; 15 Hz for A and C; 30 Hz for F and I; and 120 Hz for B, D, G, and J. Between D and E atropine (1 mg/kg i.v.) was injected, and between G and H hexamethonium (13 mg/kg i.v.) was given. Panels H, I, and J were obtained 46, 21, and 4 min after hexamethonium, respectively. The duration of stimulation as indicated by the event marker was 15 sec. Calibrations in D for perfusion pressure and time and in G for tension of the nictitating membrane apply to all panels. Note that a high frequency stimulation of preganglionic nerve elicits a two-wave response comprised of early and late components in both the perfused ear (D) and the nictitating membrane (F and G), and that the late responses are resistent to atropine (F and G) and hexamethonium (I and J). (From Chen, 1972.)

1966; Brown, 1967), and the caudal cervical and stellate ganglia of the dog (Brown, 1967; Flacke and Gillis, 1968). It should be added, however, that Alkadhi and McIsaac (1971) have observed a noncholinergic late response in the cat superior cervical ganglion partially blocked by chlorisondamine.

Chen (1971) further observed that choline chloride restores only the early response, not the late response, of a ganglion which has been subjected to hemicholinium and prolonged preganglionic stimulation. Close arterial injection of KCl to the dog superior cervical ganglion also caused the early and late responses (Chen, 1974). The late response was quite similar in time course and pharmacological characteristics to the late response elicited by preganglionic stimulation but disappeared completely after a chronic preganglionic denervation.

All these findings are compatible with the idea that the late response of the superior cervical and lumbosacral ganglia of the dog is produced by a noncholinergic synaptic mechanism. The chemical transmitter responsible for this transmission is not known. However, it is certain that K ion is not directly involved. In addition to its direct depolarizing action, the injected KCl can activate the ganglion cells indirectly through the release of a noncholinergic substance from the presynaptic nerve terminals (Chen, 1974).

C.   Inhibitory Adrenoceptive Site

1.   Synaptic Activation and Response

The LN wave of a curarized sympathetic ganglion is always preceded by a positive (P) wave (Eccles, 1952; Eccles and Libet, 1961) (Figure 12a) which is preferentially depressed by dibenamine, an α-adrenoceptive blocking agent (Eccles and Libet, 1961), and by reserpine (Libet, 1962). Eccles and Libet (1961) postulated that an adrenergic substance liberated from the intraganglionic chromaffin cells encounters an α-adrenoceptive site on ganglion cells, and that this interaction results in hyperpolarization of the ganglion cell membrane—the P wave.

Intracellular recordings from curarized ganglia of both frog and rabbit support the hypothesis that the P wave is a hyperpolarizing postsynaptic potential, which can be generated in the absence of any cell discharge (Libet and Tosaka, 1966). The P wave has, therefore, been referred to as the slow IPSP. Although the depressant action of the slow IPSP on the excitability of mammalian ganglion cells has not been clearly shown, it has been demonstrated in frog sympathetic ganglia that a marked inhibition of afterdischarge occurs at the same time as the generation of P wave (Koketsu and Nishi, 1967). The slow IPSP (Figure 12b) induced by a train of preganglionic stimuli

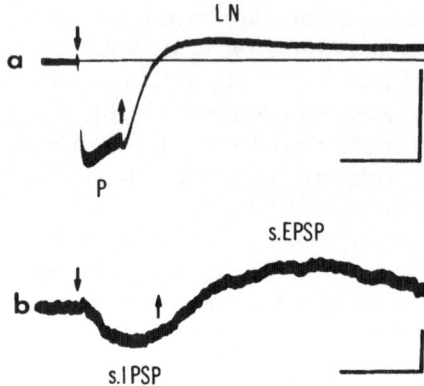

Figure 12. a: P and LN potentials, the extracellular counterparts of the slow IPSP and slow EPSP, respectively, recorded from the surface of a nicotinized bullfrog sympathetic ganglion. b: Slow IPSP and slow EPSP recorded intracellularly from a nicotinized bullfrog sympathetic ganglion cell. In both records, a train of tetanic stimuli (arrows) was applied to the preganglionic B fibers at a frequency of 10 Hz. Calibrations: 5 mV and 10 sec.

(10–40 Hz for 1 sec) shows a synaptic delay of 30–100 msec, amplitude of 2–8 mV (with intracellular recording), and duration of 10–30 sec; a single orthodromic volley elicits a very small or hardly detectable slow IPSP (Eccles and Libet, 1961; Libet, 1967, 1970; Libet et al., 1968; Nishi and Koketsu, 1968b).

2. Ionic Mechanism of Slow IPSP

Like the slow EPSP, the slow IPSP does not behave as one would expect for an IPSP generated by an increased postsynaptic permeability to ions (Kobayashi and Libet, 1968; Koketsu and Nishi, 1967; Nishi and Koketsu, 1968b). The slow IPSP recorded from the surface of nicotinized frog ganglia is diminished and eventually abolished by depolarization, whereas it is markedly enhanced by moderate hyperpolarization. When the applied hyperpolarization is strong enough to nullify or reverse the afterhyperpolarization of a ganglionic action potential, the slow IPSP tends to decrease. A much stronger hyperpolarization eventually abolishes the slow IPSP but cannot reverse the polarity of the response (Koketsu and Nishi, 1967; Nishi and Koketsu, 1968b). In curarized rabbit ganglion cells (Kobayashi and Libet, 1968), the slow IPSP is decreased in amplitude by progressive reduction of membrane potential and is nullified by a 20-mV depolarization. On the other hand, the amplitude of the slow IPSP is increased by moderate hyperpolarization of 10–30 mV, although further hyperpolarization consistently produces a decrease in amplitude and the IPSP can usually be nullified by hyperpolarization somewhat greater than 30 mV. It should be pointed out that no alteration in membrane conductance is detected during the slow IPSP in both frog and rabbit ganglion cells (Kobayashi and Libet, 1968; Nishi and Koketsu, 1968c).

Koketsu and Nishi (1967) and Nishi and Koketsu (1968b) found in nicotinized frog sympathetic ganglia that alteration of the external Cl has little effect on the slow IPSP but also reported that the slow IPSP is depressed or abolished by ouabain, low temperature, or the removal of the external K ions and is enhanced markedly after loading the ganglia with Na. On the basis of these results, they suggested that the slow IPSP is caused by synaptic activation of an electrogenic Na pump. Kobayashi and Libet (1968), on the other hand, reported that removal of the extracellular K does not depress the slow IPSP; and further the depressant action of ouabain on the slow IPSP is not specific because there is also depression of the fast EPSP (Kobayashi and Libet, 1968). They are of the opinion that the electrogenetic mechanism of the slow IPSP may involve active transport, but that ouabain-sensitive Na–K pump or a Cl pump are excluded as the generator (Kobayashi and Libet, 1968; Libet, 1970). Weight and Padjen (1972) proposed an alternative hypothesis that the slow IPSP is generated by a fall in Na conductance induced by transmitter action.

It should be added that although the slow IPSP (P wave) can be readily recorded from the surface of a curarized ganglion, the intracellular recording of this response is difficult owing to its occurrence in a limited number of cells and its smallness in amplitude. In addition, the slow IPSP generally occurs concomitantly with the slow EPSP. These properties have hampered the study of the slow IPSP and also contributed to the diversity of suggestions on its electrogenesis. It is desirable to devise a new experimental approach for determining whether the response is a result of electrogenic ion transport or some other process.

3. Disynaptic Mediation Through Dopaminergic Cells

The hypothesis of an intervening adrenergic step in mediating the slow IPSP (Eccles and Libet, 1961; see Section II-C-1) is linked to the observations that epinephrine exerts an inhibitory action on sympathetic ganglion cells (Marrazzi, 1939a; Lundberg, 1952) and that the chromaffin cells in the ganglion probably are responsible for the output of epinephrine produced by preganglionic volleys (Bülbring, 1944). It has been shown that norepinephrine and epinephrine do elicit hyperpolarizing responses in mammalian sympathetic ganglia (De Groat and Volle, 1966; Libet and Kobayashi, 1968, 1969), and recent histological evidence is consistent with the disynaptic hypothesis of Eccles and Libet (1961). Matthews and Raisman (1969) demonstrated that the chromaffin-like cells make efferent synaptic contacts with the dendrites and somata of ganglion cells and that they also make afferent synaptic contacts with presynaptic boutons filled with nongranulated vesicles.

Libet (1970) has shown more recently that dopamine can elicit hyper-polarizing responses in mammalian sympathetic ganglia as effectively as norepinephrine and epinephrine and that dopamine is the only catecholamine able to restore the slow IPSP of the ganglia in which catecholamines of chromaffin cells were believed to be depleted by bethanechol. He found, moreover, that incubation of ganglia with diethyldithiocarbamate, which inhibits the enzymatic conversion of dopamine to norepinephrine, specifically enhances the slow IPSP. On the basis of these findings, Libet (1970) proposed that dopamine is probably the major, if not the exclusive, second transmitter in the disynaptic sequence that physiologically mediates the slow IPSP.

By means of formaldehyde histochemistry and cytospectrofluorometry, Libet and Owman (1974) were able to identify dopamine localized to the intraganglionic "small intensely fluorescent" cells in the rabbit's superior cervical ganglion, and also to the characteristically beaded fibers forming a network in close contact with virtually all ganglion cell bodies. They measured the changes in the dopamine content of these interneurons (small intensely fluorescent cells) in conjunction with changes in the slow IPSP of the ganglion under various experimental conditions. The measurements indicated that (1) preganglionic impulses, by a cholinergic muscarinic synaptic action, can induce a release of dopamine from dopamine interneurons; (2) the ability of the ganglion to respond with a slow IPSP to orthodromic input is dependent on the supply of functionally releasable dopamine in these interneurons; and (3) the functionally releasable transmitter *in vitro* appears to comprise roughly 50% of the total dopamine content of the interneurons. The results well support the hypothesis (Libet, 1970) that a dopamine interneuron is activated muscarinically by preganglionic nerve impulses and mediates the production of slow IPSP in sympathetic ganglion cells.

III. PRESYNAPTIC RECEPTOR SITES

A. Cholinoceptive Site

The first demonstration of a specific reactivity of cholinergic nerve terminals not shared by their associated nerve axon was made by Masland and Wigton (1940) who reported that intravenous administration of neostigmine causes propagated antidromic activity in motor nerve fibers. Riker and

Szreniawski (1959) showed in the cat superior cervical ganglion that close arterial injection of ACh induces antidromic firing in the preganglionic fibers. Antidromic responses were observed also by Volle and Koelle (1961) but only in a limited number of experiments on the cat superior cervical ganglion. Douglas *et al.* (1960), on the other hand, proposed that the ACh-induced firing of the preganglionic nerve trunk of the rabbit cervical sympathetic ganglia was explicable on the grounds that it represented the postganglionic discharge in the aberrant recurrent fibers.

When an anticholinesterase is applied to the superior cervical ganglion of the cat by close arterial injection, it evokes a prolonged postganglionic discharge (Volle and Koelle, 1961; Takeshige and Volle, 1962; Volle, 1962*a*). Because this discharge does not occur in the chronically denervated ganglion and since acetylcholinesterase is located on presynaptic nerve terminals of the ganglion (Koelle and Koelle, 1959), it is suggested that this discharge is initiated by the action of ACh liberated from the preganglionic nerve terminals (Koelle, 1961, 1962; Volle and Koelle, 1961). The rat superior cervical ganglion infected with pseudorabies shows periodic bursts of impulse discharge (Dempsher *et al.*, 1955; Dempsher and Riker, 1957). Dempsher and Riker (1957) suggested that the virus-induced impulses have their origin in the synaptic endings and that ACh plays a role in the genesis and spread of this periodic activity over both pre- and postganglionic trunks.

By means of a sucrose-gap technique (Kosterlitz and Wallis, 1966), Koketsu and Nishi (1968) have shown that the intraganglionic portion of the presynaptic nerve is depolarized when the ganglia are exposed to ACh or when tetanic stimulation is given to the preganglionic nerve trunk, particularly in the presence of an anticholinesterase. They suggested that the terminal region of the preganglionic nerve is endowed with a cholinoceptive site which is sensitive to a nicotinic action of ACh. The following sections will describe the general characteristics of the presynaptic depolarization induced by endogenous, as well as extrinsically applied, ACh and the influence of ACh on the excitability of presynaptic nerve terminals and the release of transmitter therefrom.

1. Depolarization of Preganglionic End Fibers by Tetanic Stimulation and ACh

Perfusion of a bullfrog paravertebral ganglion placed in the sucrose-gap chamber with a solution containing 0.5–2.5 mM ACh produces in the intraganglionic portion of presynaptic nerve fibers a slow depolarization that is markedly enhanced by previous application of an anticholinesterase (Figure 13a,b). The *inter*ganglionic portion of preganglionic trunk is not depolarized by ACh. Nicotine (0.02–0.1 mM) applied to the ganglion induces a large and

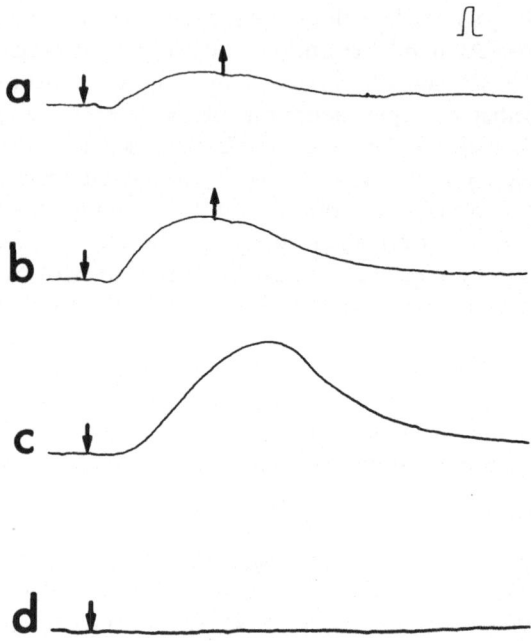

Figure 13. Depolarization of the terminal portion of preganglionic nerve fibers by direct application of ACh. a: depolarization produced by application of 2.4 mM ACh (the moment of addition and withdrawal of ACh is marked by downward and upward arrows, respectively. b: Depolarization induced by the same amount of ACh but 20 min after addition of 0.02 mM physostigmine. c: Transient depolarization following addition of 0.1 mM nicotine. d: no response to 2.4 mM ACh in the presence of physostigmine and nicotine. All records were obtained by a sucrose-gap method from a bullfrog paravertebral sympathetic ganglion preparation. Calibration: square pulse of 1 mV for 10 sec. (From Koketsu and Nishi, 1968.)

transient depolarization of the *intra*ganglionic presynaptic nerve; this depolarization lasts for several minutes (Figure 13c). After nicotinization of the ganglion, no detectable presynaptic depolarization is observed when ACh is added to the superfusing solution (Figure 13d). Atropine (up to 0.2 mM) does not show any effect on the ACh depolarization, while *d*-tubocurarine in a concentration of 0.2 mM depresses or blocks the latter. Similar to the nicotinic depolarization, the ACh depolarization is transient and subsides within several minutes if ACh is continuously applied to the ganglion.

ACh (0.5–2.5 mM) causes a transient reduction in the amplitude of action potentials of the preganglionic end fibers; the reduction measured 2–3 min after addition of ACh (2.5 mM) being about 8% of the original peak amplitude and more pronounced in the presence of an anti-ChE. A marked (30–60%) attenuation of the intraganglionic presynaptic spike is induced by nicotine (0.1 mM). This nicotine action is also a transient phenomenon, as the amplitude of the action potentials is restored spontaneously if nicotine application is continued (Figure 14). The time course of the spike attenuation is in good agreement with that of nicotine depolarization.

However, these results obtained by the sucrose-gap technique do not serve to clarify the exact site of the ACh depolarization within the intraganglionic portion of presynaptic nerve. This site may be the membrane of the presynaptic nerve terminals or the membrane of a more proximal part of the terminals. To acquire more detailed information about the ACh-sensitive locus, Ginsborg (1971) recorded extracellularly the action potentials from individual preganglionic nerve terminals in the lumbar sympathetic chain of frogs (*Rana pipiens*) in various experimental conditions. He showed that the terminal action potentials were unaffected by changes in external Mg or Ca concentration, but were attenuated or even abolished by ACh (1.0–2.4 mM) or carbachol (0.6–4.8 mM). In the presence of tubocurarine (5 × 10⁻⁵ M), ACh and carbachol had no effect on the presynaptic action potential. Thus Ginsborg demonstrated clearly that the terminals of preganglionic nerves are indeed endowed with a cholinoceptive site sensitive to the nicotinic depolarizing action of ACh and carbachol.

These findings indicate that the endogenous ACh liberated by nerve impulses may also depolarize the presynaptic cholinoceptive site. This possibility of ACh depolarization, concomitant with the preganglionic nerve activity, can be tested by comparing the action potential recorded from the terminal portion of presynaptic nerve trunk. With single stimulation there is no significant difference between the terminal and axonal action potentials. Their spike is followed by a very small, slow positive afterpotential. In contrast, a characteristic difference of the two potentials is noted following a train of tetanic stimulation. In the case of the terminal action potential, the

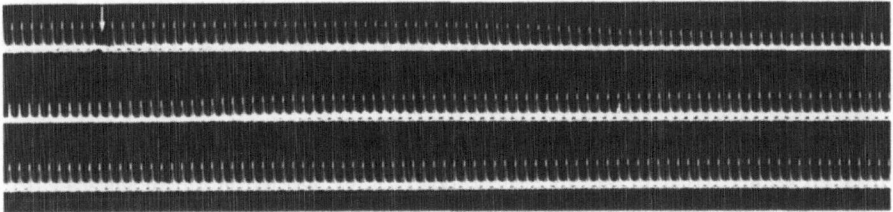

Figure 14. **The decrease in the amplitude of the action potential of the preganglionic nerve terminals under the effect of nicotine.** The moment of addition of nicotine (0.1 mM) is shown by arrow. Preganglionic nerve was stimulated successively at intervals of 2 sec, and the potentials were recorded with an ac amplifier. Note the transient reduction in the amplitude of the action potential. (From Koketsu and Nishi, 1968.)

enhanced positive afterpotential, which is also seen following the axonal action potential, does not return to the original level but overshoots it by forming a slow negative afterpotential (Figure 15a, c), while the enhanced positive axonal afterpotential simply returns to the original level without forming a slow negative potential (Figure 15f). The slow negative potential recorded from the terminal portion becomes more prominent when the membrane of the nerve terminals is hyperpolarized by an extrinsically applied anodal current (Figure 15b). Physostigmine (0.02 mM) and tetraethylpyrophosphate (TEPP) (0.005 mM) markedly enhance the slow negative afterpotential (Figure 15d), but never affect the *inter*ganglionic axonal responses (Figure 15g). The slow negative potential is markedly depressed by nicotine (0.1 mM), *d*-tubocurarine (0.2 mM), or ACh (0.5–2.5 mM; Figure 15e), but is not appreciably affected by atropine (0.2 mM). Thus, the pharmacological nature of the slow negative potential is similar to the presynaptic depolari-

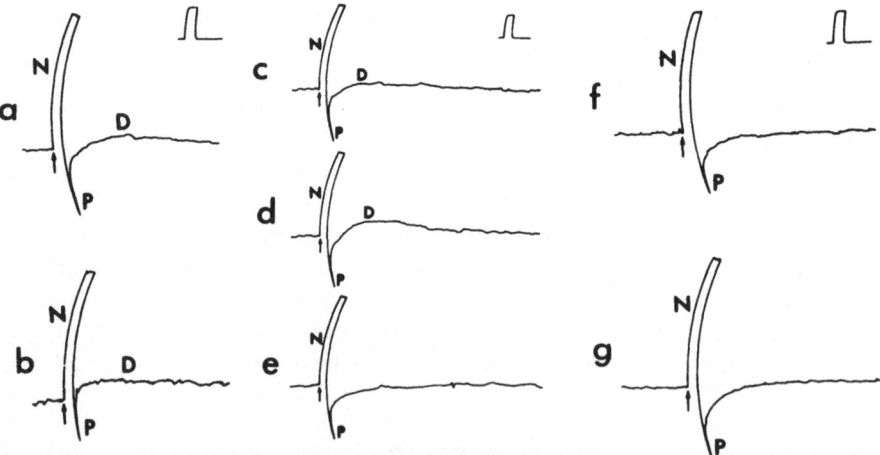

Figure 15. Electrical responses of the terminal (a–e) and axonal (f, g) portions of the preganglionic nerve following repetitive preganglionic nerve stimulation. The responses in the left, middle, and right column were obtained by a sucrose-gap method from three different preparations of the bullfrog paravertebral sympathetic ganglion. a and b: Potentials by repetitive stimulation without (a) and with (b) application of an anodal current to the ganglion. c, d, and e: Potentials obtained before (c) and 10 min after application of 0.005 mM tetraethylpyrophosphate (d) and 20 min after application of 2.5 mM ACh (e). f and g: Potentials elicited without (f) and with (g) previous application of 0.002 mM physostigmine; note the absence of any effect by the anticholinesterase. In each record, beginning of repetitive stimulation (50 Hz for approximately 10 sec) is shown by an arrow. The negative and positive afterpotentials and the slow negative potential are marked as N, P and D, respectively. The peak amplitude of the negative afterpotential is out of scale in all records. Calibration pulse: 1 mV in amplitude and 10 sec in duration. (From Koketsu and Nishi, 1968.)

zation induced by direct application of ACh. Apparently, the endogenous ACh is also capable of depolarizing the presynaptic cholinoceptive sites.

2. Alteration of Terminal Threshold by ACh and by Tetanic Stimulation

When a stimulating microelectrode is placed near the presynaptic nerve terminals (cf. Hubbard and Schmidt, 1961), a short cathodal current pulse evokes a fast EPSP which has the minimum latency of 1.5–2.0 msec. Frequently, the stimulating current also elicits the soma action potential which masks the evoked EPSP. However, a constant hyperpolarizing current applied through the recording microelectrode can suppress the soma spike and thereby isolate the EPSP. With a stimulating electrode in this position, a long cathodal current, which is subliminal to the terminal membrane firing, induces a burst of miniature EPSPs. The terminal threshold can be determined by the smallest short-current pulse to evoke an EPSP which has comparable amplitude to that of the EPSP elicited by stimulation of preganglionic nerve trunk.

Superfusion of the ganglion with 0.01–0.05 mM ACh does not significantly change the threshold of terminal membrane. With 0.5 mM ACh a fall in terminal threshold can be recognized although the observable fall is relatively small (6 $\pm$ 0.6% SE; Nishi, 1970). Figure 16 represents a typical series of records showing the lowering of the terminal threshold by 0.5 mM ACh applied for 1 min. In this experiment, subthreshold current pulses (90% of threshold strength) were delivered repetitively at intervals of 2 sec through the stimulating electrode to the terminals. About 10 sec after the beginning of ACh superfusion, current pulses started to excite the terminals, as judged by the appearance of orthodromic responses which were characterized by the step formed by the EPSP. At the beginning, the terminal firing was intermittent, probably because of critical amplitude of terminal membrane depolarization. During the plateau phase of postsynaptic depolarization, each pulse without exception evoked an orthodromic response, indicating that the presynaptic depolarization was also sustained. As the postsynaptic depolarization subsided after cessation of ACh superfusion, the terminal excitation became again intermittent and finally disappeared at the time when the postsynaptic membrane potential was almost completely restored. The result indicates that the presynaptic terminal membrane is really depolarized by ACh and that the time course of the terminal depolarization is almost parallel to that of postsynaptic depolarization insofar as the duration of ACh perfusion is limited to less than 1 min. However, if ACh was applied for a much longer period of time, the lowering of terminal threshold was not maintained but disappeared in a few minutes, while the postsynaptic depolarization persisted. This may rule out the possibility that the nerve terminal might have

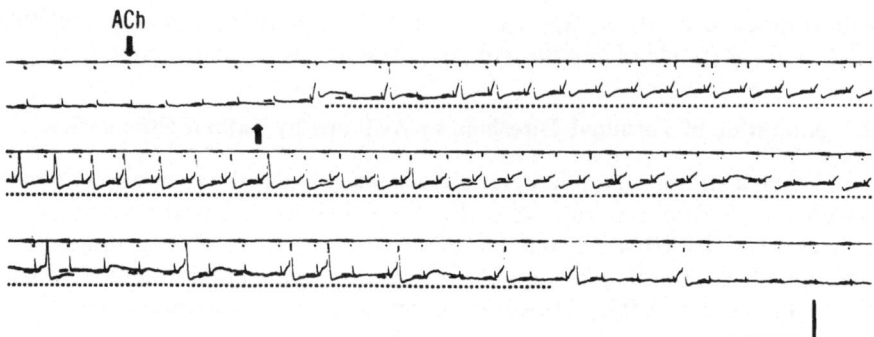

ACh

Figure 16. Effect of ACh on the threshold of presynaptic nerve terminals. The terminal membrane was stimulated successively by current pulses which were subliminal (90% of threshold intensity) before application of ACh. Recordings were taken from a bullfrog sympathetic ganglion cell. Direct stimulation of ganglion cell membrane by the current pulses was prevented by applying an anodal current through the intracellular recording microelectrode. The moments of addition and withdrawal of ACh (0.5 mM) are marked by downward and upward arrows, respectively. Pulses in the upper traces represent cathodal current pulses (1.5 msec in duration) applied to the terminals at intervals of 2 sec. Lower traces represent the postsynaptic membrane potential recorded intracellularly. The dotted line indicates the level of the cell membrane potential before application of ACh. Upper and lower traces were displayed with a fast sweep (see calibration) on an oscilloscope and photographed on a slowly moving film. Calibrations: 100 mV and 50 msec (From Nishi, 1970.)

been depolarized, not directly by ACh, but secondarily by an increase of extracellular K concentration resulting from the postsynaptic depolarization.

As stated earlier, the reduction of the intraganglionic presynaptic spikes by nicotine (0.1 mM) was also transient, lasting only for 3 min in spite of the continued presence of the drug (Figure 14). Similar results have been obtained with the presynaptic terminal spikes under the influence of ACh or carbachol (Ginsborg, 1971). All these results suggest that the presynaptic cholinoceptive sites are desensitized after a few minutes of activation by a nicotine drug. In contrast, the desensitization of postsynaptic nicotinic receptors develops at a much slower rate. For example, the depolarization of ganglion cells induced by perfusion with 0.1 mM nicotine tends to decline in about 10 min and disappears in 20–30 min (cf. Nishi and Koketsu, 1968a).

Curarization of the ganglion with 0.01–0.05 mM *d*-tubocurarine, which partially depresses the evoked EPSP, markedly reduces or completely eliminates the lowering of the terminal threshold by ACh. When the ganglion is pretreated with physostigmine (0.01 mM), the percentage of the cell population that responded with a fall of the terminal threshold is not appreciably increased, but the induced threshold changes are considerably enhanced (the mean fall, $15 \pm 0.15\%$ SE) and prolonged.

Tetanic stimulation (10 Hz for 10 sec) of preganglionic nerve trunk induces monophasic or biphasic changes in threshold of the terminal membrane. Normally, the terminal threshold is raised by more than 20% immediately following the cessation of stimulation. The elevated threshold decreases rapidly for the first few seconds and then returns slowly to the control level; still later, there is sometimes, but not always, a phase of lowered threshold level (Figure 17, curve A). The biphasic change is clearly recognized in about 30% of cells, although the threshold fall in the second phase is as small as $4 \pm 0.6\%$ SE. Addition of 0.01 mM d-tubocurarine, which partially depresses the EPSP, completely eliminates the second phase, i.e., the fall of the terminal threshold (curve B). In the cells which do not show the second phase, the recovery from the elevated threshold is considerably delayed by d-tubocurarine. When the preparation is pretreated with 0.01 mM physostigmine for over 30 min, approximately 50% of cells show biphasic changes. In those cells, the initial phase (elevated threshold) is markedly smaller and shorter, while the second phase (lowered threshold) is enhanced (the mean fall, $11 \pm 1.1\%$ SE) and prolonged (curve C).

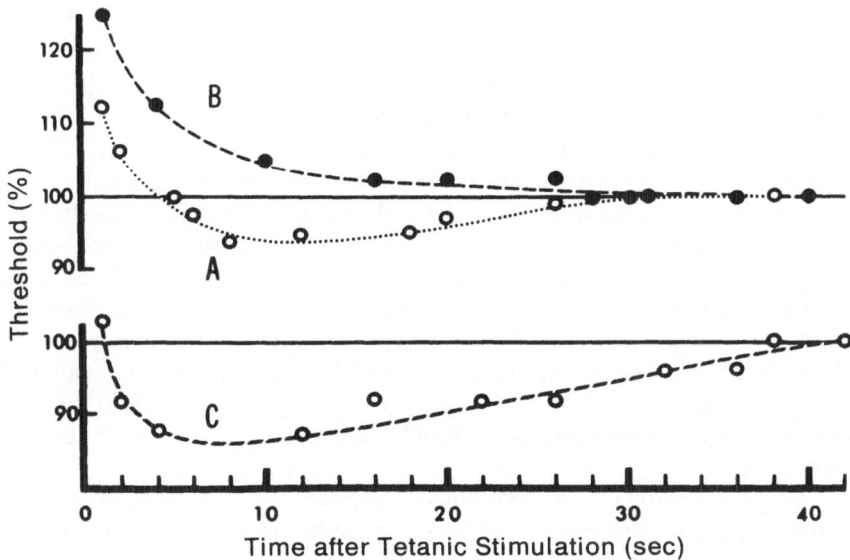

Figure 17. **Changes in threshold of the presynaptic terminal membrane following a train of orthodromic stimuli (10 Hz for 10 sec).** Curves A and B were obtained from a bullfrog sympathetic ganglion cell before and 10 min after addition of d-tubocurarine (0.01 mM) to perfusing solution. Curve C was obtained from a ganglion cell of a different preparation approximately 50 min after addition of physostigmine (0.01 mM). (From Nishi, 1970.)

The rise and fall of terminal threshold appear to correspond temporally to the enhanced positive afterpotential and slow negative potential, respectively, which follow the tetanic firing of the intraganglionic portion of the presynaptic nerve. This implies that the repetitive firing of terminal membrane is also followed by a prominent afterhyperpolarization and that the liberated ACh is capable of producing a terminal membrane depolarization which counteracts the posttetanic hyperpolarization.

3. Effects of ACh on Spontaneous Transmitter Release

In regard to the *raison d'être* of the presynaptic cholinoceptive site, it is important to determine whether the ACh depolarization of terminal membrane is large enough to release endogenous ACh. This may be tested by recording miniature EPSP before and during superfusion of the ganglion with solutions containing ACh (cf. Liley, 1956). However, ACh in concentrations (over 0.5 mM) that effectively depolarize the presynaptic terminal membrane greatly reduces the amplitude of miniature EPSP because of the concomitant large depolarization of the postsynaptic membrane. Furthermore, fine control of the amplitude as well as of the duration of postsynaptic depolarization, by changing the concentration of applied ACh, is difficult to achieve owing to the individual variations in postsynaptic ACh sensitivity and the slowness of ACh depolarization. In addition, repetitive trials of ACh superfusion will desensitize the pre- and postsynaptic receptors.

Such complications will be minimized if minute amounts of ACh are applied iontophoretically close to the presynaptic nerve terminals during intracellular recording of miniature EPSP. With this method, the size and duration of the induced response can be well controlled, and ACh application can be repeated without causing significant desensitization of ACh receptors. By proper adjustment of the tip position of the ACh-filled electrode, the diffusion distance of ejected ACh to the subsynaptic membrane can be made less than 10 μm, calculated from the peak time of induced ACh potential (del Castillo and Katz, 1955; Koketsu *et al.*, 1968). At such a short distance, ACh released iontophoretically should reach the presynaptic terminal membrane.

Since the frequency of spontaneous miniature EPSP of bullfrog paravertebral sympathetic neurons is very low (only 3.0 $\pm$ 0.5 SE per min), the evoked miniature EPSP can be easily detected. However, ACh applied iontophoretically close to the presynaptic nerve terminals does not consistently evoke miniature EPSP except in a few eserinized cells (Nishi, 1970). A series of records taken from one of these eserinized cells in which the ACh injection elicited miniature EPSP is shown in Figure 18. In control recordings (A) only a single miniature EPSP spontaneously generated is seen. Ejection of relatively small amounts of ACh (as evidenced by small ACh potentials in

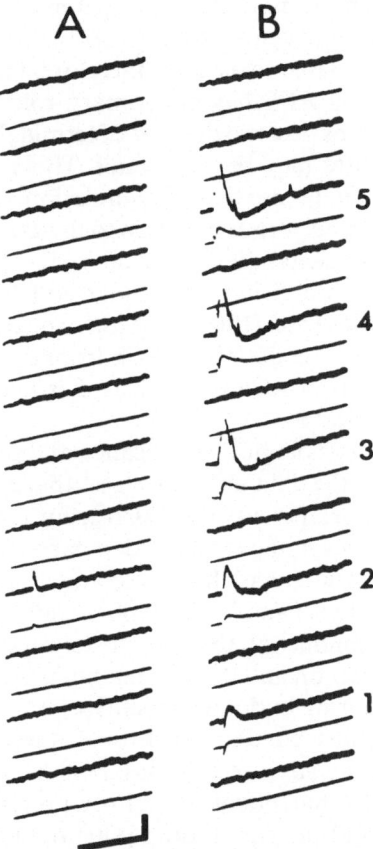

Figure 18. Miniature EPSP evoked by ACh iontophoretically applied to the presynaptic nerve terminals. A and B are a series of paired ac (upper, thick traces) and dc (lower, thin traces) recordings obtained from a bullfrog sympathetic ganglion cell. The ganglion was perfused with a solution containing physostigmine (0.01 mM). A spontaneous miniature EPSP is seen in control recordings (A). The ACh was ejected from an ACh-filled electrode near the presynaptic nerve terminals in records 1–5. The ejection current was increased stepwise in records 1–3 and maintained at the same increased intensity in records 3–5. Note the appearance of miniature EPSP as ACh ejection was intensified (records 3–5). Paired traces were photographed on a moving film at intervals of 2 sec. The recording proceeds from bottom to top. Calibration: vertical bar, 2 mV for ac recordings and 10 mV for dc recordings; horizontal bar, 500 msec. (From Nishi, 1970.)

traces 1 and 2) did not evoke any miniature responses, but when the ACh ejection was intensified, as it evoked ACh potentials more than 10 mV in amplitude (traces 3, 4, 5), two to three miniature EPSPs were clearly induced on the falling phase of ACh potentials. Thus after eserinization, close application of ACh could evoke miniature EPSP, although in a limited number of cells. It appears that in the majority of presynaptic fibers the amplitude of ACh depolarization is insufficient for transmitter liberation even after eserinization. It would be reasonable to assume, therefore, that the depolarization of terminal membrane by ACh has no primary role for liberation of the transmitter. This is perhaps because the area of terminal membrane occupied by the cholinoceptive sites may be very small. This is in keeping with the experimental facts that an intense tetanic stimulation of preganglionic fibers or application of a high concentration of ACh to the ganglion cannot increase the terminal membrane excitability more than 10–15%, nor is it able to elicit antidromic presynaptic firing (Dempsher and Riker, 1957). Furthermore, according to Collier et al. (1969) only high concentrations of ACh are capable of releasing labeled endogenous ACh from the cat superior cervical ganglion, and the amount of ACh thus released is markedly less than that liberated by nerve stimulation.

Although the real physiological significance of the presynaptic nicotinic receptors is still unclear, the data do not suggest that endogenous ACh activates effectively or releases percussively ACh from the nerve terminals (cf. Koelle, 1961, 1962). However, the terminal depolarization elicited by endogenous ACh effectively counteracts the posttetanic hyperpolarization of the terminal membrane (Koketsu and Nishi, 1968; Nishi, 1970). This counteraction might aid impulse conduction through the terminal arborization during posttetanic hyperpolarization and thereby maintain indirectly the constancy of transmitter output during and after repetitive presynaptic firing. In fact, the safety factor of impulse conduction through the terminal arborization should be low even in the absence of posttetanic hyperpolarization. For a further elucidation of the functional role of the presynaptic cholinoceptor, its ionic requirements and the equilibrium potential during active state are yet to be investigated.

B. Adrenoceptive Site

The blocking action of epinephrine on ganglionic transmission, initially reported by Marrazzi (1939a), has been described by many investigators (Bülbring, 1944; Matthews, 1956; Eccles and Libet, 1961; Pardo et al., 1963). Lundberg (1952) suggested that epinephrine hyperpolarizes the postsynaptic membrane, but this change in membrane potential is not always present when transmission is depressed by epinephrine. Paton and Thompson (1953) proposed that epinephrine has a dual action on the ganglion cells; it may not only reduce the ACh output from presynaptic terminals but also depress the postsynaptic sensitivity to the transmitter. Contrary to their common blocking action, an enhancement of transmission has also been found when lower doses of catecholamines were administered (Bülbring and Burn, 1942;

Bülbring, 1944; Malméjac, 1955; Trendelenburg, 1956). Furthermore, blocking doses of catecholamines have been observed to potentiate the ganglionic responses to ACh (Konzett, 1950; Kewitz and Reinert, 1952). Costa *et al.* (1961) showed that ganglionic transmission is enhanced following administration of dibenamine or after depletion of ganglionic catecholamines with reserpine. De Groat and Volle (1966) reported that sympathetic ganglia contain two pharmacologically distinctive sites; one, which is blocked by α-adrenoceptor blocking agents, mediates catecholamine-induced inhibition and ganglionic hyperpolarization, and the other, which is blocked by β-adrenoceptor blocking agents, mediates catecholamine-evoked facilitation and ganglionic depolarization. Christ and Nishi (1969, 1971a, b) have shown that epinephrine does not significantly hyperpolarize the ganglion cell membrane in concentrations which block transmission. They reached the conclusion that epinephrine blockade is primarily caused by the decrease in transmitter output and that this action of epinephrine is exerted through an α-adrenoceptive site at the presynaptic nerve terminals. This concept is based on the following evidence obtained from the isolated rabbit superior cervical ganglia by means of the intracellular microelectrode method.

1. Depression of EPSP by Catecholamines

Superfusion of the ganglion with a solution containing 0.01 mM epinephrine causes in many cells a rapid and reversible blockade of the orthodromic action potential. As illustrated in Figure 19, the orthodromic response

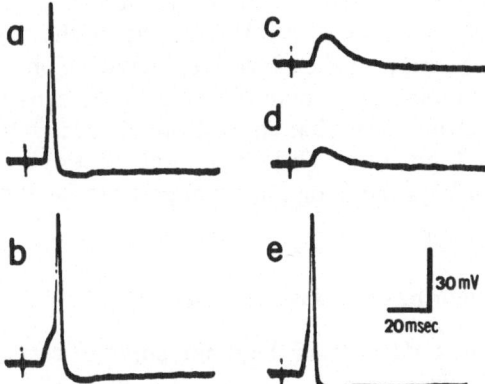

Figure 19. Effect of epinephrine on the orthodromic response of a rabbit superior cervical ganglion cell. Record a was taken in control solution. Records b, c and d were obtained 50 s, 60 s, and 120 s after beginning epinephrine (0.01 mM) perfusion, respectively. Record e was obtained 240 s after completion of epinephrine perfusion. (From Christ and Nishi, 1969).

is reduced to an EPSP with a markèdly attenuated amplitude and rate of rise. The minimum effective concentration of epinephrine ranges between 0.001 mM and 0.005 mM among different cells. With 0.01 mM epinephrine a 30–70% reduction of EPSP amplitude is consistently observed. Norepinephrine and isoproterenol applied at a concentration of 0.01 mM also depress the EPSP amplitude. However, their blocking action is much weaker and slower than that of epinephrine. The order of depressant potency is epinephrine, norepinephrine, and isoproterenol. The α-adrenoceptor blocking agents, such as phenoxybenzamine or dihydroergotamine, which do not affect the EPSP itself at a concentration of 0.01 mM, effectively antagonize the blocking action of epinephrine. For example, pretreatment of the ganglion with phenoxybenzamine (0.01 mM) for 10 min renders the ganglion cells completely insensitive to the blocking action of epinephrine for more than 2 hr. In contrast, the β-adrenoceptor blocking agents, such as propranolol (0.03 mM) or dichloroisoproterenol (0.01 mM), show no antagonistic influence on the epinephrine action.

Blockade of ganglion cell response with 0.01 mM epinephrine is not accompanied by any noticeable change in the membrane potential nor the threshold for the membrane excitation. Only when epinephrine concentration is raised to 1.0 mM is there a consistent slow depolarization varying 5–15 mV in amplitude which is occasionally preceded by a short period of hyperpolarization of less than 5 mV in amplitude. It appears, therefore, that a lowering of membrane excitability is an unlikely mechanism of epinephrine blockade. Also, epinephrine does not appear to reduce the EPSP amplitude by virtue of increasing the cell membrane conductance, since there is no change in electrotonic potentials.

Epinephrine does not alter the amplitude and time course of the postsynaptic depolarization induced by ACh applied either by superfusion or iontophoresis. An example of the effect of epinephrine on the EPSP and the iontophoretically-induced ACh potential of a single ganglion cell is shown in Figure 20. It is clearly seen that epinephrine decreases the EPSP but has no effect on the ACh potential. This differential effect of epinephrine is most easily explained by hypothesizing a presynaptic site for the blocking action of epinephrine.

2. Effect of Epinephrine on Transmitter Release

The spontaneous MEPSPs in the rabbit superior cervical ganglion cells occur at a very low frequency (1–5/min), although their amplitude is comparable to miniature potentials of other synapses. If the ganglion is superfused with a solution containing 20 mM KCl, the frequency of MEPSPs increases in most ganglion cells to 1–10/sec. Table 1 summarizes the frequency and

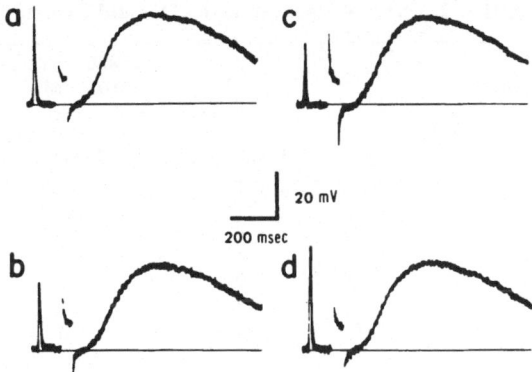

Figure 20. Effect of epinephrine on the fast EPSP and ACh-potential recorded from a rabbit superior cervical ganglion cell. Records a and b were obtained, respectively, before and 2 min after control solution was switched to an epinephrine (0.01 mM) solution. Note the selective depression of the EPSP by epinephrine. Immediately after record b was taken, control solution was introduced again. Records c and d were taken 1 and 3 min after completion of epinephrine perfusion. The resting membrane potential was maintained at approximately -80 mV by applying a continuous anodal current to prevent spike generation by the EPSP and ACh-potential. The ACh was iontophoretically applied to the cell membrane from an ACh-filled microelectrode by current pulses of 0.5 μA with 50-msec duration. (From Nishi, 1970.)

amplitude of MEPSPs in 5 cells recorded for 80 sec, before and after addition of epinephrine (0.01 mM). As seen in the table, epinephrine markedly decreases the frequency of MEPSPs but only slightly affects their amplitude. The data unequivocally suggests that epinephrine reduces the spontaneous release of the transmitter with almost no effect on the quantal size. Table 2 shows the quantal contents of evoked EPSP of the rabbit superior cervical ganglion cells superfused with high Mg–low Ca solutions before and after

TABLE 1. Effect of Epinephrine on Miniature EPSPs

Frequency			Amplitude		
Control (n/sec)	Epinephrine (n/sec)	(% decrease)	Control (mV)	Epinephrine (mV)	(% decrease)
0.97	0.88	9	0.76	0.73	4
0.89	0.73	18	0.63	0.63	0
1.68	0.72	57	0.65	0.62	5
6.20	2.01	68	1.27	1.01	3
1.61	0.61	62	1.04	1.11	13
		43 ± 11^a			5 ± 1.9^a

[a] Mean $\pm$ 1 SE (From Nishi, 1970.)

TABLE 2. Effect of Epinephrine on Quantal Content [a]

Control				Epinephrine (0.01 mM)			
Failures	[Ca] (mM)	[Mg] (mM)	m	Failures	m	% decrease	q'/q
89	0.5	5.5	0.81	161	0.22	73	1.07
94	0.5	3.5	0.76	113	0.57	25	1.02
60	0.5	5.5	1.21	182	0.10	92	0.95
132	0.5	2.5	0.42	150	0.29	31	0.92
119	0.5	2.5	0.52	133	0.41	21	1.06
83	0.5	2.5	0.88	188	0.06	93	0.85
						56 ± 12 [b]	0.98 ± 0.03 [b]

[a] Failures: number of failures in 200 stimuli; m: quantal content; q'/q: relative quantal size in epinephrine.
[b] Mean $\pm$ 1 SE (From Nishi, 1970.)

addition of 0.01 mM epinephrine. The table indicates that epinephrine decreases the quantal content as much as 56%, on average. This marked decrease in quantal release is accompanied by no significant change in quantal size. Thus, in good agreement with its effect on the spontaneous release of transmitter, epinephrine impairs the quantal release by nerve impulses but shows no prominent postsynaptic effects.

3. Mechanism of Presynaptic Depression

The above evidence taken together suggests that the main action of epinephrine on the isolated superior cervical ganglion is to decrease the transmitter output from the presynaptic nerve terminals. This is consistent with the previous observations of Paton and Thompson (1953) and Birks and MacIntosh (1961) that epinephrine can decrease the ACh output. The prevention of epinephrine blockade by α-adrenoceptor blocking agents indicate that the presynaptic action of epinephrine is exerted via an α-adrenoceptive site. Furthermore, the order of depressant potency of catecholamines is what would be anticipated for an α-receptor.

Facilitation of ganglionic transmission by epinephrine observed by some investigators (Bülbring and Burn, 1942; Bülbring, 1944; Trendelenburg, 1956) is difficult to explain; however, it is possible that in some conditions the postsynaptic depolarizing action of epinephrine might overcome its presynaptic depressant action. De Groat and Volle (1966) found that epinephrine facilitates the ganglionic transmission in the presence of an α-adrenoceptor blocking agent. This facilitation is probably a result, in part, of the enhancement of epinephrine depolarization as a result of the selective abolition of epinephrine hyperpolarization by the drug (De Groat and Volle, 1966), and in part, of the blockade of the presynaptic depressant effect of epinephrine (Christ and Nishi, 1969, 1971a, b).

It was reported that epinephrine (Krnjevic and Miledi, 1958) and norepinephrine (Jenkinson et al., 1968) increase the end-plate potential at the neuromuscular junction by increasing the release of transmitter. Bowman and Nott (1969) suggested that epinephrine may be producing its effect at the neuromuscular junction by increasing the level of free calcium ions in the motor nerve endings. If the ganglionic blocking action is related to calcium action on transmitter release, epinephrine may depress the influx of calcium ions during the nerve terminal excitation or impede the activation of transmitter release by calcium ions. However, Christ and Nishi (1971a, b) have shown in the rabbit superior cervical neurons that epinephrine does not appreciably change the probability of quantal release which is intimately related to the action of calcium ions on transmitter release (Katz and Miledi, 1968). They also found that epinephrine does not alter the excitability of the presynaptic terminal membrane. What appears most likely is that epinephrine decreases reversibly the quanta of transmitter immediately available for release.

4. Dopamine and Presynaptic Inhibition

Dopamine, which is, as mentioned before, the most likely transmitter mediating the slow IPSP in the mammalian sympathetic ganglion (Libet, 1970), depresses ganglionic transmission (Weir and McLennan, 1963). Dun and Nishi (1974) have found that the depressant action of dopamine is characteristically similar to that of epinephrine and norepinephrine (Christ and Nishi, 1971a) in that its primary action is to decrease the quantal liberation of ACh from the presynaptic nerve terminals. The postsynaptic effect of dopamine, i.e., a weak hyperpolarization which is not associated with any significant conductance change (Kobayashi and Libet, 1968), seems to play a secondary role, if any, in the blockade of ganglionic transmission via nicotinic postsynaptic site. It is conceivable, therefore, that the primary role of endogenous dopamine would be to mediate presynaptic inhibition rather than the postsynaptic inhibition.

IV. TRANSMITTER LIBERATION

A. Quantal Liberation of ACh from Preganglionic Nerve Terminals

Miniature fast EPSPs appear spontaneously and randomly in both amphibian (Blackman et al., 1963; Hunt and Nelson, 1965; Nishi and Koketsu, 1960) and mammalian sympathetic ganglion cells (Blackman et al., 1969;

Nishi and Christ, 1971a). The size of these potentials is usually about 1 mV or less with a frequency that varies considerably (0.05–10 Hz) in different cells. Hunt and Nelson (1965) estimated in frog sympathetic ganglion cells that the maximum shunt conductance of the subsynaptic membrane (G_s) during a miniature EPSP is approximately $1.7 \times 10^{-9} \, \Omega^{-1}$. Nishi et al. (1967) estimated in toad sympathetic ganglion cells that the average G_s during a miniature EPSP is $6.6 \times 10^{-9} \, \Omega^{-1}$ for B neurons and $2.5 \times 10^{-9} \, \Omega^{-1}$ for C neurons, and that the average G_s during an evoked EPSP is $0.85 \times 10^{-6} \, \Omega^{-1}$ for B neurons and $0.2 \times 10^{-6} \, \Omega^{-1}$ for C neurons. These values estimate the quantal content of an evoked EPSP to be approximately 130 for B neurons and 80 for C neurons. Using bioassay of the liberated ACh from the toad sympathetic ganglia, Nishi et al. (1967) estimated that a single preganglionic volley releases approximately 2.6×10^{-16} g of ACh per ganglion cell. Comparison of this ACh output and the quantal content of an evoked EPSP estimates a single quantum of transmitter to contain about 8000–12,000 molecules of ACh. If the electron microscopic vesicle represents a quantum, these estimates indicate that the ACh in the sympathetic synaptic vesicles may be stored hypertonically, because if the transmitter is present in the vesicles as an isotonic solution of an ACh salt, there would be about 6000 molecules in a spherical vesicle about 500 Å in diameter.

With an electron microscopic observation of the ganglionic synapses, Nishi et al. (1967) estimated that there would be about 55 synaptic knobs on a B neuron and about 15 knobs on a C neuron of the toad. By dividing the quantal content of an EPSP by the number of synaptic knobs on a single cell, it appears that a single knob in a B neuron would liberate at least 2 quanta of the transmitter per impulse, and a single knob on a C neuron about 5 quanta. Provided that the synaptic cleft is a cylinder 200 Å in height and 3 μm in diameter, the maximum concentration of liberated ACh in a cleft per impulse in the presence of an antiacetylcholinesterase would be 2.3×10^{-4} M for B neurons and 8.4×10^{-4} M for C neurons.

B. Facilitation and Depression of Transmitter Liberation

There are several reports on facilitation and depression of synaptic transmission in sympathetic ganglia (Eccles, 1935; Larrabee and Bronk, 1947; Gebber, 1968; Brimble et al., 1972). In the mammalian ganglion preparations, however, direct assessment of the pre- and postsynaptic factors contributing to facilitation and depression of synaptic response is very difficult because of the multiple presynaptic innervation and axodendritic type of synaptic arrangements. On the other hand, the amphibian sympathetic ganglia afford a suitable preparation to investigate these synaptic modulations because of the simplicity of the neuronal and synaptic arrangements.

When pairs of fast EPSPs are recorded from bullfrog sympathetic ganglion cells at intervals of 20–30 msec, the second EPSP in a pair averages 1.5 times the amplitude of the first EPSP (Gallagher et al., 1973). This facilitation gradually decreases as the interval between the pair of EPSPs is prolonged and subside as the interval is lengthened to 400 msec. At intervals greater than 500 msec, the second EPSP of a pair becomes depressed; this depression peaks at the interval of 1 sec and gradually subsides in 10 sec. Both facilitation and depression are very sensitive to the alteration of the extracellular concentration of Ca, $[Ca]_o$. Lowering $[Ca]_o$ increases the peak facilitation ratio and minimizes the peak phase of depression, while raising $[Ca]_o$ decreases the peak facilitation and increases depression.

Comparison of the amplitude of pairs of presynaptic terminal spikes shows little variability at the stimulus intervals between 5 msec and 20 sec. Furthermore, the amplitudes of MEPSPs recorded before and after the evoked EPSP demonstrate no significant variation between them. These findings indicate that the facilitation and depression are solely owing to a presynaptic event in nature, as reported for neuromuscular transmission (del Castillo and Katz, 1954; Katz and Miledi, 1965, 1968).

There is much evidence that influx of calcium through the axon membrane (Hodgkin and Keynes, 1957; Baker et al., 1971) is the first step to release quanta of transmitter from a nerve terminal (Katz and Miledi, 1967). It has been suggested that the amplitude of end-plate potential which is corrected for nonlinear summation or the quanta of transmitter released is proportional to the concentration of extracellular Ca (Bracho and Orkand, 1970; Ortiz and Bracho, 1972) or the nth power of the concentration (Jenkinson, 1957; Dodge and Rahamimoff, 1967; Hubbard et al., 1968; Katz and Miledi, 1970). One can expect the following relations:

$$[Ca]_o^n \propto (Ca_a)^n \propto (ACh)$$

where $[Ca]_o$ is the concentration of extracellular Ca, (Ca_a) is the "active Ca," which acts to release transmitter from nerve terminal, and (ACh) is the amount of released ACh. Depression of transmitter release is largely owing to depletion of available store of ACh (Otsuka et al., 1962; Thies, 1965; Mallart and Martin, 1968). This implies that the amount of ACh liberated by a single impulse is proportional to the product of the amount of readily available ACh, C, and the nth power of the amount of intracellular ionized, active Ca; $(ACh) = \rho C(Ca_a)^n$, where ρ is a proportionality constant.

Since the conductance of the subsynaptic membrane, G_{tr}, is thought to be proportional to the amount of transmitter released, the maximum G_{tr} produced by the first impulse is given by G_{tr_1}:

$$G_{tr_1} = \gamma\rho \, C_r(X_0)^n \tag{1}$$

where C_r is the readily available ACh in the resting state: X_0, is the maximum amount of active calcium that is involved with the release resulting from an initial impulse: and γ is a proportionality constant. At a resting state the amount of ionized, active calcium in a presynaptic terminal seems to be negligible since the frequency of spontaneous MEPSPs is very low (approximately 3/min), then X_0 following a presynaptic excitation is thought to be largely due to the external calcium.

After activating the transmitter release, the Ca that entered a presynaptic terminal should be extruded slowly against electrochemical gradient (cf. Hodgkin and Keynes, 1957; Baker *et al.*, 1971). Assuming that this residual Ca decays exponentially with a time constant of $1/b$, the residual Ca at a time t, after the first impulse, is expected to be $X_0 e^{-bt}$, where the boundary condition is that $t = 0$ when $(Ca_a) = X_0$. The amount of active Ca immediately after the second impulse is given by $(1 + e^{-bt})X_0$ on the assumption that the second impulse carries the same amount of Ca into the nerve terminals. The subsynaptic conductance by the second impulse, G_{tr_2}, is then given by the equation;

$$G_{tr_2} = \gamma \rho C_t (1 + e^{-bt})^n X_0^n \tag{2}$$

where C_t is the amount of readily available transmitter at a time t.

Birks and MacIntosh (1961) proposed that there are two kinds of releasable ACh stored: depot ACh and readily available ACh, and the kinetics between these two compartments has been postulated by Liley and North (1953). According to this hypothesis, the amount of available ACh at a time t after an initial release of ACh is given by

$$C_t = C_r(1 - \rho_1 e^{-ht}) \tag{3}$$

where ρ_1 and $1/h$ are a fractional release by an initial impulse and a recovery time constant of readily available ACh, respectively. From equations (1–3), the ratio of the second G_{tr} to the first is expressed as

$$G_{tr_2}/G_{tr_1} = (1 - \rho_1 e^{-ht})(1 + e^{-bt})^n \tag{4}$$

The amplitude of EPSP corrected for nonlinear summation is given by $E = (E_s - V_m)G_{tr}/G_m$, where V_m and G_m are, respectively, the resting potential and conductance of postsynaptic membrane (Martin, 1955). Since E_s, V_m and G_m are constant, E is proportional to G_{tr}, then

$$E_2/E_1 = (1 - \rho_1 e^{-ht})(1 + e^{-bt})^n \tag{5}$$

As seen in Figure 21, the E_2/E_1 ratio and its time course, obtained directly from EPSCs by the voltage-clamp method and from the maximum conductances during EPSPs in the normal and high $[Ca]_o$ media, fit fairly well the curves obtained theoretically from equation (5). The experimental values in a low Ca medium, although not shown in this figure, also agree well with the calculated curve.

The best fit of the experimental curve and theoretical curves resulted when n was taken to be one. This is consistent with the conclusion of Lipicky et al. (1963), who suggested a less than one-for-one exchange of ACh for calcium at nerve terminals of the rabbit superior cervical ganglia. On the other hand, at the neuromuscular junction as many as four calcium ions have been suggested to be necessary to cause ACh release sites to be activated (Dodge and Rahamimoff, 1967).

It is apparent from the figure that an elevation of $[Ca]_o$ increases the value of $1/b$ and p_1. The recovery time constant, h, of readily available ACh, is, however, independent of the elevation of $[Ca]_o$. This latter result is in agreement with the observations at the neuromuscular junction by Lundberg and Quilisch (1953), Takeuchi (1958), and Thies (1965), where the time course of depression is independent of the extracellular Ca concentration.

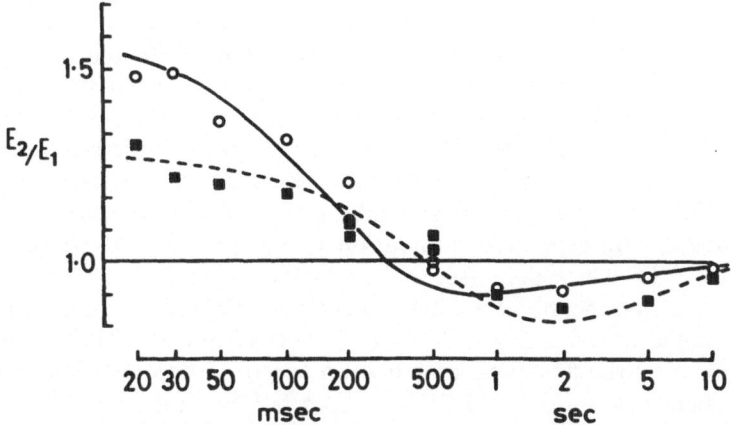

Figure 21. Comparison of the time course of experimentally obtained E_2/E_1 ratios (the second of a pair of EPSC divided by the first) with that of theoretically expected values of the ratio. The latter are derived from the equations, $E_2/E_1 = (1 - p_1 e^{-ht})(1 + e^{-bt})^n$ where $n = 1$, $p_1 = 0.13$, $h = 0.22$ sec^{-1}, and $b = 6.30$ sec^{-1} in normal calcium solution (continuous curve), and where $n = 1$, $p_1 = 0.33$, $h = 0.22$ sec^{-1}, and $b = 1.80$ sec^{-1} in 5× calcium solution (dotted curve), respectively. E_2/E_1 ratios at intervals of 1–10 sec were obtained from the maximum conductance during the rising phase of EPSP.

The analysis of pairs of EPSPs in sympathetic ganglion cells demonstrates that facilitation and depression are simultaneously occurring processes, which are a result of normal nerve terminal activity. One or the other process will predominate, depending upon the interval between impulses as well as the relative concentration of extracellular calcium ion.

C. Effects of Ganglionic Blocking Agents

Of ganglion-blocking drugs which are commonly used, tetraethylammonium (Mason and Wien, 1955; Corne and Edge, 1958; Douglas and Lywood, 1961, Matthews and Quilliam, 1964; Riker, 1965, Matthews, 1966) and mecamylamine (Lees and Nishi, 1972) have been shown to have a presynaptic action in addition to their blocking action on nicotinic receptors in autonomic ganglia.

Hexamethonium (C_6) and d-tubocurarine (d-TC) have no effect on the resting membrane potential, on the threshold for generation of the ganglion action potential elicited by direct stimulation of the cell, on the amplitude of the direct spike or of the antidromically-conducted action potential, nor on the recovery of excitability of the postganglionic neuron. Thus it may be safely concluded that the principal postsynaptic mechanism by which these drugs inhibit ganglionic transmission is a nondepolarizing type of occupation of nicotinic receptors (Lees and Nishi, 1972). Since posttetanic potentiation is predominantly due to a presynaptic facilitation of transmission, it may be used as a screening test for possible presynaptic action of drugs. In confirmation of the idea that C_6 and d-TC do not have a presynaptic blocking effect, Lees and Nishi (1972) found that there is no reduction in posttetanic potentiation; furthermore, there is no inhibition of release of neurotransmitter substance during repetitive stimulation in the presence of concentration of C_6 and d-TC which depresses the amplitude of EPSPs.

Mecamylamine, however, has a more complex mode of action in inhibiting ganglionic transmission. In common with C_6 and d-TC, mecamylamine does not affect the postganglionic neuron except to depress its response to ACh. When the amplitude of EPSPs is depressed, even minimally, posttetanic potentiation is inhibited by mecamylamine (Lees and Nishi, 1972). In addition mecamylamine causes a rapid and progressive decline in amplitude of EPSPs during the conditioning tetanus (Figure 22A); this is not observed with d-TC (Figure 22B) or C_6. On the other hand, the amplitude of the ACh potential in the presence of mecamylamine (10 μM) is not reduced when the potential is elicited immediately after the early tetanic run-down (Figure 23A). Moreover, the amplitude of ACh potential with the repeated application of ACh does not show run-down (Figure 23B). These findings indicate that the inhi-

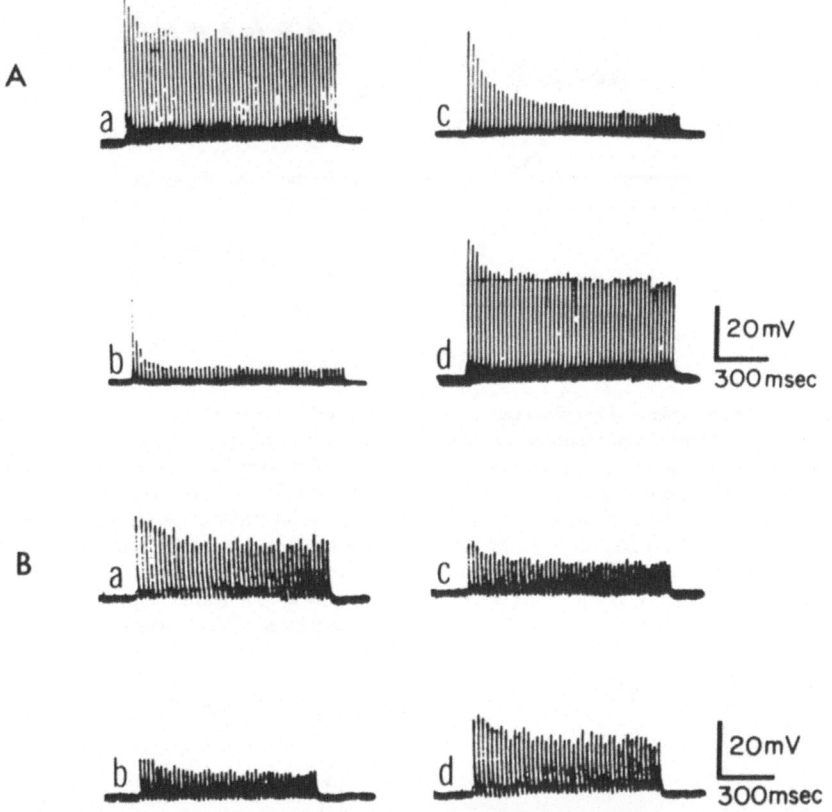

Figure 22. A: Effect of mecamylamine on amplitude of successive EPSP in a train (40 Hz): a, control; b, after exposure to mecamylamine (10 μM) for 7 min; c and d, recovery at 15 and 60 min, respectively, after cessation of exposure to mecamylamine. All records were taken from the same cell in rabbit superior cervical ganglion; calibrations: 20 mV and 300 msec. **B: Lack of effect of d-tubocurarine on amplitude of successive EPSP in a train (40 Hz):** a, control; b, after exposure to d-tubocurarine (10 μM) for 3 min; c and d, recovery at 7 and 20 min, respectively, after cessation of exposure to d-tubocurarine. All records were taken from the same cell in rabbit superior cervical ganglion; calibrations: 20 mV and 300 msec. (From Lees and Nishi, 1972.)

bition of posttetanic potentiation and the excessive run-down of tetanically induced EPSPs must be due to a reduction in amount of ACh released.

By means of the variance method (Elmqvist and Quastel, 1965), Lees and Nishi (1972) estimated the quantum content of each EPSP in a tetanic train before and after application of mecamylamine. It can be seen in Figure 24 that, under control conditions, the quantal content (m), falls rapidly, but

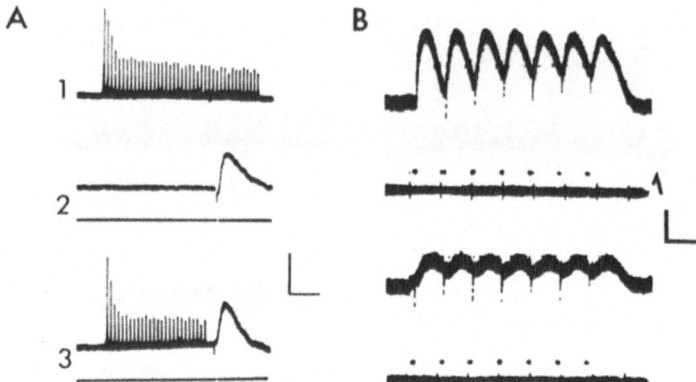

Figure 23. A: Response of ganglion cell to ACh in presence of mecamylamine (10 μM): 1, tetanus at 40 Hz; 2, control cell response to iontophoretic application of ACh; 3, tetanus at 40 Hz followed by iontophoretic application of ACh at time of maximal depression of amplitude of EPSP. Lower trace in records 2 and 3 show the current pulse (55 nA for 10 msec) for ACh ejection. All records were taken from the same cell in rabbit superior cervical ganglion; calibrations: 10 mV and 200 msec. **B: Membrane response to rapid repetitive application of ACh.** ACh potentials (upper traces) induced at 2 Hz by applying current pulses (lower traces) of 61 nA for 20 msec through the ACh electrode. 1, before, and 2, 10 min after, exposure of ganglion to mecamylamine (10 μM); calibrations: 10 mV and 200 msec. (From Lees and Nishi, 1972.)

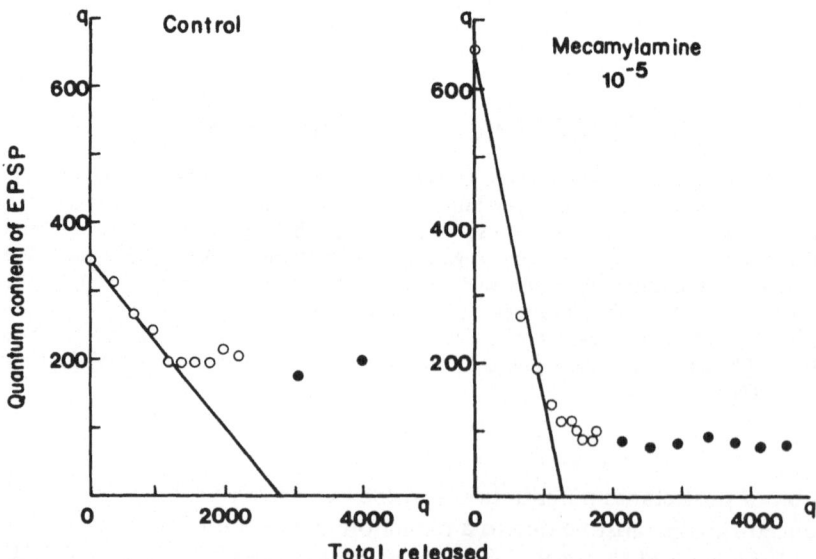

Figure 24. Effect of mecamylamine (10 μM) on quantal content of EPSP in a train (40 Hz). Ordinates, quantal content of EPSP (quanta). Abscissa, sum of quantal contents of all previous EPSP (quanta). Open circles, initial 10 EPSPs of train; closed circles, groups of 5 consecutive EPSPs. (From Lees and Nishi, 1972.)

TABLE 3. Effects of Mecamylamine on Quantal Content of EPSPs in Rabbit Superior Cervical Ganglion[a]

	Quantal content (m) of first EPSP (quanta)	Available store (n) (quanta)	Fractional release (p)	Quantal size (q) (mV)	Mobilization rate (quanta/msec)
Control	340	3144	0.11	0.15	4.68
Mecamylamine					
10 μM (10 min)	494[c]	1854[b]	0.28[b]	0.04[c]	2.65[b]
	(+46 %)	(−41 %)	(+157 %)	(−72%)	(−43 %)
Recovery (30 min)	414[c]	2494[b]	0.20	0.09	3.47[b]
	(+22 %)	(−21 %)	(+85 %)	(−40%)	(−27 %)

[a] Mean values of 6 experiments (From Lees and Nishi, 1972.)
[b] Difference is significant at $P = 0.01$ as compared to control.
[c] Difference is significant at $P = 0.05$ as compared to control.

only to a small extent, before the value is maintained relatively constant, probably because mobilization of ACh then matches release. A surprising, but consistent finding is that, in the presence of mecamylamine, the quantal content of the first EPSP in a train is greatly increased. Thereafter, m is less than in the corresponding control EPSP and declines much more rapidly. It should be added that the increase in m of the first EPSP of a train is not usually recognizable with intervals of less than 2 min between trains. The data obtained by further statistical analysis are shown in Table 3. It is shown that the fractional release is increased by nearly 160%, while the available store of the transmitter is decreased by about 40% in the presence of mecamylamine (10 μM). Furthermore, the mobilization rate which is obtained by dividing the mean quantal content by the stimulus interval is decreased by 40%. No such alterations are observed with C_6 (Table 4) or d-TC (Table 5). These characteristic effects of mecamylamine on the quantal liberation of ACh well

TABLE 4. Effects of Hexamethonium on Quantal Content of EPSPs in Rabbit Superior Cervical Ganglion[a]

	Quantal content (m) of first EPSP (quanta)	Available store (n) (quanta)	Fractional release (p)	Quantal size (q) (mV)	Mobilization rate (quanta/msec)
Control	256	3139	0.09	0.10	3.88
Hexamethonium					
50 μM (10 min)	269	3561	0.08	0.05[b]	3.93
Recovery (20 min)	272	3486	0.08	0.09[c]	3.86

[a] Mean values of 4 experiments (From Lees and Nishi, 1972.)
[b] Difference is significant at $P = 0.01$ as compared to control.
[c] Difference is significant at $P = 0.05$ as compared to control.

TABLE 5. Effect of d-Tubocurarine on Quantal Content of EPSPs in Rabbit Superior Cervical Ganglion[a]

	Quantal content (m) of first EPSP (quanta)	Available store (n) (quanta)	Fractional release (p)	Quantal size (q) (mV)	Mobilization rate (quanta/msec)
Control	222	2940	0.08	0.09	4.02
d-Tubocurarine					
10 μM (10 min)	252	2924	0.08	0.05[b]	3.58
Recovery (20 min)	234	2970	0.08	0.08[b]	4.06

[a] Mean values of 4 experiments (From Lees and Nishi, 1972.)
[b] Difference is significant at $P = 0.01$ as compared to control.
[c] Difference is significant at $P = 0.05$ as compared to control.

explain the marked run-down of a tetanic train of EPSPs and the disappearance of posttetanic potentiation by this compound.

V. SOME SPECIFIC PHYSIOPHARMACOLOGIC CHARACTERISTICS OF POSTSYNAPTIC NEURON MEMBRANE

A. Effects of Alkaline Earth Cations

1. Calcium, Barium, and Strontium Spikes of Amphibian Sympathetic Neurons

Bullfrog sympathetic ganglion cells are capable of producing action potentials (Ca spikes; Figure 25) in a Na-free isotonic $CaCl_2$ solution when they are directly stimulated by cathodal currents applied through an intracellular microelectrode (Koketsu and Nishi, 1968, 1969). This is a unique characteristic of ganglion cells which differentiates them from other neurons of the vertebrate. The resting membrane potential in an isotonic $CaCl_2$ solution is higher than that in Ringer solution; the former ranges from -80 to -110 mV, whereas the latter ranges -50 to -70 mV, depending on individual cells. The effective resistance of the resting cell membrane in an isotonic $CaCl_2$ solution is also considerably larger than that in Ringer solution; the mean value of the former is about 200 MΩ, whereas that of the latter is about 40 MΩ.

The threshold for initiation of Ca spikes ranges from -5 to -15 mV, and the peak potential of Ca spikes ranges from $+40$ to $+55$ mV, with the

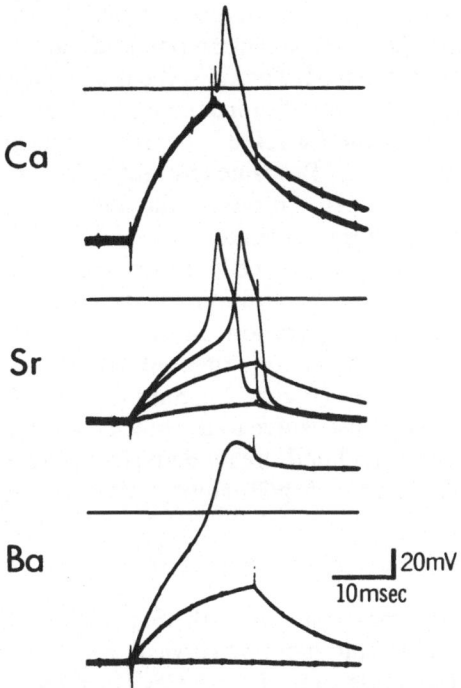

Figure 25. Intracellularly recorded action potentials of bullfrog sympathetic ganglion cells perfused with Na-free isotonic solutions of CaCl$_2$ (top), SrCl$_2$ (middle), and BaCl$_2$ (bottom). Action potentials were elicited by depolarizing current pulses applied through the cell membrane.

spike duration 3–5 msec. The maximum rate of rise of Ca spikes varies largely between individual cells; its mean value (ca. 60 V/sec) is approximately 40% of that of Na spikes.

The maximum rate of rise of the Ca spikes decreases when the resting membrane is depolarized by a cathodal current, while it does not show any appreciable change when the membrane is hyperpolarized by an anodal current, indicating that Ca inactivation, similar to Na inactivation, takes place when the membrane is depolarized. The inactivation curve, which represents the relationship between the maximum rate of rise of the Ca spikes and the membrane potential level, shows that inactivation of the Ca-carrying system is almost completely removed when the membrane potential is maintained at a level higher than −80 mV in a solution containing more than 8.4 mM Ca.

The value of the peak potential of the Ca spike is almost linearly proportional to the Ca concentration in the external solution, the increment for a 10-fold increase in Ca concentration being about 30 mV. This suggests that the inward movement of Ca ions across the membrane is responsible for the production of the Ca spike. No action potentials are produced with Ca at a concentration less than 5 mM. The Ca spike is more resistant to TTX than is the Na spike. The Na spike disappears within 5 min in the presence of 1.6 μM of TTX, whereas the Ca spike is depressed but not abolished in the presence of 15.7 μM of TTX. Procaine (18 mM, which blocks the Na spike within a few minutes, markedly prolongs the falling phase and slightly depresses the rising phase of the Ca spike.

Bullfrog sympathetic ganglion cells are also capable of producing action potentials in an isotonic $SrCl_2$ solution (Sr Spikes; Figure 25) which are similar to Ca spikes in configuration. In an isotonic $BaCl_2$ solution they produce markedly prolonged action potentials (Ba spikes), which often lasts for more than a few seconds (Figure 25). Similar to the Ca spikes, both the Sr and Ba spikes are very insensitive to the blocking action of TTX and procaine. The cells, on the other hand, are rendered inexcitable when the ganglion is superfused with an isotonic $MgCl_2$ solution for more than 10 min.

2. Barium Spike of Mammalian Sympathetic Neurons

In contrast to the amphibian sympathetic ganglion cells, the mammalian sympathetic neurons (rabbit superior cervical ganglion cells; Tashiro and Nishi, 1972) are inexcitable in a Na-free $CaCl_2$ or $SrCl_2$ medium, but can produce a prolonged action potential in a Na-free $BaCl_2$ medium. The preganglionic fibers also have this property (Greengard and Straub, 1959). This difference between the amphibian and mammalian neurons might imply that along with the phylogenic evolution of the animal, the autonomic cell membrane alters its physicochemical properties and becomes more selective in its permeability to ions in the generation of the action potential.

B. Effects of Caffeine

1. Rhythmic Hyperpolarizations and Slow Depolarization Induced by Caffeine

Caffeine and other methylxanthines, such as theophylline and theobromine, are known to stimulate various central neurons (Libet and Gerard, 1941; Gualtierotti, 1955a, b; Hahn, 1960; Maiti and Domino, 1961; Sant' Ambrogio et al., 1962) as well as peripheral adrenergic cells (Atuk et al., 1967; Poisner, 1973). At the cellular level, methylxanthines inhibit phosphodiesterase breakdown of cyclic 3', 5'-adenosine monophosphate (AMP) (Butcher and Sutherland, 1962), and thereby potentiate its metabolic stimulating action in many tissues including brain slices (Rall and Sattin, 1970). Caffeine is also known to increase the Ca permeability of the cytoplasmic membrane (Bianchi, 1961) and release Ca from the sarcoplasmic reticulum in the skeletal muscle (Weber and Herz, 1968).

Kuba *et al.* (1972) found that caffeine induces in the amphibian sympathetic ganglion cells a slow depolarization which is intervened by rhythmic hyperpolarizations. Figure 26A shows a typical sequence of the membrane potential induced by 3 mM caffeine. Within 1 min after the beginning of a caffeine perfusion, the cell membrane shows a slow transient hyperpolarization (the initial caffeine hyperpolarization; ICH), which lasts for about

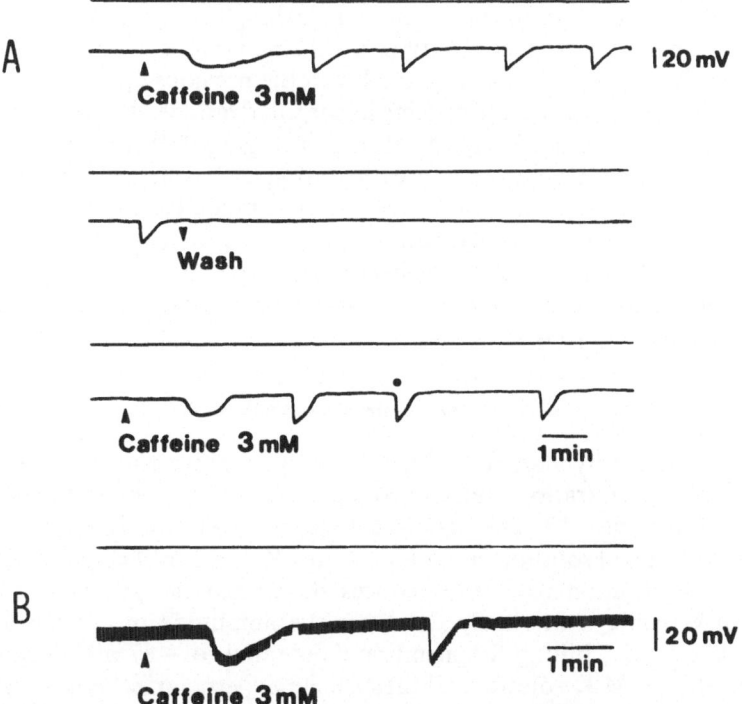

Figure 26. A: **Caffeine-induced hyperpolarizations of a single bullfrog sympathetic ganglion cell.** Caffeine (3 mM) was applied twice at the time marked by upward arrows. Before the second application, the preparation was washed with Ringer solution for 11 min. A dot indicates a hyperpolarizing response triggered by an antidromic impulse. All records were taken successively. B: **Lowering of membrane resistance during caffeine-induced hyperpolarizations, as shown by a marked reduction of electrotonic potentials.** Anodal current pulses (0.17 nA, 200 msec) were applied through the cell membrane every 2 sec. Recordings in both A and B were made by an inkwriting recorder whose response was fast enough to reproduce faithfully the caffeine-induced potentials but was not fast enough to follow action potentials. The upper line in each record represents the zero potential level.

2 min and is followed by a small and slow progressive depolarization. In 2–5 min, rhythmic hyperpolarizations (the rhythmic caffeine hyperpolarizations; RCHs) suddenly begin to take place, as seen in the record. The interval of RCHs is fairly constant in the same cell, but varies considerably in different cells from 15 sec to as long as 10 min. A hyperpolarization quite similar to the RCH can be triggered by an action potential elicited either by orthodromic, antidromic, or direct intracellular stimulation (the evoked caffeine hyperpolarization; ECH). The amplitude of all these caffeine hyperpolarizations ranges from a few mV to over 30 mV, but never exceeds the peak level of the afterhyperpolarization of the action potential.

The RCHs occur even if the caffeine perfusion is continued for several hours, while they all disappear soon after washing the ganglion with Ringer solution. Furthermore, reapplication of caffeine induces the same sequence of potential changes that was observed with the previous application.

During the generation of caffeine hyperpolarizations, the cell membrane resistance decreases markedly. As shown in Figure 26B, the amplitude of electrotonic potentials decreases greatly during each caffeine hyperpolarization. The maximum reduction in electrotonic potential amplitude is seen at the peak of each hyperpolarization, and this amounts to 30–50% of the value during the absence of a caffeine hyperpolarization. This suggests that the caffeine hyperpolarization is associated with a drastic increase in membrane permeability to certain ions.

2. Ionic Mechanism of Caffeine Hyperpolarization

The caffeine hyperpolarizations are very sensitive to a change in the external K concentration and also to a change in the membrane potential, as shown in Figure 27. The uppermost record shows the ICH, RCH, and ECHs in a control solution containing 2 mM K and 3 mM caffeine. Raising the K concentration to 8 mM reduces the membrane potential by only a few mV, while it markedly decreases the amplitude of caffeine hyperpolarizations. By shifting the membrane potential to -87 mV during perfusion with 8 mM K solution, all the caffeine hyperpolarizations—the ICH, RCHs, and ECHs—are completely reversed in polarity. At this level, the afterhyperpolarization of the action potential is also reversed. As the applied hyperpolarization is reduced to the level of -62 mV, the caffeine hyperpolarizations are almost nullified, and so is the afterpotential of the action potential. Upon returning to the original membrane potential of -51 mV, both the polarity and the amplitude of caffeine potentials are restored. This series of observations indicates that the caffeine hyperpolarizations have an equilibrium potential which is the same or very close to the K equilibrium potential. It should be added that replacement of the NaCl of Ringer solution with

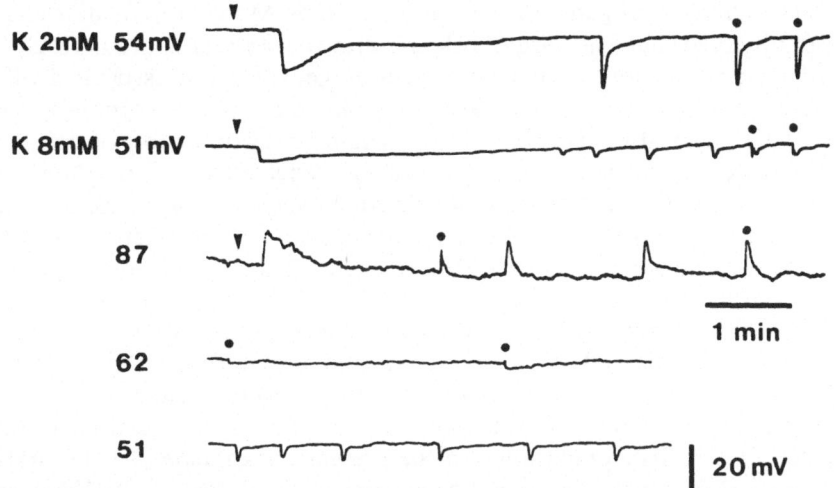

Figure 27. Effects of high K concentration and continuous hyperpolarization on caffeine-induced hyperpolarizations. The first and second records show the initial, the rhythmic, and the evoked caffeine potentials in the 2 and 8 mM K Ringer solutions both containing 2 mM caffeine. Before and after obtaining the second record, the preparation was perfused with a caffeine-free 8 mM K Ringer solution. At the beginning of the third record, caffeine (2 mM) was added again to the 8 mM K Ringer solution. The cell membrane was artificially hyperpolarized during the third and fourth records, but not during the fifth record. All records were obtained from the same cell in bullfrog sympathetic ganglion. Arrows mark beginning of caffeine application, and dots indicate responses evoked by antidromic stimulation. Membrane potential levels at the beginning of each record are shown in mV on the left.

sucrose or tris-chloride does not noticeably affect the amplitude of the caffeine hyperpolarizations. These findings strongly suggest that all the caffeine hyperpolarizations are generated by the same mechanism, namely an increased membrane permeability to K ions.

3. Role of Ca in the Production of Caffeine Hyperpolarizations

The occurrence of caffeine hyperpolarizations is profoundly dependent upon the external Ca concentration. As the Ca concentration of the perfusing solution is decreased, the frequency of RCHs is reduced markedly. Futhermore, removal of the external Ca causes a complete blockade of all caffeine hyperpolarizations which is swiftly reversible after return to the normal Ringer solution.

Since caffeine is well known to release calcium from the sarcoplasmic reticulum into the sarcoplasm (Weber and Herz, 1968), it is conceivable that caffeine exerts a similar action on some intraneuronal organelles or the plasma membrane of ganglion cells. Furthermore, Meech and Strumwasser (1970) observed that injection of calcium into the *Aplysia* neurons resulted in a hyperpolarization of the neuron membrane which was associated with an increased membrane conductance for potassium ions. According to the observation and also to the possible calcium releasing action of caffeine, the increased potassium conductance of the caffeine-treated ganglion cell membrane might be attributed to an elevated concentration of the internal free calcium. Disappearance of caffeine hyperpolarizations after removal of the external calcium is consistent with this idea. In such a calcium-deprived condition, the elevation of the internal calcium concentration by caffeine would be hardly achieved because, as Bianchi (1961) reported, caffeine increases the influx as well as the efflux of calcium and the accelerated calcium efflux can take place even in the absence of the external calcium.

Endo *et al.* (1970) observed spontaneous repeated contractions of the skinned muscle fiber preparation in the presence of caffeine (0.2–1.0 mM). They also demonstrated evidence suggesting that the free Ca itself has an action on the sarcoplasmic reticulum which promotes the release of Ca leading to a regenerative release of Ca. If a similar regenerative release process for Ca occurs in the sympathetic ganglion cells under the influence of caffeine, the rhythmicity of RCHs might be explained as follows: When caffeine reaches the cell, it releases Ca regeneratively from some specific sites until the storage of Ca is fully depleted. The consequent increase in the internal Ca concentration elicits an increase in K permeability of the membrane. The depleted storage sites then resume an uptake of Ca with a slow time course, decreasing the free Ca concentration in the cell and restoring the K permeability. Once the Ca concentration of the storage sites attains a critical level for the action of caffeine, a new response will again be initiated.

It has been shown that Ca enters the cell during an action potential (Hodgkin and Keynes, 1957); above all, the amphibian sympathetic ganglion cells are endowed with a specific capability of producing a "Ca spike" (Koketsu and Nishi, 1969). Owing to this entry of Ca, together with the possible freeing of Ca from the cell membrane by virtue of depolarization, an action potential might cause a temporary increase in the internal free Ca. This would trigger, in the presence of caffeine, a regenerative release of Ca from its storage sites (Endo *et al.*, 1970) and would eventually cause a hyperpolarization—the evoked caffeine potential.

4. Mechanism of Caffeine Depolarization

The depolarization of ganglion cells after exposure to 2–3 mM caffeine slowly attains its plateau level (10–15 mV) in 10 min. This caffeine depolarization is not significantly affected in either amplitude or time course when the Cl in Ringer solution is totally replaced by glutamate. This implies that Cl permeability of the cell membrane is not involved in the production of the caffeine depolarization. Replacement of Na with tris reduces the caffeine depolarization approximately 20%. When the superfusing Ringer solution is changed to Ca-free Ringer, the membrane potential shows a slow decrease. This depolarization is completely prevented by the total replacement of Na with tris. If the preparation had been pretreated with a Na-free, Ca-free solution for over 5 min, addition of caffeine (2–3 mM) does not induce any depolarization at all. It is most likely then that the caffeine depolarization is primarily caused by an increased entry of Ca ions across the cell membrane. This hypothesis is consistent with one of the characteristic effects of caffeine to increase the Ca permeability of the cell membrane (Bianchi, 1961). The small reduction of the caffeine depolarization by the removal of Na indicates that Na contributes only partially to this depolarization. It appears that the depolarization caused by Ca entry, as well as the unbinding of membrane Ca in the presence of caffeine, gives rise to a small increase in Na conductance.

The accumulation of cyclic 3',5'-AMP in the neurons owing to the depressant action of caffeine on phosphodiesterase activity (Butcher and Sutherland, 1962) might possibly influence the ionic conductance of the cell membrane. However, perfusion of the ganglion with a solution containing 2 mM dibutyryl cyclic AMP does not induce any recognizable changes in the membrane potential. This may rule out direct involvement of cyclic AMP in the generation of caffeine depolarization or caffeine hyperpolarization.

It should be added that the caffeine depolarization is not mediated by any synaptic mechanism such as the liberation of ACh from the presynaptic terminals or direct stimulation of the postsynaptic cholinoceptive sites; both d-TC and atropine are ineffective in preventing the caffeine depolarization. Furthermore, the late slow EPSP which is generated at a noncholinergic site (Nishi and Koketsu, 1968a) shows no appreciable changes after a prolonged exposure to caffeine.

C. Hyperpolarization Owing to Activity of an Electrogenic Sodium Pump

It has been shown by several workers (Pascoe, 1956; Brown, 1966; Kosterlitz, et al., 1968, 1970; Brown et al., 1969, 1972; Lees and Wallis, 1974) that after superior cervical ganglia from rabbit, rat, or kitten have been depolarized by acetylcholine, carbachol or choline acting on nicotinic receptors, removal of the depolarizing agent results in a hyperpolarization of the ganglion cells. For convenience, this is termed "afterhyperpolarization." That the afterhyperpolarization is a property of the ganglion cells and not of the postganglionic axons coursing through the ganglion is shown by the failure of an afterhyperpolarization to occur in the postganglionic axons of the internal carotid nerve of the rabbit (Kosterlitz et al., 1968). Furthermore, the afterhyperpolarization is not a consequence of a large depolarization of the cells because depolarization induced by altering $[K]_0$ is never followed by hyperpolarization (Lees and Wallis, 1974). Since the amplitude and time course of the afterhyperpolarization is not dependent on the Cl concentration in the bathing fluid, an increased Cl conductance cannot be involved.

If the afterhyperpolarization were caused by an increased K conductance, a reduction in $[K]_0$ would result in an increase in amplitude of the afterhyperpolarization. Correspondingly, as the membrane potential approaches E_K, an increase in K permeability would be accompanied by a progressively smaller hyperpolarization. It is found, however, that when K ions are omitted from the bathing solution, the amplitude of the afterhyperpolarization is never increased and is usually greatly diminished after about 35 min in this medium (Lees and Wallis, 1974). When 12.5 mM K–Krebs solution is used, the resting potential of rabbit superior cervical ganglion cells is close to E_K. Under these conditions, the amplitude of the afterhyperpolarization is unchanged or even increased, and its rate of development, which is always reduced in K-free Krebs solution, is greatly increased. Thus, the explanation for the mechanism of the afterhyperpolarization cannot be in terms of an increased K conductance.

It can be readily demonstrated that the amplitude of the afterhyperpolarization is related more closely to the duration of depolarization than to the magnitude of depolarization; furthermore, reduction in $[Na]_0$ results in a smaller afterhyperpolarization. These observations are consistent with the view that the afterhyperpolarization is related to, or a consequence of, the amount of Na entering the cells during the preceding depolarization. Further support comes from the results of the following type of experiment: in K-free solutions, acetylcholine causes a depolarization which declines slowly to be followed by a small afterhyperpolarization. If, at this time $[K]_0$ is raised to the control value, a large, rapid hyperpolarization immediately ensues (Kosterlitz et al., 1970). These results can be explained only by the acivity of an electrogenic sodium pump which requires K extracellularly for its operation (Rang and Ritchie, 1968). The additional important findings that ouabain and glucose-free solutions inhibit the development of the afterhyperpolarization point to this potential being caused by the metabolically dependent extrusion of Na by a pumping mechanism with a coupling ratio which is not unity for Na–K exchange. A very similar electrogenic sodium pump is thought to be present in rat superior cervical ganglia (Brown et al., 1972) and in the membrane of the nonmyelinated axons of the rabbit vagus nerve (Rang and Ritchie, 1968).

ACKNOWLEDGMENT

The author wishes to thank Dr. G. M. Lees for his help and criticism in the preparation of the manuscript. Most of the investigations carried out in the author's laboratory at Loyola University Medical Center, Illinois, were supported by NIH Research Grant NS06672 and NSF Research Grant GB 30360.

REFERENCES

Ambache, N., 1949, The nicotinic action of substances supposed to be purely smooth muscle stimulating. (B) Effect of $BaCl_2$ and pilocarpine on the superior cervical ganglion, *J. Physiol. (London)* 110:164.

Ambache, N., Perry, W. L. M., and Robertson, P. A., 1956, The effect of muscarine on perfused superior cervical ganglia of cats, *Br. J. Pharmacol.* 11:442.

Alkadhi, K. A., and McIsaac, R. J., 1971, Non-nicotinic ganglionic transmission during partial ganglionic blockade with chlorisondamine, *Fed. Proc.* 30:655.

Araki, T., and Otani, T., 1955, Response of single motoneurons to direct stimulation in toad's spinal cord, *J. Neurophysiol.* 18:472.

Atuk, N. O., Blaydes, M. C., Westervelt, F. B., Jr., and Wood, J. E., Jr., 1967, Effect of aminophylline on urinary excretion of epinephrine and norepinephrine in man, *Circulation* 35:745.

Baker, P. F., Hodgkin, A. L., and Ridgeway, E. B., 1971, Depolarization and calcium entry in squid giant axons, *J. Physiol (London)* 218:709.

Bianchi, C. P., 1961, Effects of caffeine on radiocalcium movement in frog sartorius, *J. Gen. Physiol.* 44:845.

Billingsley, P. R., and Ranson, S. W., 1918, On the number of nerve cells in the ganglion cervicale superius and of nerve fibres in the cephalic end of the truncus in the cat and on the numerical relations of preganglionic and postganglionic neurones, *J. Comp. Neurol.* 29:359.

Birks, R., and MacIntosh, F. C., 1961, Acetylcholine metabolism of a sympathetic ganglion, *Can. J. Biochem. Physiol.* 39:787.

Blackman, J. G., and Purves, R. D., 1969, Intracellular recordings from ganglia of the thoracic sympathetic chain of the guinea-pig, *J. Physiol. (London)* 203:173.

Blackman, J. G., Ginsborg, B. L., and Ray, C., 1963, Spontaneous synaptic activity in sympathetic ganglion cells of the frog, *J. Physiol. (London)* 167:389.

Blackman, J. G., Crowcroft, P. J., Devine, C. E., Holman, M. E., and Yonemura, K., 1969, Transmission from preganglionic fibres in the hypogastric nerve to peripheral ganglia of male guinea-pigs, *J. Physiol. (London)* 201:723.

Bowman, W. C., and Nott, M. W., 1969, Actions of sympathomimetic amines and their antagonists on skeletal muscle, *Pharmacol. Rev.* 21:27.

Bracho, H., and Orkand, R. K., 1970, Effect of calcium on excitatory neuromuscular transmission in the crayfish, *J. Physiol. (London)* 206:61.

Brimble, M. J., Wallis, D. I., and Woodward, B., 1972, Facilitation and inhibition of cell groups within the superior cervical ganglion of the rabbit, *J. Physiol. (London)* 226:629.

Bronk, D. W., 1939, Synaptic mechanisms in sympathetic ganglia, *J. Neurophysiol.* 2:380.

Brown, A. M., 1967, Cardiac sympathetic adrenergic pathways in which synaptic transmission is blocked by atropine sulfate, *J. Physiol. (London)* 191:271.

Brown, D. A., 1966, Depolarization of normal and preganglionically denervated superior cervical ganglia by stimulant drugs, *Br. J. Pharmacol. Chemother.* 26:511.

Brown, D. A., Brownstein, M. J., and Scholfield, C. N., 1969, On the nature of the drug-induced after-hyperpolarization in isolated rat ganglia, *Br. J. Pharmacol.* **37**:511.

Brown, D. A., Brownstein, M. J., and Scholfield, C. N., 1972, Origin of the after-hyperpolarization that follows removal of depolarizing agents from the isolated superior cervical ganglion of the rat, *Br. J. Pharmacol.* **44**:651.

Brown, G. L., 1934, Conduction in the cervical sympathetic, *J. Physiol. (London)* **81**:228.

Bülbring, E., 1944, The action of adrenaline on transmission in the superior cervical ganglion, *J. Physiol. (London)* **103**:55.

Bülbring, E., and Burn, J. H., 1942, An action of adrenaline on transmission in sympathetic ganglia which may play a part in shock, *J. Physiol. (London)* **101**:289.

Butcher, R. W., and Sutherland, E. W., 1962, Adenosine 3′, 5′-phosphate in biological materials, *J. Biol. Chem.* **237**:1244.

Chen, S. S., 1969, Late contraction of nictitating membrane of the dog, *Am. J. Physiol.* **217**:1205.

Chen, S. S., 1971, Transmission in superior cervical ganglion of the dog after cholinergic suppression, *Am. J. Physiol.* **221**:209.

Chen, S. S., 1972, Late discharges in dog's sympathetic ganglia, *Can. J. Physiol.* **50**:263.

Chen, S. S., 1974, Biphasic stimulation of the canine superior cervical ganglion (SCG) by K$^+$, *Fed. Proc.* **33**:552.

Christ, D. D., and Nishi, S., 1969, Presynaptic action of epinephrine on sympathetic ganglia, *Life Sci.* **8**:1235.

Christ, D. D., and Nishi, S., 1971a, Site of adrenaline blockade in the superior cervical ganglion of the rabbit, *J. Physiol. (London)* **213**:107

Christ, D. D., and Nishi, S., 1971b, Effects of adrenaline on nerve terminals in the superior cervical ganglion of the rabbit, *Br. J. Pharmacol.* **41**:331.

Collier, B., Vickerson, F. H. L., and Varma, D. R., 1969, Effect of acetylcholine (ACh) on transmitter release in cat superior cervical ganglion, *Fed. Proc.* **28**:670.

Coombs, J. S., Curtis, D. R., and Eccles, J. C., 1957a, The interpretation of spike potentials of motoneurons, *J. Physiol. (London)* **139**:198.

Coombs, J. S., Curtis, D. R., and Eccles, J. C., 1957b, The generation of impulses in motoneurones, *J. Physiol. (London)* **139**:232.

Corne, S. J., and Edge, N. D., 1958, Pharmacological properties of pempidine (1:2:2:6:6-pentamethylpiperidine), a new ganglion blocking compound, *Br. J. Pharmacol. Chemother.* **13**:339.

Costa, E., Revzin, A. M., Kuntzman, R., Spector, S., and Brodie, B. R., 1961, Role for ganglionic norepinephrine in sympathetic synaptic transmission, *Science (New York)* **133**:1822.

Crowcroft, P. J., and Szurszewski, J. H., 1971, A study of the inferior mesenteric and pelvic ganglion of guinea-pigs with intracellular electrodes, *J. Physiol. (London)* **219**:421.

De Castro, F., 1932, Sympathetic ganglia, normal and pathological, in *Cytology and Cellular Pathology of the Nervous System* (W. Penfield, ed.), Vol. 1, p. 319, P. B., Hoeber, New York.

De Groat, W. C., and Volle, R. L., 1963, Ganglionic actions of oxotremorine, *Life. Sci.* **8**:618.

De Groat, W. C., and Volle, R. L., 1966, The actions of the catecholamines on transmission in the superior cervical ganglion of the cat, *J. Pharmacol. Exp. Ther.* **154**:1.

de Robertis, E. D. P., 1964, *Histophysiology of Synapses and Neurosecretion*, Pergamon, Oxford.

de Robertis, E. D. P., and Bennett, H. S., 1954, Submicroscopic vesicular component in the synapse, *Fed. Proc.* **13**:35.

del Castillo, J., and Katz, B., 1954, Statistical factors involved in neuromuscular facilitation and depression, *J. Physiol. (London)* **124**:574.

del Castillo, J., and Katz, B., 1955, On the localization of acetylcholine receptors, *J. Physiol. (London)* **128**:157.

Dempsher, J., and Riker, W. K., 1957, The role of acetylcholine in virus-infected sympathetic ganglia, *J. Physiol. (London)* **139**:145.

Dempsher, J., Larrabee, M. G., Bang, F. B., and Bodian, D., 1955, Physiological changes in sympathetic ganglia infected with pseudorabies virus, *Am. J. Physiol.* **182**:203.

Dodge, F. A., and Rahamimoff, P., 1967, Co-operative action of calcium ions in transmitter release at the neuromuscular junction, *J. Physiol. (London)* **193**:419.

Douglas, W. W., and Lywood, D. W., 1961, The stimulant effect of TEA on acetylcholine output from the superior cervical ganglion: Comparison with barium, *Fed. Proc.* **20**:324.

Douglas, W. W., Lywood, D. W., and Straub, R. W., 1960, On the excitant effect of acetylcholine on structure in the preganglionic trunk of the cervical sympathetic: With a note on the anatomical complexities of the region, *J. Physiol. (London)* **153**:250.

Dun, N., and Nishi, S., 1974, Effects of dopamine on the superior cervical ganglion of the rabbit, *J. Physiol. (London)* **239**:155.

Eccles, J. C., 1935, Facilitation and inhibition in the superior cervical ganglion, *J. Physiol. (London)* **85**:207.

Eccles, J. C., 1936, Synaptic and neuromuscular transmission, *Ergeb. Physiol.* **38**:339.

Eccles, J. C., 1943, Synaptic potentials and transmission in sympathetic ganglion, *J. Physiol. (London)* **101**:464.

Eccles, R. M., 1952, Responses of isolated curarized sympathetic ganglia, *J. Physiol. (London)* **117**:196

Eccles, R. M., 1955, Intracellular potentials recorded from a mammalian sympathetic ganglion, *J. Physiol. (London)* **130**:572.

Eccles, R. M., 1963, Orthodromic activation of single ganglion cells, *J. Physiol. (London)* **165**:387

Eccles, R. M., and Libet, B., 1961, Origin and blockade of the synaptic responses of curarized sympathetic ganglia, *J. Physiol. (London)* **157**:484.

Elfvin, L. G., 1963, The ultrastructure of the superior cervical sympathetic ganglion of the cat: II. The structure of the preganglionic end fibres and the synapse as studied by serial sections, *J. Ultrastruct. Res.* **8**:441.

Elfvin, L. G., 1968, A new granule-containing nerve cell in the inferior mesenteric ganglion of the rabbit, *J. Ultrastruct. Res.* **22**:37.

Elmqvist, D., and Quastel, D. M., 1965, A quantitative study of end-plate potentials in isolated human muscle, *J. Physiol. (London)* **178**:505.

Emmelin, N., and MacIntosh, F. C., 1956, The release of acetylcholine from perfused sympathetic ganglia and skeletal muscles, *J. Physiol. (London)* **131**:477.

Endo, M., Tanaka, M., and Ogawa, Y., 1970, Calcium induced release of calcium from the sarcoplasmic reticulum of skinned muscle fibres, *Nature (London)* **228**:34.

Erulkar, S. D., and Woodward, J. K., 1968, Intracellular recording from mammalian superior cervical ganglion *in situ*, *J. Physiol. (London)* **199**:189.

Fatt, P., 1957, Sequence of events in synaptic activation of a motoneurone, *J. Neurophysiol.* **20**:61.

Flacke, W., and Gillis, R. A., 1968, Impulse transmission via nicotinic and muscarinic pathways in the stellate ganglion of the dog, *J. Pharmacol. Exp. Ther.* **163**:266.

Fujimoto, S., 1967, Some observations on the fine structure of the sympathetic ganglion of the toad, *Bufo vulgaris japonicus*, *Arch. Histol. Jpn.* **28**:313.

Fuortes, M. G. F., Frank, K., and Becker, M. D., 1957, Steps in the production of motoneuron spikes, *J. Gen. Physiol.* **40**:735.

Gallagher, J. P., Tashiro, N., and Nishi, S., 1973, Facilitation and depression of fast EPSP's in bullfrog sympathetic ganglion cells, *Fed. Proc.* **32**:799.

Gebber, G. L., 1968, Prolonged ganglionic facilitation and the positive afterpotential, *Int. J. Neuropharmacol.* **7**:195.

Ginsborg, B. L., 1971, On the presynaptic acetylcholine receptors in sympathetic ganglia of the frog, *J. Physiol. (London)* **216**:237.

Greengard, P., and Straub, R. W., 1959, Restoration by barium of action potentials in sodium-deprived mammalian B and C fibres. *J. Physiol. (London)* **145**:562.

Grillo, M. A., 1966, Electron microscopy of sympathetic tissues, *Pharmacol. Rev.* **18**:387.

Gualtierotti, T., 1955a, Variations in the frog's spinal reflexes caused by the action on the brain of large doses of caffeine, *J. Physiol. (London)* **128**:320.

Gualtierotti, T., 1955b, The contribution of spinal centers to the action of caffeine on frog's spinal reflexes, *J. Physiol. (London)* **128**:326.

Gyermek, L., Sigg, E. B., and Binder, E., 1963, Ganglionic stimulant action of muscarine, *Am. J. Physiol.* **204**:68.

Hahn, R., 1960, Analeptics, *Pharmacol. Rev.* **12**:447.

Hilton, J. G., 1961, The pressor response to neostigmine after ganglionic blockade, *J. Pharmacol. Exp. Ther.* **132**:23.

Hodgkin, A. L., and Keynes, R. D., 1957, Movements of labelled calcium in squid giant axons, *J. Physiol. (London)* **138**:253.

Hubbard, J. I., and Schmidt, R. F., 1961, Stimulation of motor nerve terminals, *Nature (London)* **191**:1003.

Hubbard, J. I., Jones, S. F., and Landau, E. C., 1968, On the mechanism by which calcium and magnesium affect the release of transmitter by nerve impulses, *J. Physiol. (London)* **196**:75.

Huber, B. C., 1899, A contribution on the minute anatomy of the sympathetic ganglia of the different classes of vertebrates, *J. Morphol.* **17**:27.

Hunt, C. C., and Nelson, P. G., 1965, Structural and functional changes in the frog sympathetic ganglion following cutting of the presynaptic nerve fibres, *J. Physiol. (London)* **177**:1.

Jacobowitz, D., 1970, Catecholamine fluorescence studies of adrenergic neurons and chromaffin cells in sympathetic ganglia, *Fed. Proc.* **29**:1929.

Jenkinson, D. H., 1957, The nature of the antagonism between calcium and magnesium ions at the neuromuscular junction, *J. Physiol. (London)* **138**:434.

Jenkinson, D. H., Stamenovic, B. A., and Whitaker, B. D. L., 1968, The effect of noradrenaline on the end-plate potential in twitch fibres of the frog, *J. Physiol. (London)* **195**:743.

Jones, A., 1963, Ganglionic actions of muscarinic substances, *J. Pharmacol. Exp. Ther.* **141**:195.

Katz, B., and Miledi, R., 1965, The effect of calcium on acetylcholine release from motor nerve terminals, *J. Physiol. (London)* **161**:496.

Katz, B., and Miledi, R., 1967, The timing of calcium action during neuromuscular transmission, *J. Physiol. (London)* **189**:535.

Katz, B., and Miledi, R., 1968, The role of calcium in neuromuscular facilitation, *J. Physiol. (London)* **195**:481.

Katz, B., and Miledi, R., 1970, Further study of the role of calcium in synaptic transmission, *J. Physiol. (London)* **207**:789.

Kewitz, H., and Reinert, H., 1952, Prüfung Pharmakologischer Wirkungen oberen sympathischen Halsganglion bei verschiedenen Erregungzuständen, *Arch. Exp. Pathol. Pharmakol.* **215**:547.

Kobayashi, H., and Libet, B., 1968, Generation of slow postsynaptic potentials without increases in ionic conductance, *Proc. Natl. Acad. Sci. U.S.A.* **60**:1304.

Kobayashi, H., and Libet, B., 1970, Actions of norepinephrine and acetylcholine on sympathetic ganglion cells, *J. Physiol. (London)* **208**:353.

Koelle, G. B., 1961, A proposed dual neurohumoral role of acetylcholine: Its functions at the pre- and postsynaptic sites, *Nature (London)* **190**:208.

Koelle, G. B., 1962, A new general concept of the neurohumoral functions of acetylcholine and acetylcholinesterases, *J. Pharm. Pharmacol.* **14**:65.

Koelle, W. A., and Koelle, G. B., 1959, The location of external or functional acetylcholines-terase at the synapses of autonomic ganglia, *J. Pharmacol. Exp. Ther.* **126**:1.

Koketsu, K., 1969, Cholinergic synaptic potentials and the underlying ionic mechanisms, *Fed. Proc.* **28**:101.

Koketsu, K., and Nishi, S., 1967, Characteristics of the slow inhibitory postsynaptic potential of bullfrog sympathetic ganglion cells, *Life Sci.* **6**:1827.

Koketsu, K., and Nishi, S., 1968, Cholinergic receptors at sympathetic preganglionic nerve terminals, *J. Physiol. (London)* **196**:293.

Koketsu, K., and Nishi, S., 1969, Calcium and action potentials of bullfrog sympathetic gan-glion cells, *J. Gen. Physiol.* **53**:608.

Koketsu, K., Nishi, S., and Soeda, H., 1968, Acetylcholine-potential of sympathetic ganglion cell membrane, *Life Sci.* **7**:741.

Konzett, H., 1950, Sympathomimetica und Sympathicolytica am isoliert durchströmten Gan-glion Cervicale superius der Katze, *Helv. Physiol. Pharmacol. Acta* **8**:245.

Konzett, H., and Waser, P. G., 1956, Zur ganglionären Wirkung von Muscarin, *Helv. Physiol. Acta* **14**:202.

Koppanyi, T., 1932, Studies on the synergism antagonism of drugs. I. The non-parasympathetic antagonism between atropine and the miotic alkaloids, *J. Pharmacol. Exp. Ther.* **46**:395.

Kosterlitz, H. W., and Wallis, D. I., 1966, The use of the sucrose-gap method for recording ganglionic potentials, *J. Physiol. (London)* **183**:1p.

Kosterlitz, H. W., Lees, G. M., and Wallis, D. I., 1968, Resting and action potentials recorded by the sucrose-gap method in the superior cervical ganglion of the rabbit, *J. Physiol. (London)* **195**:39.

Kosterlitz, H. W., Lees, G. M., and Wallis, D. I., 1970, Further evidence for an electrogenic sodium pump in a mammalian sympathetic ganglion, *Br. J. Pharmacol.* **40**:275.

Krnjević, K., and Miledi, R., 1958, Some effects produced by adrenaline upon neuromuscular propagation in rats, *J. Physiol. (London)* **141**:291.

Kuba, K., and Nishi, S., 1971, Membrane current associated with the fast EPSP of sympathetic neurons, *Physiologist* **14**:176.

Kuba, K., Minota, S., and Nishi, S., 1972, Spontaneous and evoked slow hyperpolarizations in caffeine treated bullfrog sympathetic ganglion cell, *Fed. Proc.* **31**:319.

Larrabee, M. G., and Bronk, D. W., 1947, Prolonged facilitation of synaptic excitation in sympathetic ganglia, *J. Neurophysiol.* **10**:139.

Larrabee, M. G., and Posternak, J. M., 1952, Selective action of anesthetics in synapses and axons in mammalian sympathetic ganglia, *J. Neurophysiol.* **15**:91.

Lees, G. M., and Nishi, S., 1972, Analysis of the mechanism of action of some ganglion-blocking drugs in the rabbit superior cervical ganglion, *Br. J. Pharmacol.* **46**:78.

Lees, G. M., and Wallis, D. I., 1974, Hyperpolarization of rabbit superior cervical ganglion cells due to activity of an electrogenic sodium pump, *Br. J. Pharmacol.* **50**:79.

Levy, B., and Ahlquist, R. P., 1962, A study of sympathetic ganglionic stimulants, *J. Pharmacol. Exp. Ther.* **137**:219.

Libet, B., 1962, Slow synaptic responses in sympathetic ganglia, *Fed. Proc.* **21**:345.

Libet, B., 1964, Slow synaptic responses and excitatory changes in sympathetic ganglia, *J. Physiol. (London)* **174**:1.

Libet, B., 1967, Long latent periods and further analysis of slow synaptic responses in sympa-thetic ganglia, *J. Neurophysiol.* **30**:494.

Libet, B., 1970, Generation of slow inhibitory and excitatory postsynaptic potentials, *Fed. Proc.* **29**:1945.

Libet, B., and Gerard, R. W., 1941, Steady potential fields and neurone activity, *J. Neurophysiol.* **4**:438.

Libet, B., and Kobayashi, H., 1968, Electrogenesis of slow postsynaptic potentials in sympathetic ganglion cells, *Fed. Proc.* **27**:750.

Libet, B., and Kobayashi, H., 1969, Generation of adrenergic and cholinergic potentials in sympathetic ganglion cells, *Science (New York)* **164**:1530.

Libet, B., and Owman Ch., 1974, Concomitant changes in formaldehyde-induced fluoresence of dopamine interneurones and in slow inhibitory postsynaptic potentials of the rabbit superior cervical ganglion, induced by stimulation of the preganglionic nerve or by a muscarinic agent, *J. Physiol.* **237**:635.

Libet, B., and Tosaka, T., 1966, Slow postsynaptic potentials recorded intracellularly in sympathetic ganglia, *Fed. Proc.* **25**:270.

Libet, B., Chichibu, S., and Tosaka, T., 1968, Slow synaptic responses and excitability in sympathetic ganglia of the bullfrog, *J. Neurophysiol.* **31**:383.

Liley, A. W., 1956, The effects of presynaptic polarization on the spontaneous activity at the mammalian neuromuscular junction, *J. Physiol. (London)* **134**:427.

Liley, A. W., and North, K. A. K., 1953, An electrical investigation of effects of repetitive stimulation on mammalian neuromuscular junction, *J. Neurophysiol.* **16**:509.

Lipicky, R. J., Hertz, L., and Shanes, A. M., 1963, Ca^{45} transfer and acetylcholine release in the rabbit superior cervical ganglion, *J. Cell. Comp. Physiol.* **62**:233.

Lloyd, D. P. C., 1937, The transmission of impulses through the inferior mesenteric ganglia, *J. Physiol. (London)* **91**:296.

Lloyd, D. P. C., 1939, The excitability states of inferior mesenteric ganglion cells following preganglionic activation, *J. Physiol. (London)* **95**:464.

Long, J. P., and Eckstein, J. W., 1961, Ganglionic actions of neostigmine methylsulfate, *J. Pharmacol. Exp. Ther.* **133**:216.

Lundberg, A., 1952, Adrenaline and transmission in the sympathetic ganglion of the cat, *Acta Physiol. Scand.* **26**:252.

Lundberg, A., and Quilisch, H., 1953, On the effect of calcium on presynaptic potentiation and depression at the neuromuscular junction. *Acta Physiol. Scand.* **30** (Suppl. 3):121.

Maiti, A., and Domino, E. F., 1961, Effects of methylated xanthines on the neuronally isolated cerebral cortex, *Exp. Neurol.* **3**:18.

Mallart, A., and Martin, A. R., 1968, The relation between quantum content and facilitation at the neuromuscular junction of the frog, *J. Physiol. (London)* **196**:593.

Malméjac, J., 1955, Action of adrenaline on synaptic transmission and on adrenal medullary secretion, *J. Physiol. (London)* **130**:497.

Marrazzi, A. S., 1939a, Adrenergic inhibition at sympathetic synapses, *Am. J. Physiol.* **127**:738.

Marrazzi, A. S., 1939b, Electrical studies on the pharmacology of autonomic synapses. I. The action of parasympathetic drugs on sympathetic ganglia, *J. Pharmacol. Exp. Ther.* **65**:18.

Martin, A. R., 1955, A further study of the statistical composition of the endplate potential, *J. Physiol. (London)* **130**:114.

Martin, A. R., and Pilar, G., 1963a, Dual mode of synaptic transmission in the avian ciliary ganglion, *J. Physiol. (London)* **168**:443.

Martin, A. R., and Pilar, G., 1963b, Transmission through the ciliary ganglion of the chick, *J. Physiol. (London)* **168**:464.

Masland, R. L., and Wigton, R. S., 1940, Nerve activity accompanying fasciculation produced by prostigmine, *J. Neurophysiol.* **3**:269.

Mason, D. F. J., and Wien, R., 1955, The actions of heterocyclic bisquaternary compounds especially of a pyrrolidinium series, *Br. J. Pharmacol. Chemother.* **10**:124.

Matthews, E. K., 1966, The presynaptic effects of quaternary ammonium compounds on the acetylcholine metabolism of a sympathetic ganglion, *Br. J. Pharmacol. Chemother.* **26**:552.

Matthews, E. K., and Quilliam, J. P., 1964, Effects of central depressant drugs upon acetylcholine release, *Br. J. Pharmacol. Chemother.* **22**:415.

Matthews, M. R., and Raisman, G., 1968, Two cell types in the superior cervical ganglion of the rat, *J. Anat.* **103**:397.

Matthews, M. R., and Raisman, G., 1969, The ultrastructure and somatic efferent synapses of small granule-containing cells in the superior cervical ganglion, *J. Anat.* **105**:255.

Matthews, R. J., 1956, The effect of epinephrine, levarterenol and DL-isoproterenol on transmission in the superior cervical ganglion of the cat, *J. Pharmacol. Exp. Ther.* **116**:433.

Meech, R. W., and Strumwasser, F., 1970, Intracellular calcium injection activates potassium conductances in *Aplysia* nerve cells, *Fed. Proc.* **29**:834.

Nishi, S., 1970, Cholinergic and adrenergic receptors at sympathetic preganglionic nerve terminals, *Fed. Proc.* **29**:1957.

Nishi, S., 1973, Electrogenesis of muscarinic and noncholinergic slow EPSP's of amphibian sympathetic ganglion cells, in *Interneuronal Transmission in the Autonomic Nervous System* (P. Kostyuk, ed.), pp. 112–135, Naukova Dumka, Kiev (in Russian).

Nishi, S., and Christ, D. D., 1971, Electrophysiological and anatomical properties of mammalian parasympathetic ganglion cells, *Proc. Int. Union Physiol. Sci.* **IX**, P. 421.

Nishi, S., and Koketsu, K., 1960, Electrical properties and activities of single sympathetic neurons in frogs, *J. Cell. Comp. Physiol.* **55**:15.

Nishi, S., and Koketsu, K., 1966, Late after-discharge of sympathetic postganglionic fibers, *Life Sci.* **5**:1991.

Nishi, S., and Koketsu, K., 1967, Excitatory and inhibitory postsynaptic potentials of amphibian sympathetic ganglion cells, *Fed. Proc.* **26**:329.

Nishi, S., and Koketsu, K., 1968a, Eearly and late after-discharges of amphibian sympathetic ganglion cells, *J. Neurophysiol.* **31**:109.

Nishi, S., and Koketsu, K., 1968b, Analysis of slow inhibitory postsynaptic potential of bullfrog sympathetic ganglion, *J. Neurophysiol.* **31**:717.

Nishi, S., and Koketsu, K., 1968c, Underlying mechanisms of ganglionic slow IPSP and posttetanic hyperpolarization of pre- and postganglionic elements, *Proc. Int. Union Physiol. Sci.*, **VII**, P. 321.

Nishi, S., and North, R. A., 1973, Intracellular recording from the myenteric plexus of the guinea-pig ileum, *J. Physiol. (London)* **231**:471.

Nishi, S., Soeda, H., and Koketsu, K., 1965, Studies on sympathetic B and C neurons and patterns of preganglionic innervation, *J. Cell. Comp. Physiol.* **66**:19.

Nishi, S., Soeda, H., and Koketsu, K., 1967, Release of acetylcholine from sympathetic ganglionic nerve terminals, *J. Neurophysiol.* **30**:114.

Nishi, S., Soeda, H., and Koketsu, K., 1969a, Unusual nature of ganglionic slow EPSP studied by a voltage clamp method, *Life Sci.* **8**:33.

Nishi, S., Soeda, H., and Koketsu, K., 1969b, Influence of membrane potential on the fast acetylcholine potential of sympathetic ganglion cells, *Life Sci.* **8**:499.

Norberg, K. A., and Hamberger, B., 1964, The sympathetic adrenergic neuron, *Acta Physiol. Scand.* **63** (Suppl. 238):1.

Obrador, S., and Odoriz, J. B., 1936, Transmission through a lumbar sympathetic ganglion, *J. Physiol. (London)* **86**:269.

Ortiz, C. L., and Bracho, H., 1972, Effect of reduced calcium on excitatory transmitter release at the crayfish neuromuscular junction, *Comp. Biochem. Physiol.* **41**:805.

Otsuka, M., Endo, M., and Nonomura, Y., 1962. Presynaptic nature of neuromuscular depression, *Jpn. J. Physiol.* **12**:573.

Pappano, A. J., and Volle, R. L., 1962, The reversal by atropine of ganglionic blockade produced by acetylcholine or methacholine, *Life Sci.* **12**:677.

Pardo, E. G., Cato, J., Gijon, E., and Alonso de Florida, F., 1963, Influence of several adrenergic drugs on synaptic transmission through the superior cervical and the ciliary ganglia of the cat, *J. Neurophysiol.* **31**:717.

Pascoe, J. E., 1956, The effects of acetylcholine and other drugs on the isolated superior cervical ganglion, *J. Physiol. (London)* **132**:242.

Paton, W. D. M., and Thompson, J. W., 1953, The mechanism of action of adrenaline on the superior cervical ganglion of the cat, *Int. Physiol. Congr.* **19**:664.

Perri, V., Sacchi, O., and Casella, C., 1970, Electrical properties of the sympathetic neurons in the rat and guinea-pig superior cervical ganglion, *Pflugers. Arch. ges. Physiol.*, **314**:40.

Pick, J., 1963, On the submicroscopic organization of the sympathetic ganglion in the frog (Rana pipiens), *J. Comp. Neurol.* **120**:409.

Pick, J., 1970, *The Autonomic Nervous System*, pp. 103–185, J. B. Lippincott Company, Philadelphia.

Poisner, A. M., 1973, Caffeine-induced catecholamine secretion: Similarity to caffeine-induced muscle contraction, *Proc. Soc. Exp. Biol. Med.* **142**:103.

Rall, R. W., and Sattin, A., 1970, Factors influencing the accumulation of cyclic AMP in brain tissue, in *Role of Cyclic AMP in Cell Function: Advances in Biochemical Psycho-pharmacology* (P. Greengard and Costa, E., eds.) Vol. 3. pp. 113–133, Raven Press, New York.

Rang, H. P., and Ritchie, J. M., 1968, On the electrogenic sodium pump in mammalian non-myelinated nerve fibres and its activation by various external cations, *J. Physiol. (London)* **196**:183.

Riker, W. K., 1965, Effects of tetraethylammonium on synaptic transmission in the frog sympathetic ganglia, *J. Pharmacol. Exp. Ther.* **147**:161.

Riker, W. K., and Szreniawski, Z., 1959, The pharmacological reactivity of presynaptic nerve terminals in a sympathetic ganglion, *J. Pharmacol. Exp. Ther.* **126**:233.

Root, M. A., 1951, Certain aspects of the vasopressor action of pilocarpine, *J. Pharmacol. Exp. Ther.* **101**:125.

Roszkowski, A. P., 1961, An unusual type of sympathetic ganglionic stimulant. *J. Pharmacol. Exp. Ther.* **132**:156.

Sanghvi, I., Murayama, S., Smith, C. M., and Unna, K. R., 1963, Action of muscarine on the superior cervical ganglion of the cat, *J. Pharmacol. Exp. Ther.* **142**:192.

Sant'Ambrogio, G., Frazier, D. I., and Boyarsky, L. L., 1962, Effect of caffeine on spinal reflexes, *Proc. Soc. Exp. Biol. Med.* **109**:273.

Shaw, F. W., MacCallum, M., Dewhurst, D. S., and Mainland, J. F., 1951, The possibility of the dual nature of sympathetic ganglion cells III, *Aust. J. Exp. Biol. Med. Sci.* **29**:153.

Siegrist, G., DeRibaupierre, F., Dolivo, M., and Rouiller, C., 1966, Les cellules chromaffines des ganglions cervicaux superieurs du rat, *J. Microsc. (Paris)* **5**:791.

Skok, V., 1968, The electrophysiology of cat's superior cervical sympathetic ganglion neurons, *Proc. Int. Union Physiol. Sci.*, *VII*, P. 403.

Takeshige, C., and Volle, R. L., 1962, Bimodal response of sympathetic ganglia to acetylcholine following eserine or repetitive preganglionic stimulation, *J. Pharmacol. Exp. Ther.* **138**:66.

Takeshige, C., and Volle, R. L., 1963a, Asynchronous postganglionic firing from resting sympathetic ganglia treated with neostigmine, *Br. J. Pharmacol.* **20**:214.

Takeshige, C., and Volle, R. L., 1963b, Cholinoceptive sites in denervated ganglia, *J. Pharmacol. Exp. Ther.* **141**:206.

Takeshige, C., and Volle, R. L., 1964, Modification of ganglionic responses to cholinomimetic drugs following preganglionic stimulation, anticholinesterase agents, and pilocarpine, *J. Pharmacol. Exp. Ther.* **146**:335.

Takeshige, C., Pappano, A. J., De Groat, W. C., and Volle, R. L., 1963, Ganglionic blockade produced in sympathetic ganglia by cholinomimetic drugs, *J. Pharmacol. Exp. Ther.* **141**:333.

Takeuchi, A., 1958, The long-lasting depression in neuromuscular transmission of frog, *Jpn. J. Physiol.* **8**:102.

Takeuchi, A., and Takeuchi, N., 1960, On the permeability of end-plate membrane during the action of the transmitter, *J. Physiol. (London)* **154**:52.

Tashiro, N., and Nishi, S., 1972, Effects of alkali-earth cations on sympathetic ganglion cells of the rabbit, *Life Sci.* **11**:941.

Taxi, J., 1961, Étude de l'ultrastructure des zones synaptiques dans les ganglions sympathiques de la Grenouille, *C. R. Acad. Sci.* **252**:174.

Thies, R. E., 1965, Neuromuscular depression and apparent depletion of transmitter in mammalian muscles, *J. Neurophysiol.* **28**:427.

Tosaka, T., and Libet, B., 1965, Slow postsynaptic potentials recorded intracellularly in sympathetic ganglia of the frog, *Proc. Int. Union Physiol. Sci.*, *IV*, P. 386.

Trendelenburg, U., 1954, The action of histamine and pilocarpine on the superior cervical ganglion and the adrenal glands of the cat, *Br. J. Pharmacol.* **9**:481.

Trendelenburg, U., 1956, Modification of transmission through the superior cervical ganglion of the cat, *J. Physiol. (London)* **132**:529.

Trendelenburg, U., 1966, Transmission of preganglionic impulses through the muscarinic receptors of the superior cervical ganglion of the cat, *J. Pharmacol. Exp. Ther.* **154**:426.

Uchizono, K., 1964, On different types of synaptic vesicles in the sympathetic ganglion of amphibia, *Jpn. J. Physiol.* **14**:210.

Volle, R. L., 1962a, The actions of several ganglion blocking agents on the postganglionic discharge induced by diisopropyl phosphorofluoridate (DFP) in sympathetic ganglia. *J. Pharmacol. Exp. Ther.* **135**:45.

Volle, R. L., 1962b, Enhancement of postganglionic responses to stimulating agents following repetitive preganglionic stimulation, *J. Pharmacol. Exp. Ther.* **136**:68.

Volle, R. L., and Koelle, G. B., 1961, The physiological role of acetylcholinesterase (AChE) in sympathetic ganglia, *J. Pharmacol. Exp. Ther.* **133**:223.

Weber, A., and Herz, R., 1968, The relationship between caffeine contracture of intact muscle and the effect of caffeine on reticulum, *J. Gen. Physiol.* **52**:750.

Weight, F., and Padjen, A., 1972, Slow postsynaptic inhibition and sodium inactivation in frog sympathetic ganglion cells, *Abstract 1489, 5th Int. Congr. Pharmacol.*, San Francisco.

Weight, F. F., and Votava, J., 1970, Slow synaptic excitation in sympathetic ganglion cells: Evidence for synaptic inactivation of potassium conductance, *Science (New York)* **170**:755.

Weir, M. C. L., and McLennan, H., 1963, The action of catecholamines in sympathetic ganglia, *Can. J. Biochem. Physiol.* **41**:2627.

Williams, T. H., 1967a, Electron microscopic evidence for an autonomic interneuron, *Nature (London)* **214**:309.

Williams, T. H., 1967b, The question of the intraganglionic (connector) neuron of the autonomic nervous system, *J. Anat.* **101**:603.

Wolf, G. A., Jr., 1941, The ratio of preganglionic neurons to postganglionic neurons in the visceral nervous system, *Anat. Rev.* **79**:80.

Woodward, J. K., Bianchi, C. P., and Erulkar, S. D., 1969, Electrolyte distribution in rabbit superior cervical ganglion, *J. Neurochem.* **16**:289.

Yamamoto, T., 1963, Some observations on the fine structure of the sympathetic ganglion of bullfrog, *J. Cell Biol.* **16**:159.

Index